Non-CML Myeloproliferative Diseases

Guest Editor

ROSS LEVINE, MD

HEMATOLOGY/ONCOLOGY CLINICS OF NORTH AMERICA

www.hemonc.theclinics.com

Consulting Editors
GEORGE P. CANELLOS, MD
NANCY BERLINER, MD

October 2012 • Volume 26 • Number 5

SAUNDERS an imprint of ELSEVIER, Inc.

W.B. SAUNDERS COMPANY
A Division of Elsevier Inc.

1600 John F. Kennedy Blvd. ● Suite 1800 ● Philadelphia, PA 19103-2899

http://www.theclinics.com

HEMATOLOGY/ONCOLOGY CLINICS OF NORTH AMERICA Volume 26, Number 5
October 2012 ISSN 0889-8588, ISBN 13: 978-1-4557-4941-6

Editor: Patrick Manley
Developmental Editor: Donald Mumford

Hematology/Oncology Clinics (ISSN 0889-8588) is published bimonthly by Elsevier Inc., 360 Park Avenue South, New York, NY 10010-1710. Months of issue are February, April, June, August, October, and December. Business and Editorial Offices: 1600 John F. Kennedy Blvd., Ste. 1800, Philadelphia, PA 19103–2899. Customer Service Office: 3251 Riverport Lane, Maryland Heights, MO 63043. Periodicals postage paid at New York, NY and at additional mailing offices. Subscription prices are $353.00 per year (domestic individuals), $576.00 per year (domestic institutions), $173.00 per year (domestic students/residents), $401.00 per year (Canadian individuals), $705.00 per year (Canadian institutions) $477.00 per year (international individuals), $705.00 per year (international institutions), and $233.00 per year (international and Canadian students/residents). International air speed delivery is included in all *Clinics* subscription prices. All prices are subject to change without notice. **POSTMASTER:** Send address changes to *Hematology/Oncology Clinics of North America*, Elsevier Health Sciences Division, Subscription Customer Service, 3251 Riverport Lane, Maryland Heights, MO 63043. Customer Service (orders, claims, online, change of address): Elsevier Health Sciences Division, Subscription Customer Service, 3251 Riverport Lane, Maryland Heights, MO 63043. Tel: 1-800-654-2452 (U.S. and Canada); 314-447-8871 (outside U.S. and Canada). Fax: 314-447-8029. E-mail: journalscustomerservice-usa@elsevier.com (for print support); journalsonlinesupport-usa@elsevier.com (for online support).

Reprints. For copies of 100 or more, of articles in this publication, please contact the Commercial Reprints Department, Elsevier Inc., 360 Park Avenue South, New York, New York 10010-1710; Tel.: 212-633-3813, Fax: 212-462-1935, E-mail: reprints@elsevier.com.

Hematology/Oncology Clinics of North America is covered in *MEDLINE/PubMed (Index Medicus), EMBASE/ Excerpta Medica, and BIOSIS.*

Printed and bound by CPI Group (UK) Ltd, Croydon, CR0 4YY

Transferred to Digital Print 2012

Contributors

CONSULTING EDITORS

GEORGE P. CANELLOS, MD
William Rosenberg Professor of Medicine, Department of Medical Oncology, Dana-Farber Cancer Institute, Boston, Massachusetts

NANCY BERLINER, MD
Chief, Division of Hematology, Brigham and Women's Hospital; Professor of Medicine, Harvard Medical School, Boston, Massachusetts

GUEST EDITOR

ROSS L. LEVINE, MD
Associate Member, Human Oncology and Pathogenesis Program; Leukemia Service, Department of Medicine, Memorial Sloan-Kettering Cancer Center, New York, New York

AUTHORS

OMAR ABDEL-WAHAB, MD
Human Oncology and Pathogenesis Program; Leukemia Service, Department of Medicine, Memorial Sloan-Kettering Cancer Center, New York, New York

SHUBHA ANAND, PhD
Department of Haematology, Cambridge Institute of Medical Research, University of Cambridge, Cambridge, United Kingdom

KAPIL N. BHALLA, MD
The University of Kansas Medical Center, Kansas City, Kansas

KRISTINA BRUMME
Division of Hematology, Department of Medicine, Brigham and Women's Hospital, Harvard Medical School, Boston, Massachusetts

DOMENICA CARAMAZZA, MD
Division of Hematology, Department of Internal Medicine, Ospedale di Circolo e Fondazione Macchi, Varese, Italy

NICHOLAS C.P. CROSS, PhD
Professor of Human Genetics, Faculty of Medicine, University of Southampton, Southampton; Wessex Regional Genetics Laboratory, Salisbury NHS Foundation Trust, Salisbury, United Kingdom

BENJAMIN L. EBERT, MD, PhD
Division of Hematology, Department of Medicine, Brigham and Women's Hospital, Harvard Medical School, Boston, Massachusetts

ANDREA FERRARIO, MD
Division of Hematology, Department of Internal Medicine, Ospedale di Circolo e
Fondazione Macchi, Varese, Italy

WARREN FISKUS, PhD
The University of Kansas Medical Center, Kansas City, Kansas

SIDDHARTHA GANGULY, MD
Department of Hematology/Oncology, The University of Kansas Medical Center,
Westwood, Kansas

ANNA L. GODFREY, MRCP, FRCPath
Cambridge Institute for Medical Research and Department of Haematology, University
of Cambridge; Department of Haematology, Addenbrooke's Hospital, Cambridge,
United Kingdom

ANTHONY R. GREEN, PhD, FRCPath
Cambridge Institute for Medical Research and Department of Haematology, University
of Cambridge; Department of Haematology, Addenbrooke's Hospital, Cambridge,
United Kingdom

ASHOT S. HARUTYUNYAN, MD
CeMM Research Center for Molecular Medicine of the Austrian Academy of Sciences,
Vienna, Austria

BRIAN J.P. HUNTLY, MRCP, FRCPath, PhD
Department of Haematology, Cambridge Institute of Medical Research, University
of Cambridge; Cambridge University Hospitals, NHS Foundation Trust, Addenbrooke's
Hospital; Wellcome trust/MRC Cambridge Stem Cell Institute, Cambridge Institute
of Medical Research, University of Cambridge, Cambridge, United Kingdom

SUMAN KAMBHAMPATI, MD
Department of Hematology/Oncology, The University of Kansas Medical Center,
Westwood, Kansas

ROBERT KRALOVICS, PhD
CeMM Research Center for Molecular Medicine of the Austrian Academy of Sciences;
Division of Hematology and Blood Coagulation, Department of Internal Medicine I,
Medical University of Vienna, Vienna, Austria

STEVEN W. LANE, MD
Queensland Institute of Medical Research, Brisbane, Australia

ROSS L. LEVINE, MD
Associate Member, Human Oncology and Pathogenesis Program; Leukemia Service,
Department of Medicine, Memorial Sloan-Kettering Cancer Center, New York, New York

MARGHERITA MAFFIOLI, MD
Division of Hematology, Department of Internal Medicine, Ospedale di Circolo e
Fondazione Macchi, Varese, Italy

MICHELE MERLI, MD
Division of Hematology, Department of Internal Medicine, Ospedale di Circolo e
Fondazione Macchi, Varese, Italy

ANN MULLALLY, MD
Division of Hematology, Department of Medicine, Brigham and Women's Hospital, Harvard Medical School, Boston, Massachusetts

ANIMESH PARDANANI, MBBS, PhD
Division of Hematology, Department of Medicine, Mayo Clinic, Rochester, Minnesota

FRANCESCO PASSAMONTI, MD
Division of Hematology, Department of Internal Medicine, Ospedale di Circolo e Fondazione Macchi, Varese, Italy

FABIO P.S. SANTOS, MD
Hematology and Oncology Center, Hospital Israelita Albert Einstein, Sao Paulo, Sao Paulo, Brazil

JOANNAH SCORE, PhD
Research Fellow, Faculty of Medicine, University of Southampton, Southampton; Wessex Regional Genetics Laboratory, Salisbury NHS Foundation Trust, Salisbury, United Kingdom

AYALEW TEFFERI, MD
Department of Hematology, Mayo Clinic, Rochester, Minnesota

SRDAN VERSTOVSEK, MD, PhD
Department of Leukemia, The University of Texas MD Anderson Cancer Center, Houston, Texas

Contents

pathways, although the exact molecular mechanisms underlying these observations were unknown. This situation altered with the discovery of the JAK2 V617F, which presaged the ongoing description of further mutations predicted to activate canonical signaling pathways in MPN. This article covers the nature of these mutations and summarizes functional experiments in model systems and in human MPN cells to define the signaling pathways altered and how these drive and determine the MPN cellular phenotype. Also discussed are recently described, novel noncanonical signaling pathways to chromatin predicted to alter gene transcription more directly and to also contribute to the MPN phenotype.

It is thought that myeloproliferative neoplasms (MPNs) are driven by somatic mutations, although hereditary factors also play a prominent role in the pathogenesis of the disease. Hereditary thrombocytosis and erythrocytosis are not malignant disorders but are clinically similar to MPNs. Several mutations have been found that explain a proportion of hereditary thrombocytosis and hereditary erythrocytosis. Germline variants can influence the risk of leukemic transformation in MPNs and the course of the disease through interaction with acquired chromosomal aberrations. Overall, it has been shown that germline factors play an important part in MPN pathogenesis.

Since the discovery of activating mutations in *JAK2* in patients with myeloproliferative neoplasms (MPNs) in 2005, gene discovery efforts have identified additional disease alleles, which can predate or occur subsequent to acquisition of *JAK2/MPL* mutations. In 2009, somatic copy number loss and mutations in the genes *TET2* and *ASXL1* were identified in MPN patients. Genetic analysis of MPN patient cohorts with adequate sample size and clear clinical annotation are needed to understand the importance of these mutations on MPN phenotype, risk of transformation to leukemia, response to therapy, and influence on overall survival.

Myeloproliferative neoplasm (MPN) animal models accurately re-capitulate human disease in mice and have been an important tool for the study of MPN biology and therapy. Transplantation of *BCR-ABL* transduced bone marrow into irradiated syngeneic mice established the field of MPN animal modeling. Genetically engineered MPN animal models have enabled detailed characterization of the effects of specific MPN-associated genetic abnormalities on hematopoietic stem and progenitor cells (HSPCs). Xenograft models have allowed the study of primary human MPN-propagating cells in vivo. *JAK2V617F*, the most common molecular abnormality in *BCR-ABL* negative MPN, has been extensively studied using retroviral, transgenic, knock-in and xenograft models.

HEMATOLOGY/ONCOLOGY CLINICS OF NORTH AMERICA

Preface

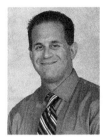

Ross L. Levine, MD
Guest Editor

In the past decade, genetic and functional studies have provided unparalleled insight into the molecular pathogenesis of myeloproliferative neoplasms (MPNs). This includes the identification of novel mutations, which contribute to disease pathogenesis, the development of genetically accurate animal models of MPNs, and the development and approval of molecularly targeted therapies for MPN patients. This has ushered in a new era for MPN researchers and patients, where genetic studies have informed efforts in the laboratory and in the clinic, which have already improved outcomes for MPN patients. In this issue we present a series of reviews by world leaders in the MPN field, which describe our current knowledge of the role of inherited and acquired disease alleles in MPN pathogenesis, the role of specific pathways in MPN disease initiation and transformation, and the continued development of novel therapeutics for MPN patients. We believe readers will find these reviews enlightening and provide a timely, broad overview of MPN biology and therapy.

Ross L. Levine, MD
Human Oncology and Pathogenesis Program
Memorial Sloan Kettering Cancer Center
1275 York Avenue, Box 20
New York, NY 10065, USA

E-mail address:
leviner@mskcc.org

Hematol Oncol Clin N Am 26 (2012) xi
http://dx.doi.org/10.1016/j.hoc.2012.08.002
0889-8588/12/$ – see front matter © 2012 Elsevier Inc. All rights reserved.

Role of Additional Novel Therapies in Myeloproliferative Neoplasms

Warren Fiskus, PhD[a], Siddhartha Ganguly, MD[b],
Suman Kambhampati, MD[b], Kapil N. Bhalla, MD[a],*

KEYWORDS

- JAK2-V617F • HDAC inhibitor • hsp90 inhibitors • PI3K/AKT inhibitor
- MEK inhibitor • Myeloproliferative neoplasms

KEY POINTS

- With the recent approval by the US Food and Drug Administration of ruxolitinib, significant progress has been made in the treatment of myeloproliferative neoplasms.
- Drug toxicity and lack of effect on janus kinase 2 (JAK2) V617F allelic burden remain a problem with JAK inhibitors in the treatment of myeloproliferative neoplasms (MPN).
- Activation of collaborating pathways downstream of JAK2 V617F strongly supports the development and testing of novel agents for the treatment of patients with MPN.
- Treatment with chromatin-modifying agents (eg, histone deacetylase inhibitors and DNA methyltransferase 1 inhibitors) targets the deregulated epigenome and shows activity against MPN cells.
- Clinical experience with JAK inhibitors supports the rationale to develop safe and effective combinations, which incorporate JAK inhibitors with other agents active against MPN cells.

INTRODUCTION

The identification of an acquired, somatic, gain-of function, point mutation at valine 617, V617F, in the janus kinase 2 (JAK2) gene was a major advance in the understanding of the clonal Philadelphia-chromosome negative myeloproliferative neoplasms (MPNs).[1–5] The JAK2-V617F mutation is present in ~90% of patients with polycythemia vera and in approximately 50% to 60% of patients with essential thrombocythemia (ET) and primary

[a] The University of Kansas Medical Center, 3901 Rainbow Boulevard, Robinson Hall 4030, Mail Stop 1027, Kansas City, KS 66160, USA; [b] Department of Hematology/Oncology, The University of Kansas Medical Center, 2330 Shawnee Mission Parkway, Mail Stop 5003, Westwood, KS 66205, USA
* Corresponding author.
E-mail address: kbhalla@kumc.edu

Hematol Oncol Clin N Am 26 (2012) 959–980
http://dx.doi.org/10.1016/j.hoc.2012.07.001
0889-8588/12/$ – see front matter © 2012 Elsevier Inc. All rights reserved.
hemonc.theclinics.com

myelofibrosis (PMF).[4] JAK2 is a cytoplasmic, non-receptor, tyrosine kinase that via its association with cytokine receptors serves as a signaling mediator for hematopoietic cytokines such as erythropoietin (Epo) and thrombopoietin (Tpo) to regulate cell proliferation and growth (**Fig. 1**).[4,6] Binding of a ligand to cytokine receptor results in phosphorylation and activation of JAK2, which is the initiating step in the signaling cascade.[6] On activation, JAK2 recruits and phosphorylates the signal transducer and activation of transcription (STAT) factors STAT5 and STAT3.[4,6] This situation results in dimerization and translocation of STAT3 and STAT5 to the nucleus, where they activate transcription of genes involved in cell proliferation, survival, and resistance to apoptosis (eg, Bcl-xL, MCL1, PIM1, and Cyclin D1).[5–7] JAK2 kinase activity is regulated by homology domains, in particular, the JH1 (catalytic kinase domain) and the JH2 (the

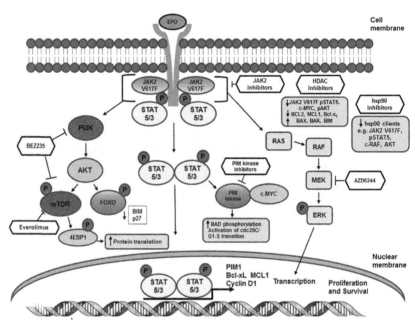

Fig. 1. JAK2 V617F signaling pathways and molecular targeted agents. Binding of cytokines (eg, Epo) to membrane-bound receptors induces dimerization of the receptor, which engages cytoplasmic kinases including JAK2. JAKs are activated through tyrosine phosphorylation by the cytoplasmic domain of the cytokine receptor. JAK2 phosphorylation results in the activation of downstream signaling through recruitment of STAT3 and STAT5. STAT5 and STAT3 are phosphorylated by JAK2, leading to the formation of stable homodimers and their subsequent localization to the nucleus. In the nucleus, STAT proteins bind promoter DNA sequences and activate transcription of genes involved in cell proliferation, differentiation, and survival (eg, Cyclin D1, PIM, Bcl-xL, and MCL-1). The V617F mutation in JAK2 causes its constitutive activation and autophosphorylation in MPN cells. Along with the membrane-bound receptor, JAK2 V617F also activates the PI3K-AKT-mammalian target of rapamycin (mTOR)-forkhead transcription factors (FOXO) as well as the RAS/RAF/MAP/ERK signaling pathway, which induces transcription and signals for survival and proliferation. Treatment with inhibitors of JAK2 attenuates JAK2 V617F phosphorylation and downstream signaling through STAT5 and STAT3 as well as signaling through PI3K/AKT, mTOR, and RAS/RAF/MAP/ERK and PIM kinase. Recently, inhibitors that target proteins in these deregulated pathways as well as HDAC and hsp90 inhibitors have been developed and tested as single agents or in multitargeted combinations with JAK2-TKI.

pseudokinase domain), which serves an autoinhibitory function.[7,8] The V617F point mutation within the JH2 domain disrupts its autoinhibitory function, resulting in constitutive activation of JAK2-mediated signaling pathways through the STAT5 and STAT3, phosphatidylinositol 3-kinase (PI3K) and extracellular signal-regulated kinase.[7–9] Studies have shown that cytoplasmic STAT5a, through GAB2, is the link between JAK/STAT signaling and activation of the PI3K/AKT/mammalian target of rapamycin (mTOR) pathways.[6,10] JAK2V617F-mediated alterations in transcription can also occur through a noncanonical pathway through which JAK2 enters the nucleus, phosphorylates histone H3 at tyrosine (Y) 41 and displaces HP1α from the chromatin.[11,12] Phosphorylation of Y41 on histone H3 leads to increased expression of oncogenes such as LMO2 in MPN cells (**Fig. 2A**).[11,12] Since the identification of JAK2V617F in MPN, additional mutations in JAK2 and other genes have been identified that also lead to constitutive activation of JAK/STAT signaling. One example is the identification of 4 novel somatic mutations in exon 12 of JAK2.[13] These mutations are located in a region

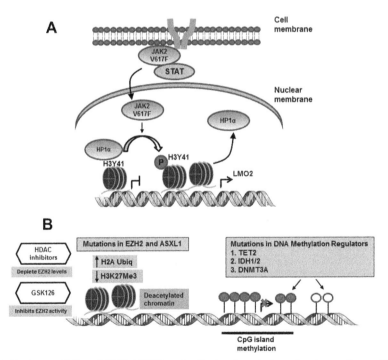

Fig. 2. Nuclear activity of JAK2 V617F and effects of mutations in chromatin-modifying enzymes in MPN. (*A*) JAK2 V617F is activated by autophosphorylation. The activated JAK2 translocates to the nucleus and phosphorylates histone H3 on tyrosine 41. Phosphorylation of tyrosine 41 disrupts HP1α association with the chromatin, leading to increased transcription of the oncogene, LMO2. (*B*) Mutations in histone regulators such as EZH2 and ASXL1 lead to a loss of lysine 27 trimethylation on histone H3 and increased ubiquitination of lysine (K)119 on histone H2A. Treatment with epigenetic drugs (eg, HDAC inhibitors) lowers the expression levels of EZH2 and specific inhibitors of EZH2 (eg, GSK126) inhibit the activity of EZH2 within the polycomb repressive complex. In addition, mutations in DNA methylation regulators (eg, TET2, IDH1/2, and DNMT3A) leads to abnormal loss of DNA methylation (indicated by open circles) as well as gains of methylation in many CpG islands (indicated by filled circles). These losses of DNA methylation can span large regions on multiple chromosomes.

between the SH2 and JH2 domain and result in the gain-of function and activation of JAK2 similar to the V617F mutation. In JAK2V617F-negative MPN, mutations have also been described in the Tpo receptor c-MPL, particularly a point mutation at codon 515, which results in the substitution of tryptophan by leucine, lysine, asparagines, or alanine (W515L/K/N/A).[4,14] Mutations in MPL are associated with spontaneous activation of MPL and downstream signaling through JAK/STAT.[4,15] Similar to the action of constitutively activated JAK2V617F, expression of MPLW515L has been shown to transform hematopoietic stem cells (HSCs), resulting in growth factor independence, deregulated signaling through STAT, mitogen-activated protein kinase, and PI3K pathways as well as upregulation of anti-apoptotic proteins such as Bcl-xL.[15,16] Previous studies have shown that expression of MPLW515L in murine models causes lethal MPN, with myelofibrosis (MF) resulting from JAK2 activation.[16] Although less common (<10% of MPN cases), additional mutations in MPN have also been described in the intracellular signaling genes (eg, Casitas B-cell lymphoma [CBL]).[17] CBL is an adapter protein that has also been shown to possess E3 ubiquitin ligase activity, and it serves to negatively regulate JAK2 signaling through ubiquitination and subsequent internalization of growth factor receptors.[17,18] Because of these factors, CBL has been considered to be a tumor suppressor gene that acts to suppress JAK2 signaling.[17,18] In MPN cells, mutations that inactivate or cause truncation of CBL result in enhanced downstream signaling through JAK/STAT and modulation of cell cycle, proliferation, and apoptosis-related proteins.[17,18] Suppressor of cytokine signaling (SOCS) proteins are also negative regulators of JAK signaling, the expression of which is inactivated by mutation or through CpG island hypermethylation of the SOCS1 or SOCS3 promoter in MPN cells, leading to excessive cytokine signaling.[19,20] Although mutations in the SOCS genes have been described in MPN, their occurrence is rare, and their role in the pathogenesis of MPN is controversial. In addition, LNK mutations have been described in MPN.[21] LNK, (also called Src homology 2 B3), is a plasma membrane-bound adapter protein with several domains including an SH2 domain that can bind to MPL and JAK2 and negatively regulate JAK/STAT signaling in response to Epo receptor or MPL signaling.[21,22] LNK mutations have been detected in 6% to 13% of chronic phase and blast phases of MPN and occur within a hot spot in the pleckstrin homology domain of exon 2.[21,22] LNK mutations in JAK2V617F-negative MPN are associated with myeloid progenitor expansion and cytokine responsive pSTAT5 and pSTAT3 expression, which phenocopies activating mutations in JAK2.[22,23]

ADDITIONAL SIGNALING PATHWAYS ACTIVATED IN MPN CELLS

In addition to the mutations activating the JAK/STAT pathway, other pro-growth and pro-survival signaling pathways downstream of the JAK/STAT pathway are also deregulated in MPN (see **Fig. 1**). These pathways includes the PI-3K/AKT/mTOR pathway, which cross talks and activates the RAS/RAF/MEK/ERK pathway, downregulating the pro-apoptotic protein BIM, in response to growth factor signaling in cancer cells.[24–26] MEK is a key protein kinase in the RAS/RAF/MEK/ERK pathway, which signals for cancer cell proliferation and survival.[25,27] MEK has been found to be frequently activated in cancer and regulates the biosynthesis of the inflammatory cytokines tumor necrosis factor, interleukin 6 (IL-6), and IL-1, which can act as growth and survival factors in cancer cells.[25,27] Because the PI3K/AKT/mTOR pathway is commonly activated in many hematologic malignancies including myeloproliferative neoplasms, inhibition of this pathway could have broad anti-MPN activity.[15,28] Constitutive, unregulated JAK/STAT activity can also result in activation of the proviral integration site (PIM) kinases.[29] Expression of PIM1 is directly regulated through JAK/STAT signaling when the FERM domain of JAK2 is intact.[29] The PIM kinases have been shown to promote the growth and survival of transformed myeloid progenitor cells.[30]

MUTATIONS IN EPIGENETIC MODIFIERS IN MPN

Similar to the other myeloid malignancies, mutations in genes regulating the epigenetic control of gene expression, the so-called epimutations, has also been noted in MPNs. These epimutations include mutations in ASXL1 (additional sex combs like 1), the polycomb group protein EZH2 and TET2 (ten-eleven-translocation 2) (see **Fig. 2**B).[23,31–33] The enhancer of zeste (EZH2) gene encodes a histone methyltransferase that along with suppressor of zeste 12 (SUZ12) and embryonic ectoderm development (EED) comprises the polycomb repressive complex (PRC) 2.[34,35] The PRC2 complex functions to epigenetically silence gene expression through trimethylation of lysine (K) 27 on histone H3, a repressive histone mark.[34,35] Mutations in EZH2 have been observed throughout the coding sequence but predominate in the C-terminal SET domain and negatively affect the histone methyltransferase activity of the PRC2 for lysine (K) 27 on histone H3.[36,37] EZH2 mutations have been identified in 5.9% of patients with PMF, 1.2% of post-PV-MF, and 9.4% of post-ET-MF and were found to coexist in ~40% of JAK2V617F-positive and ~22% of ASXL1 mutation-positive patients with MF.[37] Patients coexpressing these mutations cluster into the International Prognostic Scoring System (IPSS) high-risk category, have shorter leukemia-free survival and significantly shorter overall survival (OS) compared with EZH2 wild-type (WT) patients.[37] Patients with PMF and mutated EZH2 showed higher leukocyte and blast counts and presented with larger spleens at diagnosis than those with WT EZH2.[37] ASXL1 mutations have been identified in ~55% of PMF and 22% of post-PV/ET-MF patients.[38] Mutations in ASXL1 are most commonly located in exon 12 and result in a missense or a frameshift, resulting in a loss of function for ASXL1 and decreased ASXL1 expression.[31,32] Loss of ASXL1 function leads to a genome-wide loss of trimethylation on lysine 27 of histone H3 and increased gene expression at loci with bivalent chromatin marks.[39] ASXL1 mutations have also been observed to coexist with JAK2V617F in approximately 48% of PMF and post-PV/ET-MF patients.[40] Similar to EZH2 mutations, patients with coexistence of ASXL1 mutations and JAK2V617F cluster into the IPSS high-risk category, experience significantly shorter LFS, and significantly shorter OS.[40,41] In addition, ASXL1 mutant patients had a greater than 2-fold higher incidence of leukemia (34.9% vs 15.2%) than ASXL1 wild-type patients.[40,41] Furthermore, LFS in double ASXL1/EZH2-mutated PMF patients was significantly shorter than in patients with single ASXL1 or EZH2 mutations (25 vs 138 vs 153 months).[40] The TET2 gene is located on chromosome 4q24, a common break point involved in translocations in myeloid neoplasms.[18–20] TET2 functions to convert 5-methylcytosine to 5-hydroxymethycytosine (5hmC) and has been found to be mutated in 7% to 16% of patients with JAK2V617F MPN.[18–20,42] Mutations in TET2 compromise its catalytic activity, resulting in lower levels of 5-hmC in the genomic DNA as well as global hypomethylation of DNA.[42] TET2 mutations have been observed in both JAK2V617F-positive and JAK2V617F-negative MPN; however, because of the diverse array of the identified mutations, they provide limited prognostic relevance.[43,44] Similar to other myeloid malignancies, isocitrate dehydrogenase 1 (IDH1) and IDH2 mutations have been identified in MPNs.[18–21,23,45] Unlike WT IDH1 and IDH2, which catalyze the conversion of isocitrate to α-ketoglutarate (α-KG), mutant IDH1 and IDH2 proteins possess neomorphic enzyme activity, resulting in the production of the oncometabolite, 2-hydroxyglutarate (2-HG).[23,46] This enzymatic activity and the resulting 2-HG lead to impairment of TET2 catalytic function and global increases in DNA hypermethylation.[47,48] Recently, 2-HG produced by IDH mutant cells was also shown to competitively inhibit α-KG-dependent dioxygenases, including the histone demethylation activity of a family of Jumonji-C domain histone demethylases.[49,50] This situation led to marked increases in repressive histone methylation marks, suggesting that IDH mutations preferentially affect repressive histone methylation marks in addition to increasing DNA methylation in the transformed cells.[49,50] Mutations in IDH1/2 are believed to be independent predictors of leukemic transformation because they are frequently identified in blast-phase MPN but not chronic-phase MPN.[23,51,52] This finding suggests that IDH mutations may collaborate with JAK2V617F in transformation to leukemia. A recent study showed that IDH-mutated MPN patients showed significantly shorter LFS and OS than patients with mutated JAK2.[51] DNMT3A belongs to a family of DNA methyltransferases that includes DNMT1 and DNMT3B, which catalyze the conversion of cytosine to 5-methylcytosine.[53,54] DNMT3A mutations have been identified in MPN, although they are most commonly found in cases of MDS and acute myeloid leukemia (AML) at position R882, which lies in the methyltransferase domain.[55–57] Previous studies have shown that loss of DNMT3A in HSCs resulted in altered DNA methylation patterns at different loci.[54] DNMT3A mutations in myeloid malignancies lead to an impairment of its DNA methyltransferase activity, which may improve the response to treatment with DNA hypomethylating agents.[58] Collectively, the documentation of epimutations in MPN creates a compelling rationale to test agents that target deregulated epigenetic mechanisms in MPN.

JAK2 KINASE INHIBITORS IN THE CLINIC

Its crucial role in cytokine signaling in normal and malignant cells, and the observation that JAK2 mutations are present in most MPNs, prompted the development of several inhibitors of JAK (JAK- tyrosine kinase inhibitor [TKI]) (eg, ruxolitinib, SAR302503, CYT387, BMS911543, and CEP701) for the treatment of these neoplasms.[59] INCB018424 (ruxolitinib) is a potent, small-molecule inhibitor of JAK1 and JAK2. A phase I-II study of ruxolitinib in MF showed that 15-mg twice-daily dosing was safe and effective in decreasing circulating inflammatory cytokines and improved constitutional symptoms.[60] In 52% of treated patients, ruxolitinib caused rapid and sustained reduction in spleen size (≥50% reduction).[60] Subsequently, 2 phase III studies of ruxolitinib were completed, which led to its approval by the US Food and Drug Administration (FDA) as a therapy for the treatment of MF.[61,62] Another small molecule under clinical investigation for the treatment of MPN is SAR302503 (TG101348), a JAK2-specific inhibitor. Treatment with SAR302503 improved constitutional symptoms, and in 40% of patients with MPN caused a 50% or greater reduction in spleen size. SAR302503 treatment was also noted to significantly reduce the JAK2V617F allelic burden in patients with MPN.[63] A more complete description of the clinical experience with these and other JAK-TKIs is given elsewhere in this issue by S. Verstovsek.

Although conferring clinical benefit in patients with advanced MPN, JAK inhibitor therapy has not reduced MF and normalized bone marrow histopathology, or significantly reduced the allelic burden of JAK2V617F and improved the survival of patients with MF.[33,62,64] Suboptimal responses to JAK2 TKI may be caused by many factors, including complexity of clonal structure of the MPN, cell intrinsic mechanisms that confer JAK2 TKI resistance, additional mutations in the JAK2 domain that confer JAK2 TKI resistance, and the inability of JAK2 TKIs to target the stem cells in MPN.[65–68] In addition, mutations in epigenetic regulators may contribute to the aggressiveness and treatment refractoriness of advanced MPNs. These factors provide a compelling rationale to develop and test novel agents that are active on targets or pathways that collaborate with JAK/STAT-mediated progrowth and prosurvival signaling, or target the deregulated epigenome in advanced MPN. Clinical experience with JAK inhibitors thus far also supports the rationale to develop safe and more effective combinations of JAK-TKI with other active agents against MPN cells.

ADDITIONAL NOVEL AGENTS FOR MPN THERAPY

Recently, numerous novel agents targeting diverse signaling targets in MPN cells have been developed and tested preclinically in the in vitro and in vivo models of MPN. These agents, including mTOR (TORC1 and TORC2) inhibitor, dual PI3K/mTOR inhibitor, AKT inhibitor, MEK inhibitor, PIM kinase inhibitor, histone deacetylase (HDAC) inhibitor, DNMT1 inhibitor, and hsp90 inhibitors, have been developed and evaluated as single agents and in some cases in combination with JAK2 inhibitors, with the goal of increasing the therapeutic options for patients with MPN (**Tables 1** and **2**).

mTOR and Dual PI3K/mTOR Inhibitors

In addition to constitutive and enhanced JAK/STAT signaling, MPN cells also show activation of the mTOR pathway downstream of PI3K/AKT.[69–71] The mTOR pathway serves a critical role in multiple cellular processes including cell growth, proliferation, and survival.[28,72] These factors make targeting the mTOR pathway an attractive therapeutic strategy for MPN. Previous studies have shown that treatment with the mTOR inhibitor, everolimus (RAD001), inhibited cell proliferation and induced apoptosis of cultured MPN cells, as well as preventing the growth of hematopoietic progenitor cells (HPCs) derived from patients with PV and PMF.[70] The clinical activity of everolimus against MPN has also been documented. A phase I/II study with everolimus was

Table 1
Novel small molecule inhibitors under investigation for the treatment of MPN

Drug	Type of Inhibitor	Disease	Preclinical or Clinical	Reference
Everolimus	mTOR	JAK2 V617F and MPL MPN	Preclinical and clinical	70,71,73
BEZ235	PI3K/mTOR	JAK2 V617F MPN	Preclinical	74
MK-2206	Allosteric AKT	JAK2 V617F MPN	Preclinical	75
SGI-1776	PIM kinase	JAK2 V617F MPN	Preclinical	83
AZD1208	PIM1, PIM2, PIM3 kinase	Not tested in MPN	Preclinical	84
Selumetinib (AZD6244)	MEK1 kinase	JAK2 V617F MPN	Preclinical	74
Panobinostat	Pan-HDAC	JAK2 V617F MPN, PMF	Preclinical and clinical (phase I and phase II)	100,102–104
Givinostat (ITF2357)	Class I/II HDAC	PV, ET, PMF	Preclinical and clinical (phase II)	105–107
AUY922	hsp90	JAK2 V617F MPN	Preclinical	115
PU-H71	hsp90	JAK2 V617F and MPL MPN	Preclinical	123
PF-04449913	Hedgehog	PMF	Clinical	128
BC2059	β-catenin antagonist	JAK2V617F MPN	Preclinical	133

Table 2
Novel combinations of targeted agents with JAK inhibitors for the treatment of MPN

Combination Therapy	Type of Inhibitor	Disease	Preclinical or Clinical	Reference
BEZ235 + TG101209	PI3K/mTOR and JAK2-TKI	JAK2 V617F MPN	Preclinical	74
Selumetinib + TG101209	MEK kinase and JAK2-TKI	JAK2 V617F MPN	Preclinical	74
SGI1776 + TG101209	PIM kinase and JAK2-TKI	JAK2 V617F MPN	Preclinical	83
Panobinostat + TG101209	Pan-HDAC and JAK2-TKI	JAK2 V617F MPN	Preclinical	100
Panobinostat + ruxolitinib	Pan-HDAC and JAK1/2-TKI	JAK2 V617F MPN	Preclinical (murine models)	104
Givinostat + hydroxyurea	Class I/II HDAC and ribonucleotide reductase	PV	Clinical (phase II)	107
Decitabine + vorinostat	DNMT1 and pan-HDAC	JAK2 V617F MPN	Preclinical (murine models)	108
AUY922 + TG101209	hsp90 and JAK-TKI	JAK2 V617F MPN	Preclinical	115
BC2059 + TG101209	β-catenin antagonist and JAK2-TKI	JAK2 V617F MPN	Preclinical	133

performed in patients with JAK2V617F or MPL mutations as well as patients with WT JAK2 with intermediate-risk/high-risk scores.[71] Patients were treated with 5 to 10 mg of everolimus per day. No dose-limiting toxicity was observed up to a dose of 10 mg/d. Although everolimus had no effect on the JAK2V617F allelic burden, 69% of patients experienced a complete resolution of systemic symptoms and 80% had reduction in pruritus. According to International Working Group for MPN Research and Treatment criteria for disease response, everolimus treatment produced a 23% response rate in the 39 patients enrolled on the study. In addition, overall clinical improvement was noted in 6 of 39 patients (~20%) and 1 patient obtained a partial remission.[71,73] These findings support the rationale for determining the clinical efficacy and safety of combined treatment with everolimus and ruxolitinib in patients with MF. There has also been considerable interest in targeting both the PI3K and mTOR pathways with dual PI3K/mTOR pathway inhibitors, several of which are in clinical development.[28] Because MPN cells have aberrant activation of the PI3K and mTOR pathways downstream of JAK2, and considerable crosstalk occurs between the pathways, this makes dual targeting of PI3K and mTOR an attractive and rational strategy for the treatment of MPNs. Preclinical studies have shown that treatment of cultured and primary MF-MPN cells with the dual PI3K/mTOR inhibitor, BEZ235, induced cell cycle growth arrest and inhibited PI3K and mTOR signaling, shown by depletion of p-AKT, p-p70S6K, and p-4EBP1, as well as exerting lethal anti-MPN activity.[74] This study also showed that the combination of BEZ235 and the JAK2-TKI TG101209 exerted synergistically lethal activity against cultured and primary CD34+ MF-MPN cells and relatively spared normal CD34+ bone marrow progenitor cells.[74] These studies support the rationale to test the in vivo activity of BEZ235 alone or in combination with ruxolitinib against MPN.

AKT Inhibitors

Previous studies have shown that the PI3K/AKT pathway is activated and supports cell growth, proliferation, and survival of MPN cells.[28] For this reason, targeting the activity of AKT could exert lethal effects against MPN cells. Preclinical studies have shown that treatment with an allosteric AKT inhibitor, MK-2206, attenuates pro-growth and pro-survival activity of AKT and induced proliferation arrest and apoptosis in cultured MPN cells.[75] Treatment with MK-2206 also inhibited the in vitro colony growth of primary CD34+ MF-MPN cells. MK-2206 also showed in vivo activity against murine transplant models of MPN, manifesting as reduced peripheral blood (PB) leukocytosis and extramedullary hematopoiesis.[75] These findings support the rationale to determine the in vitro and in vivo activity of JAK-TKI with AKT inhibitor against MPN cells.

MEK Inhibitors

Several studies have documented the increased activity of the RAS/RAF/MEK/ERK pathway in promoting growth and survival of MPN cells.[26,76] Therefore, targeting MEK kinase to interrupt this signaling is likely to be a promising therapeutic strategy in MPN. Recent in vitro studies have shown that treatment with the MEK inhibitor selumetinib (AZD6244) in cultured and primary MPN cells depleted MEK1 kinase activity, as shown by reduced pERK1/2 expression.[74] Treatment with selumetinib also induced apoptosis of cultured and primary CD34+ MPN cells. In addition, cotreatment with selumetinib and JAK2-TKI exerted synergistic apoptotic effects against cultured MPN cells.[74] Recently, a phase II study with selumetinib was conducted in patients with AML.[77] The study showed that daily administration of selumetinib was tolerated and exerted modest anti-leukemic activity in patients with AML.[77] The safety profile and activity in AML support the rationale for testing selumetinib and other safe MEK inhibitors alone or in combination with JAK inhibitors in patients with MPN.

PIM Kinase Inhibitors

The oncoprotein PIM1 belongs to a family of evolutionarily conserved cytoplasmic serine/threonine kinases (PIM1, PIM2, PIM3) that have been implicated in hematologic maligancies.[30] PIM kinases have been shown to be constitutively active, downstream effectors of JAK/STAT signaling that promote cell survival and proliferation and inhibit apoptosis by phosphorylating and inactivating the pro-apoptotic proteins BAD and ASK1 and through interaction with c-MYC.[78–81] By phosphorylating PRAS40, an inhibitor of TORC1, PIM kinase activity dissociates PRAS40 from TORC1, resulting in activation of TORC1.[82] PIM kinases are frequently overexpressed in hematologic malignancies including MPN, and because they do not require post-translational modifications, their activity is largely regulated at the transcriptional or post-transcriptional level.[81] Preclinical studies have shown that the PIM kinase inhibitor SGI-1776 inhibited the activity of PIM kinase in cultured MPN cells, as shown by depletion of p-BAD (Ser112) expression, attenuation of PRAS40 phosphorylation, decreased activity of TORC1, and attenuation of p-4EBP1 levels. SGI-1776-mediated inhibition of PIM kinases also reduced c-MYC levels in MPN cells.[83] Treatment with SGI-1776, as a single agent, induced apoptosis of cultured and primary MF-MPN cells, which was associated with induction of p27 and BIM levels.[83] In addition, cotreatment with SGI-1776 was shown to enhance the anti-MPN activity of JAK2-TKI (TG101209) against cultured and primary MF-MPN cells. Another PIM kinase inhibitor, AZD1208, has shown in vitro and in vivo efficacy against other hematologic malignancies such as AML but has not yet been tested against MPN cells.[84] Given that AZD1208 is a pan-PIM inhibitor, and because of its proven activity in acute leukemia cells, it is likely that such an agent would show similar activity against MPN. Collectively, these observations also support the testing of PIM kinase inhibitor alone or in combination with JAK-TKI in the treatment of MPN.

HDAC Inhibitors

MPN cells have been shown to have increased HDAC levels and enhanced HDAC activity, especially of class I HDACs (1, 2, and 8).[85] Previous studies have shown that increased HDAC levels and activity strongly correlated with the degree of splenomegaly in MPN, particularly MF.[85,86] The 18 known HDACs are grouped into 5 phylogenetic classes according to their sequence homology and the cofactor required for their catalytic activity.[87] Class I (HDAC1-3 and HDAC1-8), class IIa (HDAC4, 5, 7, and 9), class IIb (HDAC6 and 10), and class IV (HDAC11) require a divalent metal ion (eg, zinc) for their deacetylase activity, whereas class III (also called sirtuins or SIRT1-7) are structurally and biochemically different from the other classes and are dependent on nicotine adenine dinucleotide (NAD+) for their catalytic activity.[87,88] HDACs are known to play significant roles in the epigenetic regulation of gene expression not only through lysine deacetylation of histone proteins but also through regulating the acetylation status of nonhistone proteins such as transcription factors and the expression of microRNAs.[89-91] HDAC inhibitors are novel, structurally diverse agents that can be divided into several structural classes, including hydroxamates, cyclic peptides, aliphatic acids, and benzamides.[92,93] Most of the HDAC inhibitors that have been developed are pan-HDAC inhibitors that inhibit class I, class II, and class IV, although class I and class I/II-specific inhibitors such as romidepsin and givinostat have also been developed.[92-95] By altering gene expression through chromatin-dependent and chromatin-independent mechanisms, regulating cell cycle progression, acetylation of proteins, inhibition of proliferation, and induction of cell death, HDAC inhibitors represent a promising class of agents for the treatment of hematologic malignancies including MPNs.[92-94] Panobinostat (LBH589) is a potent hydroxamate-based pan-HDAC inhibitor with nanomolar inhibitor activity against class I, II, and IV HDACs, which has been shown to induce the acetylation of both histone and nonhistone proteins in transformed cells, deplete antiapoptotic proteins (eg, Bcl-x$_L$, MCL1, and BCL-2) and induce pro-apoptotic proteins (eg, BAX, BAK, and BIM).[96-99] Recent studies have determined the in vitro activity of panobinostat against MPN cells. Treatment with panobinostat depleted the expression levels of mutant JAK2V617F and inhibited JAK/STAT intracellular signaling in cultured and primary MF-MPN cells, induced cell cycle growth arrest, and upregulated prodeath proteins (eg, BIM).[100] Panobinostat depleted JAK2V617F expression by disrupting its chaperone association with heat shock protein (hsp) 90, resulting in proteasomal degradation of JAKV617F protein.[100] In addition, panobinostat was shown to deplete the expression levels of epigenetic regulators, including polycomb group proteins, EZH2, and SUZ12, and DNA methyltransferases in other myeloid malignancies (eg, AML), resulting in disassembly of the PRC2 complex and downregulation of trimethylated lysine 27 on histone H3.[97] Panobinostat treatment was also shown to deplete the expression of the DNA methyltransferase, DNMT1, and disrupt its chaperone association with hsp90 and with EZH2 in myeloid malignancies.[101] The clinical activity of panobinostat has also been tested against hematologic malignancies, including MPN. A recent phase I clinical trial was conducted with panobinostat in patients with hematologic malignancies, of which 13 had MF.[102] Patients treated with panobinostat experienced clinical improvement, including reductions of spleen size (57%–86%). Improvement in disease-related symptoms were observed in 4 patients with MF at doses of 30 (n = 1) and 60 mg (n = 3) of administered orally 3 times a week.[102] In a separate phase I study, prolonged, low-dose panobinostat (25 mg 3 times a week) ameliorated constitutional symptoms, improved clinical features, and caused significant reductions of marrow fibrosis.[103] Preclinical studies have also shown that cotreatment with panobinostat further enhanced JAK2-TKI-mediated inhibition of JAK/STAT signaling in MPN and exerted synergistic anti-MPN activity against cultured and primary MF-MPN cells.[100] The combination of panobinostat and ruxolitinib has also been studied in vivo and showed improved efficacy over either agent alone in mouse models of JAK2-V617F-driven disease, without notable toxicity.[104] Based on these promising preclinical data, a phase I clinical trial has been initiated to test the combination of panobinostat with ruxolitinib in patients with MPN (NCT01433445). Preclinical studies have also shown the activity of other classes of HDAC inhibitors against MPN cells. Givinostat (ITF2357) is a synthetic class I/II HDAC inhibitor that has shown significant in vitro and in vivo activity against MPN cells, and that has exerted little toxicity against normal bone marrow progenitor cells, hepatocytes, and mesenchymal cells.[105,106] Givinostat activity was greatest in MPN cells with expression of JAK2V617F compared with JAK2 WT-expressing cells. Based on the promising in vitro and in vivo preclinical data, a phase II study was conducted to evaluate the safety and efficacy of givinostat in 29 patients with PV, ET, or PMF.[106] Givinostat was well tolerated and no grade IV toxicities were observed. Givinostat treatment alleviated pruritus in most patients, and 75% of patients with PV/ET and 38% of patients with MF had a reduction in spleen size. Of the 29 patients on the study, there was 1 complete response, 6 partial responses in patients with PV/ET, and 3 major responses in patients with MF.[106] A phase II study was also conducted to test the efficacy of the combination of givinostat and the ribonucleotide reductase inhibitor, hydroxyurea (HU) in patients with PV.[107] The combination of givinostat and HU was well tolerated and effective, with 50% of patients achieving a partial or complete response according to European LeukemiaNet criteria.[107] In addition, the preclinical use of novel combinations using HDAC inhibitors and chromatin-modifying agents such as the DNA methyltransferase inhibitor decitabine (5-aza-2'-deoxycytidine) has been reported.[108,109] In this epitargeted strategy for treating MF-MPN, the sequential treatment of decitabine followed by HDAC inhibitor (Zolinza [vorinostat]) or trichostatin A resulted in greater lethality of JAK2V617F+ PMF cells and spared normal CD34+ cells. These studies also identified that the combination of DNMT1 inhibitor and HDAC inhibitor led to significant reductions in the proportions of JAK2V617F HPCs as well as reductions in HPCs with chromosomal abnormalities.[108] This combination also upregulated expression of the chemokine receptor CXCR4 on CD34+ cells, which restored their ability to respond to CXCL12 stimulation and home to the bone marrow rather than remain aberrantly mobilized.[109] This epitargeted treatment strategy also reduced the short-term and long-term SCID repopulating cells and JAK2V617F+ HSCs in murine transplant models.[108] These preclinical data create the rationale for epigenetic targeted therapy in the treatment of MPN. A phase II study was conducted with 5-azacytidine alone in patients with relapsed or refractory MF.[110] The overall response rate on this study was 37%, and 2 patients obtained a partial or complete response. In addition, in the responders, a 61% mean reduction in circulating CD34+ cells was observed.[110] Collectively, these preclinical and clinical data represent a novel therapeutic strategy for targeting MPN progenitor (HSCs) or potentially MPN stem cells. Recently, a novel inhibitor of EZH2 methyltransferase activity (GSK-126) was reported to inhibit the methyltransferase activity of WT EZH2 and EZH2 with activating mutations at Tyr641.[111] Treatment with this inhibitor resulted in global reduction of H3K273Me and increased expression of EZH2 target genes as well as dose-dependent inhibition of tumor growth in mouse models of lymphoma.[111] Although the spectrum of mutations in MPN differ from those in lymphomas, studies to determine the activity of GSK-126 alone or in combination with other agents such as HDAC inhibitors have yet to be conducted against MPN cells.

Hsp90 Inhibitors

Hsp90 is a highly conserved, homodimeric, ATP-dependent, abundantly expressed protein, which forms the core of a super chaperone complex.[112–114] Hsp90 promotes the stabilization and folding of client proteins into their active conformation.[112–114] Each monomer of hsp90 has a highly conserved amino terminal adenosine triphosphate-binding domain, a middle client protein-binding domain, and a carboxy terminal dimerization domain.[112–114] Previous studies have shown that many oncoprotein kinases, including JAK2, FLT-3, and BCR-ABL, are client proteins of hsp90.[98–100] Furthermore, previous studies have suggested that the mutant oncoprotein kinases are more dependent on the chaperone function of hsp90 than their unmutated counterparts.[98–100] Many of the proteins that are deregulated and confer a pro-growth and pro-survival advantage to MPN cells (c-RAF, AKT, pSTAT5, and PIM) are also client proteins of hsp90.[98–100,115–119] Several hsp90 inhibitors, tanespimycin (17-AAG), alvespimycin (17-DMAG), AUY922, and ganetespib (STA9090), have been developed and are in various stages of clinical development in the treatment of hematologic and epithelial malignancies.[120–122] Preclinical studies have shown that inhibition of hsp90 in MPN cells also inhibits JAK2 expression and downstream signaling.[115,122,123] A recent study determined the in vitro and in vivo effects of treatment with PU-H71, a novel, nonquinone-based hsp90 inhibitor against JAK2V617F-expressing and MPLW515L-expressing cells.[123] Treatment with PU-H71 induced cell growth arrest and apoptosis of cultured and primary MPN cells. This finding was associated with inhibition of hsp90 chaperone function and loss of binding of JAK2 to hsp90. PU-H71 also depleted JAK2 expression levels and potently inhibited JAK2 downstream signaling in cultured and primary MPN cells. In vivo treatment of JAK2V617F or MPLW515L expressing mice with PU-H71 resulted in normalization of blood counts, decreased extramedullary hematopoiesis, and improved survival compared with vehicle control mice.[123] Similar effects on JAK2V617F expression levels, downstream signaling and anti-MPN activity were also observed with another hsp90 inhibitor, ganetespib.[122] Preclinical studies with AUY922, a third-generation hsp90 inhibitor, showed that hsp90 inhibition attenuated JAK2 V617F expression and inhibited JAK/STAT signaling in cultured and primary MPN cells.[115] Treatment with AUY922 caused dose-dependent apoptosis of cultured and primary MPN cells. Furthermore, the combination of AUY922 and the JAK2-TKI, TG101209, increased JAK2 inhibitor-mediated depletion of JAK/STAT signaling and exerted superior anti-MPN cytotoxic activity against cultured and primary MF-MPN cells. In addition, this study also showed that the combination of AUY922 and TG101209 could overcome JAK-TKI resistance in cultured human MPN cells isolated under the selection pressure of a JAK inhibitor.[115] AUY922 was also shown to be effective against JAK-TKI-resistant Ba/F3 cells expressing JAK2V617F in cis with other kinase domain mutations (eg, R683G, G935R, Y931C, and E864K) isolated by random mutagenesis in bacteria.[124] Collectively, these studies support the rationale to test hsp90 inhibitors alone, or in combination with JAK-TKI for the treatment of MPN. Testing of hsp90 inhibitors is also merited in patients who develop resistance or intolerance to JAK-TKIs.

Hedgehog Inhibitor

Hedgehog (HH) signaling pathway is involved in the self-renewal of stem cells and hematopoiesis.[125] HH signaling is activated by the HH ligand Sonic, Indian, or Desert, which negatively regulate the activity of the 12-span membrane receptor protein Patched (PTCH).[125] In turn, PTC inhibits the 7-span transmembrane protein Smoothened (SMO). HH ligands bind to PTC, leading to its internalization and degradation, thereby releasing SMO to promote the dissociation of Suppressor of Fused (SUFU)-GLI complex.[125] This situation results in nuclear localization and activity of GLI transcription factors (GLI1 and GLI2) and degradation of the repressor form GLI3. GLI1 and GLI2 induce the expression of the HH pathway target genes, including Cyclin D, Cyclin B, PTCH1, GLI1, GLI2, and BCL-2.[125,126] HH signaling is normally silenced in adult cells but becomes activated and deregulated in myeloid malignancies, including MPN.[127,128] Several HH inhibitors have been developed that target SMO, including GDC-0449 (Vismodegib), LDE225, and PF-04449913.[127,128] Recently, a first-in-man, phase Ia dose escalation study was conducted with PF-04449913, an oral SMO antagonist HH inhibitor in patients with hematologic malignancies, including MF.[128] Patients with MF treated with PF-04449913 attained stable disease, and 1 patient treated for more than 385 days, achieved a clinical improvement, with 50% reduction in spleen size that was sustained for more than 8 weeks. This study showed that PF-04449913 was safe to administer, was well tolerated, and displayed promising activity in treating MPN.[128] These findings support the rationale to further test Hh signaling inhibitors alone and in combination with JAK-TKI against MPN cells.

β-Catenin Antagonist

The canonical WNT-β-catenin signaling is essential to the self-renewal and growth of myeloid leukemia stem and MPN progenitor cells.[129,130] In transformed myeloid stem and progenitor cells with activating tyrosine kinase mutations, deregulated WNT signaling has been noted to inhibit polyubiquitylation and proteasomal degradation of β-catenin by the SCF-like complex comprising Siah-1, SIP, Skp1, and TBL1.[129,130] The multiprotein degradation complex for β-catenin is often inactivated in transformed HPCs. This situation results in the preservation, nuclear translocation, and interaction of β-catenin with the T-cell factor (TCF)/lymphoid enhancer factor transcription factor, which regulates the expression of genes such as Cyclin D1, MYC, and Survivin.[129–132] In a recent study, the activity of BC2059 (β-Cat Pharmaceuticals, Gaithersburg, MD), a potent small-molecule, anthraquinone oxime-analogue inhibitor of the WNT-β-catenin pathway, was determined in human cultured and primary MPN cells derived from patients with MF versus normal CD34+ bone marrow progenitor cells.[133] Treatment with BC2059 mediates the degradation and attenuated levels of β-catenin. Exposure to 100 nM of BC2059 induced cell cycle G1 phase accumulation and apoptosis of the cultured MPN HEL92.1.7 (HEL) and UKE1 cells expressing the mutant JAK2V617F. BC2059 treatment also induced apoptosis of CD34+ primary MPN cells from patients with advanced MPN expressing mutant JAK2. In contrast, BC2059 did not induce significant apoptosis of normal CD34+ progenitor cells. Exposure to BC2059 attenuated both β-catenin protein levels (significantly restored by cotreatment with the proteasome inhibitor) and the activity of the LEF1/TCF4 transcription factor, associated with reduced levels of Cyclin D1, MYC, and survivin in the cell lysates of BC2059-treated MPN cells. In a xenograft model of HEL cells in NOD/SCID mice, treatment with BC2059 showed significantly improved survival ($P<.001$). Compared with treatment with each agent alone, cotreatment with BC2059 (20–50 nM) and JAK2-TKI TG101209 (200–1000 nM) synergistically induced apoptosis of HEL and primary CD34+ MPN cells, but was remarkably less toxic against normal CD34+ progenitor cells ($P<.01$).[133] These preclinical studies highlight the therapeutic potential of β-catenin antagonists alone and in combination with JAK-TKI against MPN, which needs to be further explored clinically.

ALLOGENEIC STEM CELL TRANSPLANT

Despite significant advances in the therapy for MPN with the introduction and approval of JAK inhibitors, the only therapeutic modality that has been shown to be capable of inducing complete hematologic, cytogenetic, and molecular remissions in patients with MPN is allogeneic HSC transplantation (AHSCT).[134,135] Because of the risk involved, AHSCT is indicated primarily for intermediate-2-risk or high-risk patients with MPN with the goal of prolonging survival.[134,135] However, with the development of reduced intensity conditioning (RIC), AHSCT can be used to treat more patients with MF, particularly those with advanced age and additional comorbidities.[134] A multicenter phase II trial determined the efficacy of 2 regimens of RIC with fludarabine (30 mg/m² for 6 days), busulphan (1 mg/kg; 10 doses over 3 days) and antithymocyte globulin 3 × 10 mg/kg (matched sibling donor [MSD]) or 3 × 20 mg/kg (unrelated donor [URD]) in patients with MF before transplantation. RIC before transplantation was associated with low incidences of relapse at 3 and 5 years (22% and 29%, respectively). In addition, estimated 5-year disease-free survival (51%) and OS (67%) rates for patients with MF were encouraging.[134] In the MSD regimen, the overall clinical response at 6 months was 79% compared with 49% in the URD setting.[134] Other large studies of AHSCT have shown lower treatment-related mortality, particularly in HLA identical-sibling transplants (18%) and alternative related donors (19%) and 5-year disease-free survival rates ranging between 27% and 33%, depending on whether the donors were matched related or unrelated.[68,135,136] The overall goal of AHSCT therapy in MF is the achievement of JAK2V617F negativity after transplant. A recent study observed that patients who achieved JAK2V617F negativity after AHSCT had a significantly lower incidence of relapse (hazard ratio = 0.22, $P = .04$).[137] Furthermore, patients whose PB cleared of JAK2V617F had a significantly lower risk of relapse than patients whose PB had not cleared JAK2V617F (5% vs 35%, $P = .03$).[137] RIC represents a more feasible alternative for elderly patients than myeloablative transplantation for the treatment of MF.

SUMMARY

The recent recognition of clinical benefit conferred by JAK inhibitors and the FDA approval of ruxolitinib represent a significant leap forward in the therapy for MF. Already with the expanded use of these agents, limitations of this class of agents are being identified. These limitations include the potential for hematologic toxicity, lack of significant impact on the bone marrow histopathology (including MF), and reduction in the allelic burden of the activating mutations in JAK2 and other proteins that result in the constitutive activation of the JAK/STAT pathway. In the advanced stages of MPN, there is also the distinct possibility of the presence of a founder clone with mutations in the epigenetic modifiers possessing leukemia-initiating capacity and treatment refractoriness to JAK inhibitors. To address these challenges, novel agents targeting deregulated pro-growth and pro-survival kinases (eg, PI3K, AKT, mTOR, MEK and PIM), as well as other pathways involved in the self-renewal of progenitor cells (eg, HH and WNT/β-catenin) are rapidly being developed and preclinically tested alone and in combination with JAK-TKI. In addition, HDAC inhibitors or DNMT1 inhibitors have shown preclinical activity against MPN. Findings from these preclinical studies are promising and support the rationale for conducting well-designed clinical studies of the novel agents including analyses of the predictive biomarkers of response to these agents. For example, clinical studies are under way combining HDAC inhibitors with JAK-TKI in MF. Also, testing of hsp90 inhibitors for the treatment of MF is supported by several studies that have shown the ability of hsp90 inhibitors not only to deplete JAK2V617F levels and its downstream signaling but also to overcome acquired resistance to JAK-TKIs, which may emerge in patients continuously treated with JAK inhibitors. Taken together, the promising potential of these targeted single agents or their combinations with JAK-TKI represent exciting new avenues for testing as therapy for advanced MPN. The goal is to change the natural history of the disease similar to what has been observed after treatment with BCR-ABL-targeted TKIs in CML.

REFERENCES

1. Baxter EJ, Scott LM, Campbell PJ, et al. Acquired mutation of the tyrosine kinase JAK2 in human myeloproliferative disorders. Lancet 2005;365:1054–61.
2. James C, Ugo V, Le Couedic JP, et al. A unique clonal JAK2 mutation leading to constitutive signalling causes polycythaemia vera. Nature 2005;434:1144–8.
3. Levine RL, Wadleigh M, Cools J, et al. Activating mutation in the tyrosine kinase JAK2 in polycythemia vera, essential thrombocythemia, and myeloid metaplasia with myelofibrosis. Cancer Cell 2005;7:387–97.
4. Levine RL, Gilliland DG. Myeloproliferative disorders. Blood 2008;112:2190–8.
5. Levine RL, Pardanani A, Tefferi A, et al. Role of JAK2 in the pathogenesis and therapy of myeloproliferative disorders. Nat Rev Cancer 2007;7:673–83.
6. Baker SJ, Rane SG, Reddy EP. Hematopoietic cytokine receptor signaling. Oncogene 2007;26:6724–37.
7. Oku S, Takenaka K, Kuriyama T, et al. JAK2 V617F uses distinct signalling pathways to induce cell proliferation and neutrophil activation. Br J Haematol 2010;150:334–44.
8. Ungureanu D, Wu J, Pekkala T, et al. The pseudokinase domain of JAK2 is a dual-specificity protein kinase that negatively regulates cytokine signaling. Nat Struct Mol Biol 2011;18:971–6.
9. Sanz A, Ungureanu D, Pekkala T, et al. Analysis of Jak2 catalytic function by peptide microarrays: the role of the JH2 domain and V617F mutation. PLoS One 2011;6:e18522.
10. Friedbichler K, Kerenyi MA, Kovacic B, et al. Stat5a serine 725 and 779 phosphorylation is a prerequisite for hematopoietic transformation. Blood 2010;116:1548–58.
11. Dawson MA, Bannister AJ, Gottgens B, et al. JAK2 phosphorylates histone H3Y41 and excludes HP1alpha from chromatin. Nature 2009;461:819–22.
12. He J, Zhang Y. Janus kinase 2: an epigenetic 'writer' that activates leukemogenic genes. J Mol Cell Biol 2010;2:231–3.
13. Scott LM, Tong W, Levine RL, et al. JAK2 exon 12 mutations in polycythemia vera and idiopathic erythrocytosis. N Engl J Med 2007;356:459–68.
14. Pardanani AD, Levine RL, Lasho T, et al. MPL515 mutations in myeloproliferative and other myeloid disorders: a study of 1182 patients. Blood 2006;108:3472–6.
15. Levine RL, Wernig G. Role of JAK-STAT signaling in the pathogenesis of myeloproliferative disorders. Hematology Am Soc Hematol Educ Program 2006;1:233–9.
16. Koppikar P, Abdel-Wahab O, Hedvat C, et al. Efficacy of the JAK2 inhibitor INCB16562 in a murine model of MPLW515L-induced thrombocytosis and myelofibrosis. Blood 2010;115:2919–27.

17. Makishima H, Cazzolli H, Szpurka H, et al. Mutations of the e3 ubiquitin ligase cbl family members constitute a novel pathogenic lesion in myeloid malignancies. J Clin Oncol 2009;27:6109–16.

18. Tefferi A. Novel mutations and their functional and clinical relevance in myeloproliferative neoplasms: JAK2, MPL, TET2, ASXL1, CBL, IDH and IKZF1. Leukemia 2010;24:1128–38.

19. Delhommeau F, Jeziorowska D, Marzac C, et al. Molecular aspects of myeloproliferative neoplasms. Int J Hematol 2010;91:165–73.

20. Vainchenker W, Delhommeau F, Constantinescu SN, et al. New mutations and pathogenesis of myeloproliferative neoplasms. Blood 2011;118:1723–35.

21. Pardanani A, Lasho T, Finke C, et al. LNK mutation studies in blast-phase myeloproliferative neoplasms, and in chronic-phase disease with TET2, IDH, JAK2 or MPL mutations. Leukemia 2010;24:1713–8.

22. Oh ST, Simonds EF, Jones C, et al. Novel mutations in the inhibitory adaptor protein LNK drive JAK-STAT signaling in patients with myeloproliferative neoplasms. Blood 2010;116:988–92.

23. Abdel-Wahab O. Genetics of the myeloproliferative neoplasms. Curr Opin Hematol 2011;18:117–23.

24. Quintas-Cardama A, Kantarjian H, Cortes J, et al. Janus kinase inhibitors for the treatment of myeloproliferative neoplasias and beyond. Nat Rev Drug Discov 2011;10:127–40.

25. Chappell WH, Steelman LS, Long JM, et al. Ras/Raf/MEK/ERK and PI3K/PTEN/Akt/mTOR inhibitors: rationale and importance to inhibiting these pathways in human health. Oncotarget 2011;2:135–64.

26. Steelman LS, Franklin RA, Abrams SL, et al. Roles of the Ras/Raf/MEK/ERK pathway in leukemia therapy. Leukemia 2011;25:1080–94.

27. Chung E, Hsu CL, Kondo M. Constitutive MAP kinase activation in hematopoietic stem cells induces a myeloproliferative disorder. PLoS One 2011;6: e28350.

28. Engelman JA. Targeting PI3K signalling in cancer: opportunities, challenges and limitations. Nat Rev Cancer 2009;9:550–62.

29. Wernig G, Gonneville JR, Crowley BJ, et al. The Jak2V617F oncogene associated with myeloproliferative diseases requires a functional FERM domain for transformation and for expression of the Myc and Pim proto-oncogenes. Blood 2008;111:3751–9.

30. Shah N, Pang B, Yeoh KG, et al. Potential roles for the PIM1 kinase in human cancer– a molecular and therapeutic appraisal. Eur J Cancer 2008;44:2144–51.

31. Abdel-Wahab O, Pardanani A, Patel J, et al. Concomitant analysis of EZH2 and ASXL1 mutations in myelofibrosis, chronic myelomonocytic leukemia and blast-phase myeloproliferative neoplasms. Leukemia 2011;25:1200–2.

32. Carbuccia N, Murati A, Trouplin V, et al. Mutations of ASXL1 gene in myeloproliferative neoplasms. Leukemia 2009;23:2183–6.

33. Tefferi A, Vainchenker W. Myeloproliferative neoplasms: molecular pathophysiology, essential clinical understanding, and treatment strategies. J Clin Oncol 2011;29:573–82.

34. Chase A, Cross NC. Aberrations of EZH2 in cancer. Clin Cancer Res 2011;17: 2613–8.

35. Martin-Perez D, Piris MA, Sanchez-Beato M. Polycomb proteins in hematologic malignancies. Blood 2010;116:5465–75.

36. Ernst T, Chase AJ, Score J, et al. Inactivating mutations of the histone methyltransferase gene EZH2 in myeloid disorders. Nat Genet 2010;42:722–6.

37. Guglielmelli P, Biamonte F, Score J, et al. EZH2 mutational status predicts poor survival in myelofibrosis. Blood 2011;118:5227–34.
38. Ricci C, Spinelli O, Salmoiraghi S, et al. ASXL1 mutations in primary and secondary myelofibrosis. Br J Haematol 2012;156:404–7.
39. Levine RL. Mutations in epigenetic modifiers in MPN and MDS pathogenesis. Proceedings of the 103rd Annual Meeting of the American Association for Cancer Research; 2012 March 31-April 4. Chicago (IL), Philadelphia: AACR; 2012. Abstract NC18.
40. Guglielmelli P, Biamonte F, Score J, et al. Prognostic impact of EZH2 and ASXL1 mutation in myelofibrosis. ASH Annual Meeting Abstracts 2011;118:2811.
41. Stein BL, Williams DM, O'Keefe C, et al. Disruption of the ASXL1 gene is frequent in primary, post-essential thrombocytosis and post-polycythemia vera myelofibrosis, but not essential thrombocytosis or polycythemia vera: analysis of molecular genetics and clinical phenotypes. Haematologica 2011;96:1462–9.
42. Ko M, Huang Y, Jankowska AM, et al. Impaired hydroxylation of 5-methylcytosine in myeloid cancers with mutant TET2. Nature 2010;468:839–43.
43. Tefferi A, Pardanani A, Lim KH, et al. TET2 mutations and their clinical correlates in polycythemia vera, essential thrombocythemia and myelofibrosis. Leukemia 2009;23:905–11.
44. Martinez-Aviles L, Besses C, Alvarez-Larran A, et al. TET2, ASXL1, IDH1, IDH2, and c-CBL genes in JAK2- and MPL-negative myeloproliferative neoplasms. Ann Hematol 2012;91(4):533–41.
45. Gross S, Cairns RA, Minden MD, et al. Cancer-associated metabolite 2-hydroxyglutarate accumulates in acute myelogenous leukemia with isocitrate dehydrogenase 1 and 2 mutations. J Exp Med 2010;207:339–44.
46. Ward PS, Patel J, Wise DR, et al. The common feature of leukemia-associated IDH1 and IDH2 mutations is a neomorphic enzyme activity converting alpha-ketoglutarate to 2-hydroxyglutarate. Cancer Cell 2010;17:225–34.
47. Figueroa ME, Abdel-Wahab O, Lu C, et al. Leukemic IDH1 and IDH2 mutations result in a hypermethylation phenotype, disrupt TET2 function, and impair hematopoietic differentiation. Cancer Cell 2010;18:553–67.
48. Xu W, Yang H, Liu Y, et al. Oncometabolite 2-hydroxyglutarate is a competitive inhibitor of alpha-ketoglutarate-dependent dioxygenases. Cancer Cell 2011;19:17–30.
49. Chowdhury R, Yeoh KK, Tian YM, et al. The oncometabolite 2-hydroxyglutarate inhibits histone lysine demethylases. EMBO Rep 2011;12:463–9.
50. Lu C, Ward PS, Kapoor GS, et al. IDH mutation impairs histone demethylation and results in a block to cell differentiation. Nature 2012;483:474–8.
51. Sulai N, Jimma T, Lasho TL, et al. IDH mutations in primary myelofibrosis predict leukemic transformation and shortened survival: clinical evidence for leukemogenic collaboration with JAK2V617F. ASH Annual Meeting Abstracts 2011; 118:1751.
52. Tefferi A, Jimma T, Sulai NH, et al. IDH mutations in primary myelofibrosis predict leukemic transformation and shortened survival: clinical evidence for leukemogenic collaboration with JAK2V617F. Leukemia 2012;26:475–80.
53. Stegelmann F, Bullinger L, Schlenk RF, et al. DNMT3A mutations in myeloproliferative neoplasms. Leukemia 2011;25:1217–9.
54. Challen GA, Sun D, Jeong M, et al. Dnmt3a is essential for hematopoietic stem cell differentiation. Nat Genet 2012;44:23–31.
55. Brecqueville M, Rey J, Bertucci F, et al. Mutation analysis of ASXL1, CBL, DNMT3A, IDH1, IDH2, JAK2, MPL, NF1, SF3B1, SUZ12, and TET2 in myeloproliferative neoplasms. Genes Chromosomes Cancer 2012;51(8):743–55.

56. Abdel-Wahab O, Pardanani A, Rampal R, et al. DNMT3A mutational analysis in primary myelofibrosis, chronic myelomonocytic leukemia and advanced phases of myeloproliferative neoplasms. Leukemia 2011;25:1219–20.

57. Walter MJ, Ding L, Shen D, et al. Recurrent DNMT3A mutations in patients with myelodysplastic syndromes. Leukemia 2011;25:1153–8.

58. Metzeler KH, Walker A, Geyer S, et al. DNMT3A mutations and response to the hypomethylating agent decitabine in acute myeloid leukemia. Leukemia 2012; 26(5):1106–7.

59. Passamonti F, Maffioli M, Caramazza D. New generation small-molecule inhibitors in myeloproliferative neoplasms. Curr Opin Hematol 2012;19:117–23.

60. Verstovsek S, Kantarjian H, Mesa RA, et al. Safety and efficacy of INCB018424, a JAK1 and JAK2 inhibitor, in myelofibrosis. N Engl J Med 2010;363:1117–27.

61. Mascarenhas J, Hoffman R. Ruxolitinib: the first FDA approved therapy for the treatment of myelofibrosis. Clin Cancer Res 2012;18(11):3008–14.

62. Tefferi A. JAK inhibitors for myeloproliferative neoplasms; clarifying facts from myths. Blood 2012;119:2721–30.

63. Pardanani A, Gotlib JR, Jamieson C, et al. Safety and efficacy of TG101348, a selective JAK2 inhibitor, in myelofibrosis. J Clin Oncol 2011;29:789–96.

64. Tefferi A. Challenges facing JAK inhibitor therapy for myeloproliferative neoplasms. N Engl J Med 2012;366:844–6.

65. Deshpande A, Reddy MM, Schade G, et al. Kinase domain mutations in JAK2V617F confer resistance to the novel JAK2 inhibitor ruxolitinib. ASH Annual Meeting Abstracts 2011;118:125.

66. Kalota A, Jeschke GR, Carroll M, et al. Intrinsic resistance to JAK2 inhibition in myelofibrosis. ASH Annual Meeting Abstracts 2011;118:2825.

67. Pardanani A, Vannucchi AM, Passamonti F, et al. JAK inhibitor therapy for myelofibrosis: critical assessment of value and limitations. Leukemia 2011;25: 218–25.

68. Tefferi A. How I treat myelofibrosis. Blood 2011;117:3494–504.

69. Ugo V, Marzac C, Teyssandier I, et al. Multiple signaling pathways are involved in erythropoietin-independent differentiation of erythroid progenitors in polycythemia vera. Exp Hematol 2004;32:179–87.

70. Vannucchi AM, Bogani C, Bartalucci N, et al. The mTOR inhibitor, RAD001, inhibits the growth of cells from patients with myeloproliferative neoplasms. ASH Annual Meeting Abstracts 2009;114:2914.

71. Vannucchi AM, Guglielmelli P, Gattoni E, et al. RAD001, an inhibitor of mTOR, shows clinical activity in a phase I/II study in patients with primary myelofibrosis (PMF) and post polycythemia vera/essential thrombocythemia myelofibrosis (PPV/PET MF). ASH Annual Meeting Abstracts 2009;114:307.

72. Laplante M, Sabatini DM. mTOR signaling in growth control and disease. Cell 2012;149:274–93.

73. Guglielmelli P, Barosi G, Rambaldi A, et al. Safety and efficacy of everolimus, a mTOR inhibitor, as single agent in a phase 1/2 study in patients with myelofibrosis. Blood 2011;118:2069–76.

74. Fiskus W, Manepalli RR, Balusu R, et al. Synergistic activity of combinations of JAK2 kinase inhibitor with PI3K/mTOR, MEK or PIM kinase inhibitor against human myeloproliferative neoplasm cells expressing JAK2V617F. ASH Annual Meeting Abstracts 2010;116:798.

75. Khan I, Huang Z, Wen QJ, et al. Inhibition of AKT signaling potently inhibits the growth of JAK and MPL-mutant cells in the myeloproliferative neoplasms in vitro and in vivo. ASH Annual Meeting Abstracts 2011;118:3862.

76. Chung E, Kondo M. Role of Ras/Raf/MEK/ERK signaling in physiological hematopoiesis and leukemia development. Immunol Res 2011;49:248–68.

77. Odenike O, Curran E, Iyengar N, et al. Phase II study of the oral MEK inhibitor AZD6244 in advanced acute myeloid leukemia (AML). ASH Annual Meeting Abstracts 2009;114:2081.

78. Bachmann M, Kosan C, Xing PX, et al. The oncogenic serine/threonine kinase Pim-1 directly phosphorylates and activates the G2/M specific phosphatase Cdc25C. Int J Biochem Cell Biol 2006;38:430–43.

79. Bachmann M, Moroy T. The serine/threonine kinase Pim-1. Int J Biochem Cell Biol 2005;37:726–30.

80. Isaac M, Siu A, Jongstra J. The oncogenic PIM kinase family regulates drug resistance through multiple mechanisms. Drug Resist Updat 2011;14:203–11.

81. Nawijn MC, Alendar A, Berns A. For better or for worse: the role of Pim oncogenes in tumorigenesis. Nat Rev Cancer 2011;11:23–34.

82. Zhang F, Beharry ZM, Harris TE, et al. PIM1 protein kinase regulates PRAS40 phosphorylation and mTOR activity in FDCP1 cells. Cancer Biol Ther 2009;8: 846–53.

83. Fiskus WC, Buckley KM, Rao R, et al. Synergistic activity of co-treatment with pim1 kinase inhibitor SGI-1776 and histone deacetylase inhibitor panobinostat or heat shock protein 90 inhibitor AUY922 against human CML and myeloproliferative neoplasm (MPN) cells [abstract: 2651]. ASH Annual Meeting Abstracts 2009;114.

84. Keeton E, Palakurthi S, Alimzhanov M, et al. AZD1208, a novel, potent and selective pan PIM kinase inhibitor, demonstrates efficacy in models of acute myeloid leukemia [abstract: 1540]. ASH Annual Meeting Abstracts 2011;118.

85. Wang JC, Chen C, Dumlao T, et al. Enhanced histone deacetylase enzyme activity in primary myelofibrosis. Leuk Lymphoma 2008;49:2321–7.

86. Mithraprabhu S, Grigoriadis G, Khong T, et al. Deactylase inhibition in myeloproliferative neoplasms. Invest New Drugs 2010;28(Suppl 1):S50–7.

87. Minucci S, Pelicci PG. Histone deacetylase inhibitors and the promise of epigenetic (and more) treatments for cancer. Nat Rev Cancer 2006;6:38–51.

88. Arrowsmith CH, Bountra C, Fish PV, et al. Epigenetic protein families: a new frontier for drug discovery. Nat Rev Drug Discov 2012;11:384–400.

89. Glozak MA, Sengupta N, Zhang X, et al. Acetylation and deacetylation of non-histone proteins. Gene 2005;363:15–23.

90. Choudhary C, Kumar C, Gnad F, et al. Lysine acetylation targets protein complexes and co-regulates major cellular functions. Science 2009;325: 834–40.

91. Sampath D, Liu C, Vasan K, et al. Histone deacetylases mediate the silencing of miR-15a, miR-16, and miR-29b in chronic lymphocytic leukemia. Blood 2012; 119:1162–72.

92. Lane AA, Chabner BA. Histone deacetylase inhibitors in cancer therapy. J Clin Oncol 2009;27:5459–68.

93. Dokmanovic M, Clarke C, Marks PA. Histone deacetylase inhibitors: overview and perspectives. Mol Cancer Res 2007;5:981–9.

94. Dickinson M, Johnstone RW, Prince HM. Histone deacetylase inhibitors: potential targets responsible for their anti-cancer effect. Invest New Drugs 2010;28: 3–20.

95. Leoni F, Fossati G, Lewis EC, et al. The histone deacetylase inhibitor ITF2357 reduces production of pro-inflammatory cytokines in vitro and systemic inflammation in vivo. Mol Med 2005;11:1–15.

96. Bali P, Pranpat M, Bradner J, et al. Inhibition of histone deacetylase 6 acetylates and disrupts the chaperone function of heat shock protein 90: a novel basis for antileukemia activity of histone deacetylase inhibitors. J Biol Chem 2005;280: 26729–34.

97. Fiskus W, Pranpat M, Balasis M, et al. Histone deacetylase inhibitors deplete enhancer of zeste 2 and associated polycomb repressive complex 2 proteins in human acute leukemia cells. Mol Cancer Ther 2006;5:3096–104.

98. Fiskus W, Pranpat M, Bali P, et al. Combined effects of novel tyrosine kinase inhibitor AMN107 and histone deacetylase inhibitor LBH589 against Bcr-Abl-expressing human leukemia cells. Blood 2006;108:645–52.

99. George P, Bali P, Annavarapu S, et al. Combination of the histone deacetylase inhibitor LBH589 and the hsp90 inhibitor 17-AAG is highly active against human CML-BC cells and AML cells with activating mutation of FLT-3. Blood 2005;105: 1768–76.

100. Wang Y, Fiskus W, Chong DG, et al. Cotreatment with panobinostat and JAK2 inhibitor TG101209 attenuates JAK2V617F levels and signaling and exerts synergistic cytotoxic effects against human myeloproliferative neoplastic cells. Blood 2009;114:5024–33.

101. Fiskus W, Buckley K, Rao R, et al. Panobinostat treatment depletes EZH2 and DNMT1 levels and enhances decitabine mediated de-repression of JunB and loss of survival of human acute leukemia cells. Cancer Biol Ther 2009;8:939–50.

102. DeAngelo DJ, Spencer A, Fischer T, et al. Activity of oral panobinostat (LBH589) in patients with myelofibrosis [abstract: 2898]. ASH Annual Meeting Abstracts 2009;114.

103. Mascarenhas J, Mercado A, Rodriguez A, et al. Prolonged low dose therapy with a pan-deacetylase inhibitor, panobinostat (LBH589), in patients with myelo-fibrosis [abstract: 794]. ASH Annual Meeting Abstracts 2011;118.

104. Baffert F, Evrot E, Ebel N, et al. Improved efficacy upon combined JAK1/2 and pan-deacetylase inhibition using ruxolitinib (INC424) and panobinostat (LBH589) in preclinical mouse models of JAK2V617F-driven disease. ASH Annual Meeting Abstracts 2011;118:798.

105. Guerini V, Barbui V, Spinelli O, et al. The histone deacetylase inhibitor ITF2357 selectively targets cells bearing mutated JAK2(V617F). Leukemia 2008;22: 740–7.

106. Rambaldi A, Dellacasa CM, Finazzi G, et al. A pilot study of the Histone-Deacetylase inhibitor Givinostat in patients with JAK2V617F positive chronic myeloproliferative neoplasms. Br J Haematol 2010;150:446–55.

107. Rambaldi A, Finazzi G, Vannucchi AM, et al. A phase II study of the HDAC inhibitor givinostat in combination with hydroxyurea in patients with polycythemia vera resistant to hydroxyurea monotherapy. ASH Annual Meeting Abstracts 2011;118:1748.

108. Wang X, Zhang W, Tripodi J, et al. Sequential treatment of CD34+ cells from patients with primary myelofibrosis with chromatin-modifying agents eliminate JAK2V617F-positive NOD/SCID marrow repopulating cells. Blood 2010;116: 5972–82.

109. Shi J, Zhao Y, Ishii T, et al. Effects of chromatin-modifying agents on CD34+ cells from patients with idiopathic myelofibrosis. Cancer Res 2007;67:6417–24.

110. Mascarenhas J, Hoffman R. Myeloproliferative neoplasms: new translational therapies. Mt Sinai J Med 2010;77:667–83.

111. Creasy CL, McCabe MT, Korenchuk S, et al. A novel selective EZH2 inhibitor exhibits anti-tumor activity in lymphoma with EZH2 activating mutations. Proceedings

of the 103rd Annual Meeting of the American Association for Cancer Research; 2012 March 31-April 4. Chicago (IL), Philadelphia: AACR; 2012. Abstract 4700.

112. Picard D. Heat-shock protein 90, a chaperone for folding and regulation. Cell Mol Life Sci 2002;59:1640–8.

113. Trepel J, Mollapour M, Giaccone G, et al. Targeting the dynamic HSP90 complex in cancer. Nat Rev Cancer 2010;10:537–49.

114. Taipale M, Jarosz DF, Lindquist S. HSP90 at the hub of protein homeostasis: emerging mechanistic insights. Nat Rev Mol Cell Biol 2010;11:515–28.

115. Fiskus W, Verstovsek S, Manshouri T, et al. Heat shock protein 90 inhibitor is synergistic with JAK2 inhibitor and overcomes resistance to JAK2-TKI in human myeloproliferative neoplasm cells. Clin Cancer Res 2011;17:7347–58.

116. George P, Bali P, Cohen P, et al. Cotreatment with 17-allylamino-demethoxygel-danamycin and FLT-3 kinase inhibitor PKC412 is highly effective against human acute myelogenous leukemia cells with mutant FLT-3. Cancer Res 2004;64: 3645–52.

117. Pearl LH, Prodromou C, Workman P. The Hsp90 molecular chaperone: an open and shut case for treatment. Biochem J 2008;410:439–53.

118. Whitesell L, Lindquist SL. HSP90 and the chaperoning of cancer. Nat Rev Cancer 2005;5:761–72.

119. Shay KP, Wang Z, Xing PX, et al. Pim-1 kinase stability is regulated by heat shock proteins and the ubiquitin-proteasome pathway. Mol Cancer Res 2005;3:170–81.

120. Lancet JE, Gojo I, Burton M, et al. Phase I study of the heat shock protein 90 inhibitor alvespimycin (KOS-1022, 17-DMAG) administered intravenously twice weekly to patients with acute myeloid leukemia. Leukemia 2010;24:699–705.

121. Samuel TA, Sessa C, Britten C, et al. AUY922, a novel HSP90 inhibitor: final results of a first-in-human study in patients with advanced solid malignancies [abstract: 2528]. J Clin Oncol 2010;28(Suppl):15s.

122. Proia DA, Foley KP, Korbut T, et al. Multifaceted intervention by the Hsp90 inhibitor ganetespib (STA-9090) in cancer cells with activated JAK/STAT signaling. PLoS One 2011;6:e18552.

123. Marubayashi S, Koppikar P, Taldone T, et al. HSP90 is a therapeutic target in JAK2-dependent myeloproliferative neoplasms in mice and humans. J Clin Invest 2010;120:3578–93.

124. Weigert O, Lane AA, Bird L, et al. Genetic resistance to JAK2 enzymatic inhibitors is overcome by HSP90 inhibition. J Exp Med 2012;209:259–73.

125. Lin TL, Matsui W. Hedgehog pathway as a drug target: smoothened inhibitors in development. OncoTargets Ther 2012;5:47–58.

126. Harris LG, Samant RS, Shevde LA. Hedgehog signaling: networking to nurture a promalignant tumor microenvironment. Mol Cancer Res 2011;9:1165–74.

127. Irvine DA, Copland M. Targeting hedgehog in hematologic malignancy. Blood 2012;119:2196–204.

128. Jamieson C, Cortes JE, Oehler V, et al. Phase I dose-escalation study of PF-04449913, an oral Hedgehog (Hh) inhibitor, in patients with select hematologic malignancies [abstract: 424]. Blood (ASH Annual Meeting Abstracts) 2011;118.

129. Mosimann C, Hausmann G, Basler K. Beta-catenin hits chromatin: regulation of Wnt target gene activation. Nat Rev Mol Cell Biol 2009;10:276–86.

130. Gehrke I, Gandhirajan RK, Kreuzer KA. Targeting the WNT/beta-catenin/TCF/LEF1 axis in solid and haematological cancers: multiplicity of therapeutic options. Eur J Cancer 2009;45:2759–67.

131. Curtin JC, Lorenzi MV. Drug discovery approaches to target Wnt signaling in cancer stem cells. Oncotarget 2010;1:552–66.

132. Liu YC, Lai WC, Chuang KA, et al. Blockade of JAK2 activity suppressed accumulation of β-catenin in leukemic cells. J Cell Biochem 2010;111:402–11.

133. Fiskus W, Smith J, Mudunuru U, et al. Treatment with β-catenin antagonist BC2059 exerts single agent efficacy and exerts improved activity with tyrosine kinase inhibitor (TKI) or pan-histone deacetylase (HDAC) inhibitor against human CML and myeloproliferative neoplasm (MPN) progenitor cells [abstract: 65]. Blood (ASH Annual Meeting Abstracts) 2011;118.

134. McLornan DP, Mead AJ, Jackson G, et al. Allogeneic stem cell transplantation for myelofibrosis in 2012. Br J Haematol 2012;157:413–25.

135. Tefferi A. Primary myelofibrosis: 2012 update on diagnosis, risk stratification, and management. Am J Hematol 2011;86:1017–26.

136. Ballen KK, Shrestha S, Sobocinski KA, et al. Outcome of transplantation for myelofibrosis. Biol Blood Marrow Transplant 2010;16:358–67.

137. Alchalby H, Badbaran A, Zabelina T, et al. Impact of JAK2V617F mutation status, allele burden, and clearance after allogeneic stem cell transplantation for myelofibrosis. Blood 2010;116:3572–81.

Acquired Uniparental Disomy in Myeloproliferative Neoplasms

Joannah Score, PhD[a,b], Nicholas C.P. Cross, PhD[a,b],*

KEYWORDS

- Myeloproliferative neoplasm • Uniparental disomy • SNP array • TET2 • CBL
- EZH2 • JAK2

KEY POINTS

- Uniparental disomy is where both copies of a chromosome pair or parts of chromosomes have originated from one parent.
- Acquired uniparental disomy in cancer is a mechanism by which adventitious mutations are amplified leading to a growth advantage of these cells.
- Acquired uniparental disomy is now understood to be common in leukemia and renders a malignant or premalignant cell homozygous for a pre-existing mutation.
- Myeloproliferative neoplasms are clonal hematopoietic stem cell disorders characterized by overproliferation of one or more myeloid cell lineages in the bone marrow and increased numbers of mature and immature myeloid cells in the peripheral blood.
- Single nucleotide polymorphism arrays use the most frequent type of variation in the human genome and have enabled the rapid identification of uniparental disomy.
- Identification of tracts of recurrent acquired uniparental disomy, especially in hematologic malignancies, has led to identification of novel driver genes and therefore highlighted new pathways for targeted therapy.

INTRODUCTION

Cancer genomes are characterized by instability and a progressive accumulation of genetic aberrations. Loss of heterozygosity (LOH) is one such aberration and is widely recognized as a hallmark of cancer genomes.[1–8] LOH is most commonly caused by whole and partial chromosomal loss as a consequence of aneuploidy or somatically acquired deletions but in recent years it has become apparent that LOH may also be caused by uniparental disomy (UPD).

The authors have no conflict of interest to declare.

[a] Faculty of Medicine, University of Southampton, Southampton, UK; [b] Wessex Regional Genetics Laboratory, Salisbury NHS Foundation Trust, Salisbury SP2 8BJ, UK

* Corresponding author. Wessex Regional Genetics Laboratory, Salisbury NHS Foundation Trust, Salisbury SP2 8BJ, UK.

E-mail address: ncpc@soton.ac.uk

Hematol Oncol Clin N Am 26 (2012) 981–991

http://dx.doi.org/10.1016/j.hoc.2012.07.002

0889-8588/12/$ – see front matter

UPD refers to the situation in which both copies of a chromosome pair or parts of chromosomes have originated from one parent. When it occurs, UPD is often constitutional and arises from errors at meiosis I or meiosis II, the latter giving rise to isodisomy whereby the affected region is genetically identical. Constitutional isodisomy is frequently associated with developmental disorders caused by the abnormal expression of imprinted genes in the affected regions.[9] In cancer, UPD is acquired somatically and was first associated with the development of retinoblastoma.[10] It is now known that acquired UPD (aUPD; also known as acquired isodisomy or copy number neutral LOH) in cancer is a mechanism by which adventitious mutations are amplified, leading to a growth advantage of these cells.[11–13] Acquired UPD is common in solid cancers[14–20] and leukemia[6,12,21–24] and identification of tracts of recurrent aUPD, especially in hematologic malignancies, has led to identification of novel driver genes.[13,21,25–31]

This article describes how single nucleotide polymorphism (SNP) array technology has greatly facilitated the identification of regions of aUPD and led to the identification of novel mutations in myeloproliferative neoplasms (MPNs) and related disorders.

UPD AND THE IMPORTANCE OF SNP ARRAY TECHNOLOGY

Determining whether or not UPD is present is not possible using conventional cytogenetics, fluorescent *in situ* hybridization, or comparative genomic hybridization because there is no change in copy number and these techniques are usually unable to distinguish between maternal and paternal chromosomes. Before the completion of the Human Genome project and the wealth of SNP data that derived from it,[32] the identification of UPD was cumbersome, involving restriction fragment length polymorphism analysis where only small regions of the genome could be interrogated[10] or microsatellite analysis, which laboriously provided low resolution over the genome.[21] The advent of SNP array technology meant that genetic variation over the entire genome could be identified rapidly at much higher resolution than was previously possible.[33,34]

SNP arrays work by hybridizing the fragmented and fluorescently labeled sample DNA to immobilized oligonucleotide probes on glass plates or in solution. The probes are regularly spaced over the entire genome and used to identify the genotypes at specific polymorphic loci. Laser capture then identifies the ratios of fluorescent sample annealed to the probes.[35]

The first SNP array experiments looking at cancer genomes had only 600 to 1000 probes, and involved polymerase chain reactions of each SNP locus.[15,16] Now preparation of the sample can be done in one tube[35] with the number of probes exceeding 1 million. This has allowed for even higher throughput and resolution of the whole genome. SNP array technology can be used routinely to screen many patients for recurrent regions of aUPD and this information can be used in two ways: to examine if these regions are associated with prognosis,[36] and to determine the minimal affected regions (MARs) of aUPD and thereby target genes that might be mutated.[12]

ADVANTAGES AND DISADVANTAGES OF aUPD ANALYSIS BY SNP ARRAY TECHNOLOGY

For any given technique there are advantages and disadvantages, and aUPD analysis in leukemia with SNP arrays is no exception. SNP arrays, unlike metaphase cytogenetics, are not reliant on cell growth to yield detailed data on karyotype and although its throughput, resolution, and detailed mapping are vastly superior to microsatellite analysis and metaphase cytogenetics, SNP arrays cannot distinguish between one clone with several defects from several distinct clones. The technique effectively detects copy number changes (deletions or amplifications) but cannot detect balanced translocations that may, for example, be strong indicators for specific targeted therapies.[37,38] Thus, the commonly used term "SNP array karyotyping" is something of a misnomer.

Because SNP arrays were originally designed to look at population variation and germ line mutations,[39] there were several problems that needed to be overcome before successful analysis of cancer samples could be accomplished. The malignant clone size in clinical samples can be small and may be masked by a variably sized background of contaminating normal cells. This can make aUPD difficult to ascertain using conventional analysis software and therefore several algorithms were designed to enable identification of low levels of aUPD.[40,41] The resolution of these techniques depends in part on the size of the affected region, but it should be possible to detect larger regions in samples with only 20% to 30% tumor cells,[40] although a higher purity is preferred.

To unambiguously detect somatically acquired UPD it is critical to compare tumor (or tumor enriched) DNA with constitutional DNA (eg, derived from T-cells, buccal epithelia, fibroblasts, or remission samples). In the absence of constitutional DNA the possibility of an inherited region of homozygosity cannot be excluded. Indeed, analysis of lymphoblastoid cell lines derived from healthy individuals identified contiguous homozygous tracts greater than 5 Mb in nearly 10% of cases with some cases showing multiple homozygous tracts across the genome, probably as a result of consanguinity.[42] These regions were confirmed in peripheral blood samples in the subset of cases that were analyzed. In healthy individuals, runs of homozygosity greater than 20 Mb are very uncommon and therefore we have used this as a cutoff for defining likely regions of aUPD in our analysis.[25,28] Other studies have used much smaller cutoffs and in the absence of constitutional DNA it is likely that many of these regions are not derived by aUPD at all, but are simply identical by descent and of no pathogenetic significance. It is probably more appropriate to refer to these regions as copy number neutral runs of homozygosity if material is not available to prove somatic acquisition.[43]

IDENTIFICATION OF NOVEL MUTATIONS IN MPN AND MDS/MPN USING REGIONS OF aUPD

Somatically acquired UPD is now understood to be common in leukemia and renders a malignant or premalignant cell homozygous for a pre-existing mutation.[11–13,21,25–31,44–46] Reduction to homozygosity as a consequence of aUPD was initially thought to be only a mechanism for inactivation of tumor suppressor genes[10,11,19]; however, identification of aUPD in leukemia showed that oncogenic mutations are also targeted.[13,21,47]

MPNs are clonal hematopoietic stem cell disorders characterized by overproliferation of one or more myeloid cell lineages in the bone marrow and increased numbers of mature and immature myeloid cells in the peripheral blood. Excess proliferation is frequently associated with splenomegaly and cardiovascular complications and increased risk of transformation to acute leukemia. MPNs are categorized into subtypes based on specific morphologic, hematologic, and laboratory parameters, the best characterized being the four so-called classic MPNs: (1) polycythemia vera (PV), (2) essential thrombocythemia (ET), (3) primary myelofibrosis (PMF), and (4) chronic myeloid leukemia. In addition, some MPN cases have overlapping features with myelodysplastic syndromes (MDSs) and are classified separately as MDS/MPN, such as atypical BCR-ABL negative chronic myeloid leukemia and chronic myelomonocytic leukemia.

PV was the first hematologic malignancy to be associated with aUPD with the finding of a recurrently affected region at chromosome 9p.[21] However, its significance would remain obscure until this region was associated with the oncogenic V617F mutation in the *JAK2* gene in PV.[13] This acquired, single point mutation in *JAK2* was described in 95% of patients with PV, and 50% of patients with ET and PMF.[13,48–50] Acquired UPD at 9p results in a population of cells that are homozygous for V617F, and this is seen most commonly in PV and PMF but is rare in ET.[51]

SNP array analysis of MDS/MPN revealed that these were a heterogeneous group of diseases, accompanied by higher genetic instability than was previously thought. Moreover, regions of recurrent aUPD in otherwise karyotypically normal patients were a common finding, suggesting the presence of novel mutated genes in these patients.[6,52–54] Acquired UPD at 11q was one of the most common findings in these diseases, and candidate gene screening of the MAR revealed that the target in most of these cases was the Casitas B-lineage lymphoma (*CBL*) gene.[25–27] *CBL* is a negative regulator of tyrosine kinase signaling. In its positive role CBL binds to activated receptor tyrosine kinases by its N-terminal tyrosine kinase binding domain and serves as an adaptor by recruiting downstream signal transduction components, such as SHP2 and PI3K. However, the RING domain of CBL has E3 ligase activity and ubiquitinylates activated receptor tyrosine kinases on lysine residues, a signal that triggers internalization of the receptor/ligand complex and subsequent recycling or degradation.[55–57] *CBL* mutations had already been found in occasional cases of acute myeloid leukemia[58–60] but they were much more common in MDS/MPN at a frequency of about 10% and were a new class of mutation in these diseases.[25–27]

Despite SNP array refining candidate regions of aUPD to relatively small regions of the genome, some MARs contained hundreds of genes. However, SNP array data contain information on UPD and deletions. Combining both of these data sets allowed identification of additional targets. The first example of this approach focused on 4q aUPD in MDS/MPN, where focal microdeletions led to the identification of the *TET2* gene on 4q24 and further analysis showed this to be commonly mutated in many different subtypes of MDS and MPN.[29,31] Although its function at the time was unknown, TET2 is involved in epigenetic regulation; specifically, TET2 mediates the hydroxylation of 5-methylcytosine to 5-hydroxymethylcytosine in DNA.[61–63] *TET2* mutations are inactivating and often seem to be early events in the development of MPN and MDS/MPN.[31] Their prognostic value, if any, remains a matter of debate and may depend on the precise disease subtype.

In contrast, acquired UPD of 7q, found in 10% of MDS/MPN, was linked with a poor prognosis before mutation identification.[36,53] Enhancer of zeste 2 (*EZH2*) was subsequently identified as the target, again by the finding of focal microdeletions involving this gene.[28,30] EZH2 interacts with EED, SUZ12, and RBBP4 (also known as RbAp48) to form the polycomb repressive complex (PRC)-2, which functions to initiate epigenetic silencing of genes involved in cell fate decisions.[64,65] EZH2 is the catalytic component of PRC2 and specifically methylates lysine 27 of histone H3.[66–69] Trimethylated H3 (H3K27me3) serves as a signal for recruitment of further proteins, including PRC1, which maintains a silenced state. Although EZH2 had been implicated in a variety of cancers, inactivation of the gene through mutation had not before been observed. Mutations in *EZH2*, like the aUPD of 7q that amplifies it, is a poor prognostic marker in MPN and MDS/MPN.[28,30,70] Identification of *EZH2* mutations in these diseases has led to other members of PRC2 to be identified as mutated in MPN[46,71] and other leukemias,[72] underscoring the importance of genes involved in epigenetics in the genesis of leukemia. Indeed, next-generation sequencing has taken this work forward and identified other mutated epigenetic genes in MDS/MPN, such as *UTX* and *DNMT3A*.[73–75] Several other regions of aUPD have been identified in MDS/MPN[28] and it is likely that the putative targets of these events will be identified soon by next-generation sequencing approaches.

In addition to reducing mutations to homozygosity, it is possible that aUPD is associated with changes in expression levels of the genes in the affected region because some genes have expression dependent on the parent of origin,[76] whereas others are monoallelically expressed.[77,78] Acquired UPD may therefore have other as yet uncharacterized consequences that might, for example, give rise to interindividual differences within patient subgroups that could be dependent on individual genetic variation and the position of the mitotic recombination breakpoint that led to aUPD.[79]

MECHANISMS UNDERLYING aUPD

There are two mechanisms by which aUPD is thought to occur, broadly based on the type of aUPD. Segmental aUPD is thought to occur because of a reciprocal exchange of chromosomal material during mitosis, known as "mitotic recombination," which is often evident by homozygosity from the point of crossing over to the telomere (**Fig. 1**) but may give rise to interstitial aUPD if there are two points of recombination. Whole chromosome aUPD is likely to arise from nondisjunction, where an attempt is made to correct for loss of the chromosome material using the remaining chromosome copy as a template. The net result, however, is that the two chromosomes harboring the mutation segregate into the same daughter cell and provide it with a growth advantage.

In vitro studies on mouse fibroblast and normal human lymphocytes show that mitotic recombination (and therefore aUPD) is the most common mechanism of LOH with a background rate of about 1 in 100,000 cells.[80,81] Acquired UPD may be selectively preferable over large homozygous deletions because the cells may lose viability as a result of the loss of neighboring genes required for survival of the cell. There may also be reasons whereby aUPD is not adventitious to a leukemic or other cancerous cell. For instance, if the cell needs a normal functioning copy of the mutated gene for cell viability or if the mutation is already fully dominant in a heterozygous state and amplification through aUPD does not provide the cell with a further selective advantage. Mutations associated with regions of aUPD are predicted to be codominant (ie, they provide the cell with a selective advantage when heterozygous and a further advantage when homozygous).

Acquired UPD in leukemia and other cancers may be a random and spontaneous event, only evident because of the selective advantage it provides the cell. However, MDS/MPN seem to have a higher frequency of aUPD than other hematologic malignancies[25] and it is possible that aUPD is promoted by an early oncogenic mutation or genetic predisposition. Bloom and Werner syndromes exhibit increased mitotic recombination, which is caused by mutations in the RecQ helicase family of genes.[82] DNA helicases relax the tightly coiled structure of DNA and thus perform vital roles in DNA replication, DNA repair, transcription, and mitotic recombination[83,84] and it has been proposed that certain alleles or similar mutations may predispose to MPN.[85] The finding that homozygous V617F is common in PV and PMF but rare in ET might be a consequence of predisposition factors in PV and PMF that increase the probability of aUPD occurring. Alternatively, it might be that homozygous V617F does not have a selective advantage over heterozygous V617F in the context of ET but it does in the context of PV and PMF.

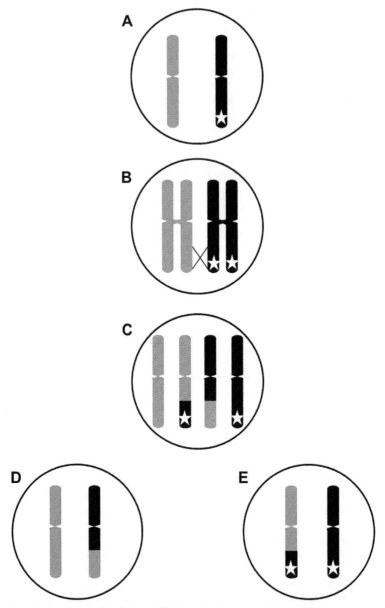

Fig. 1. Acquired uniparental disomy. (*A*) The chromosome with a *star* acquires a mutation that provides a selective advantage to that cell. (*B*) At mitosis the chromosomes undergo recombination. (*C*) The sister chromatids are pulled apart and when the daughter cells are formed one cell is wild-type (*D*) and the other is homozygous for the mutation (*E*). This mutant homozygous cell now has a proliferative/survival advantage over the wild-type and the heterozygous cell from which it was derived.

SUMMARY

SNPs are the most frequent type of variation in the human genome and can therefore be used as genomewide genetic markers.[32,86] SNP arrays swiftly became the tool of choice by which recurrent tracts of aUPD could be identified. In MPN and MDS/MPN this led to the elucidation of MARs harboring previously unsuspected mutational targets.

This important association between aUPD in MPN and MDS/MPN and amplification of mutations has increased the understanding of their pathogenesis. This has already led to important observations about prognosis,[28,30,70] disease progression,[7] and mechanisms underlying genomic instability,[85] and crucially the identification of novel pathways may lead to novel therapies.

REFERENCES

1. Fults D, Pedone CA, Thomas GA, et al. Allelotype of human malignant astrocytoma. Cancer Res 1990;50(18):5784–9.
2. Reid BJ, Barrett MT, Galipeau PC, et al. Barrett's esophagus: ordering the events that lead to cancer. Eur J Cancer Prev 1996;5(Suppl 2):57–65.
3. Thrash-Bingham CA, Greenberg RE, Howard S, et al. Comprehensive allelotyping of human renal cell carcinomas using microsatellite DNA probes. Proc Natl Acad Sci U S A 1995;92(7):2854–8.
4. Vogelstein B, Fearon ER, Kern SE, et al. Allelotype of colorectal carcinomas. Science 1989;244(4901):207–11.
5. Yamaguchi T, Toguchida J, Yamamuro T, et al. Allelotype analysis in osteosarcomas: frequent allele loss on 3q, 13q, 17p, and 18q. Cancer Res 1992;52(9):2419–23.
6. Gondek LP, Dunbar AJ, Szpurka H, et al. SNP array karyotyping allows for the detection of uniparental disomy and cryptic chromosomal abnormalities in MDS/MPD-U and MPD. PloS One 2007;2(11):e1225.
7. Klampfl T, Harutyunyan A, Berg T, et al. Genome integrity of myeloproliferative neoplasms in chronic phase and during disease progression. Blood 2011;118(1):167–76.
8. Tuna M, Knuutila S, Mills GB. Uniparental disomy in cancer. Trends Mol Med 2009;15(3):120–8.
9. Engel E. A new genetic concept: uniparental disomy and its potential effect, isodisomy. Am J Med Genet 1980;6(2):137–43.
10. Cavenee WK, Dryja TP, Phillips RA, et al. Expression of recessive alleles by chromosomal mechanisms in retinoblastoma. Nature 1983;305(5937):779–84.
11. Flotho C, Steinemann D, Mullighan CG, et al. Genome-wide single-nucleotide polymorphism analysis in juvenile myelomonocytic leukemia identifies uniparental disomy surrounding the NF1 locus in cases associated with neurofibromatosis but not in cases with mutant RAS or PTPN11. Oncogene 2007;26(39):5816–21.
12. Fitzgibbon J, Smith LL, Raghavan M, et al. Association between acquired uniparental disomy and homozygous gene mutation in acute myeloid leukemias. Cancer Res 2005;65(20):9152–4.
13. Kralovics R, Passamonti F, Buser AS, et al. A gain-of-function mutation of JAK2 in myeloproliferative disorders. N Engl J Med 2005;352(17):1779–90.
14. Chao LY, Huff V, Tomlinson G, et al. Genetic mosaicism in normal tissues of Wilms' tumour patients. Nat Genet 1993;3(2):127–31.
15. Lindblad-Toh K, Tanenbaum DM, Daly MJ, et al. Loss-of-heterozygosity analysis of small-cell lung carcinomas using single-nucleotide polymorphism arrays. Nat Biotechnol 2000;18(9):1001–5.

16. Mei R, Galipeau PC, Prass C, et al. Genome-wide detection of allelic imbalance using human SNPs and high-density DNA arrays. Genome Res 2000;10(8):1126–37.
17. Hoque MO, Lee CC, Cairns P, et al. Genome-wide genetic characterization of bladder cancer: a comparison of high-density single-nucleotide polymorphism arrays and PCR-based microsatellite analysis. Cancer Res 2003;63(9):2216–22.
18. Zhao X, Li C, Paez JG, et al. An integrated view of copy number and allelic alterations in the cancer genome using single nucleotide polymorphism arrays. Cancer Res 2004;64(9):3060–71.
19. Fearon ER, Vogelstein B, Feinberg AP. Somatic deletion and duplication of genes on chromosome 11 in Wilms' tumours. Nature 1984;309(5964):176–8.
20. Garraway LA, Widlund HR, Rubin MA, et al. Integrative genomic analyses identify MITF as a lineage survival oncogene amplified in malignant melanoma. Nature 2005;436(7047):117–22.
21. Kralovics R, Guan Y, Prchal JT. Acquired uniparental disomy of chromosome 9p is a frequent stem cell defect in polycythemia vera. Exp Hematol 2002;30(3):229–36.
22. Raghavan M, Lillington DM, Skoulakis S, et al. Genome-wide single nucleotide polymorphism analysis reveals frequent partial uniparental disomy due to somatic recombination in acute myeloid leukemias. Cancer Res 2005;65(2):375–8.
23. Kawamata N, Ogawa S, Zimmermann M, et al. Molecular allelokaryotyping of pediatric acute lymphoblastic leukemias by high-resolution single nucleotide polymorphism oligonucleotide genomic microarray. Blood 2008;111(2):776–84.
24. Lehmann S, Ogawa S, Raynaud SD, et al. Molecular allelokaryotyping of early-stage, untreated chronic lymphocytic leukemia. Cancer 2008;112(6):1296–305.
25. Grand FH, Hidalgo-Curtis CE, Ernst T, et al. Frequent CBL mutations associated with 11q acquired uniparental disomy in myeloproliferative neoplasms. Blood 2009;113(24):6182–92.
26. Sanada M, Suzuki T, Shih LY, et al. Gain-of-function of mutated C-CBL tumour suppressor in myeloid neoplasms. Nature 2009;460(7257):904–8.
27. Dunbar AJ, Gondek LP, O'Keefe CL, et al. 250K single nucleotide polymorphism array karyotyping identifies acquired uniparental disomy and homozygous mutations, including novel missense substitutions of c-Cbl, in myeloid malignancies. Cancer Res 2008;68(24):10349–57.
28. Ernst T, Chase AJ, Score J, et al. Inactivating mutations of the histone methyltransferase gene EZH2 in myeloid disorders. Nat Genet 2010;42(8):722–6.
29. Langemeijer SM, Kuiper RP, Berends M, et al. Acquired mutations in TET2 are common in myelodysplastic syndromes. Nat Genet 2009;41(7):838–42.
30. Nikoloski G, Langemeijer SM, Kuiper RP, et al. Somatic mutations of the histone methyltransferase gene EZH2 in myelodysplastic syndromes. Nat Genet 2010;42(8):665–7.
31. Delhommeau F, Dupont S, Della Valle V, et al. Mutation in TET2 in myeloid cancers. N Engl J Med 2009;360(22):2289–301.
32. Sherry ST, Ward MH, Kholodov M, et al. dbSNP: the NCBI database of genetic variation. Nucleic Acids Res 2001;29(1):308–11.
33. Chee M, Yang R, Hubbell E, et al. Accessing genetic information with high-density DNA arrays. Science 1996;274(5287):610–4.
34. Wang DG, Fan JB, Siao CJ, et al. Large-scale identification, mapping, and genotyping of single-nucleotide polymorphisms in the human genome. Science 1998;280(5366):1077–82.
35. Kennedy GC, Matsuzaki H, Dong S, et al. Large-scale genotyping of complex DNA. Nat Biotechnol 2003;21(10):1233–7.

36. Gondek LP, Tiu R, O'Keefe CL, et al. Chromosomal lesions and uniparental dis-omy detected by SNP arrays in MDS, MDS/MPD, and MDS-derived AML. Blood 2008;111(3):1534–42.

37. Jones AV, Cross NC. Oncogenic derivatives of platelet-derived growth factor receptors. Cell Mol Life Sci 2004;61(23):2912–23.

38. David M, Cross NC, Burgstaller S, et al. Durable responses to imatinib in patients with PDGFRB fusion gene-positive and BCR-ABL-negative chronic myeloprolifer-ative disorders. Blood 2007;109(1):61–4.

39. Ardlie KG, Kruglyak L, Seielstad M. Patterns of linkage disequilibrium in the human genome. Nat Rev Genet 2002;3(4):299–309.

40. Yamamoto G, Nannya Y, Kato M, et al. Highly sensitive method for genomewide detection of allelic composition in nonpaired, primary tumor specimens by use of affymetrix single-nucleotide-polymorphism genotyping microarrays. Am J Hum Genet 2007;81(1):114–26.

41. Lieberfarb ME, Lin M, Lechpammer M, et al. Genome-wide loss of heterozygosity analysis from laser capture microdissected prostate cancer using single nucleo-tide polymorphic allele (SNP) arrays and a novel bioinformatics platform dChipSNP. Cancer Res 2003;63(16):4781–5.

42. Simon-Sanchez J, Scholz S, Fung HC, et al. Genome-wide SNP assay reveals structural genomic variation, extended homozygosity and cell-line induced alter-ations in normal individuals. Hum Mol Genet 2007;16(1):1–14.

43. Stegelmann F, Bullinger L, Griesshammer M, et al. High-resolution single-nucleotide polymorphism array-profiling in myeloproliferative neoplasms iden-tifies novel genomic aberrations. Haematologica 2010;95(4):666–9.

44. Griffiths M, Mason J, Rindl M, et al. Acquired isodisomy for chromosome 13 is common in AML, and associated with FLT3-itd mutations. Leukemia 2005; 19(12):2355–8.

45. Wouters BJ, Sanders MA, Lugthart S, et al. Segmental uniparental disomy as a recurrent mechanism for homozygous CEBPA mutations in acute myeloid leukemia. Leukemia 2007;21(11):2382–4.

46. Score J, Hidalgo-Curtis C, Jones AV, et al. Inactivation of polycomb repressive complex 2 components in myeloproliferative and myelodysplastic/myeloprolifera-tive neoplasms. Blood 2012;119(5):1208–13.

47. Raghavan M, Smith LL, Lillington DM, et al. Segmental uniparental disomy is a commonly acquired genetic event in relapsed acute myeloid leukemia. Blood 2008;112(3):814–21.

48. James C, Ugo V, Le Couedic JP, et al. A unique clonal JAK2 mutation leading to constitutive signalling causes polycythaemia vera. Nature 2005;434(7037): 1144–8.

49. Levine RL, Loriaux M, Huntly BJ, et al. The JAK2V617F activating mutation occurs in chronic myelomonocytic leukemia and acute myeloid leukemia, but not in acute lymphoblastic leukemia or chronic lymphocytic leukemia. Blood 2005; 106(10):3377–9.

50. Baxter EJ, Scott LM, Campbell PJ, et al. Acquired mutation of the tyrosine kinase JAK2 in human myeloproliferative disorders. Lancet 2005;365(9464):1054–61.

51. Scott LM, Scott MA, Campbell PJ, et al. Progenitors homozygous for the V617F mutation occur in most patients with polycythemia vera, but not essential throm-bocythemia. Blood 2006;108(7):2435–7.

52. Kawamata N, Ogawa S, Yamamoto G, et al. Genetic profiling of myeloproliferative disorders by single-nucleotide polymorphism oligonucleotide microarray. Exp Hematol 2008;36(11):1471–9.

53. Heinrichs S, Kulkarni RV, Bueso-Ramos CE, et al. Accurate detection of uniparental disomy and microdeletions by SNP array analysis in myelodysplastic syndromes with normal cytogenetics. Leukemia 2009;23(9):1605–13.
54. Mohamedali A, Gaken J, Twine NA, et al. Prevalence and prognostic significance of allelic imbalance by single-nucleotide polymorphism analysis in low-risk myelodysplastic syndromes. Blood 2007;110(9):3365–73.
55. Thien CB, Langdon WY. Negative regulation of PTK signalling by Cbl proteins. Growth Factors 2005;23(2):161–7.
56. Swaminathan G, Tsygankov AY. The Cbl family proteins: ring leaders in regulation of cell signaling. J Cell Physiol 2006;209(1):21–43.
57. Schmidt MH, Dikic I. The Cbl interactome and its functions. Nat Rev Mol Cell Biol 2005;6(12):907–18.
58. Sargin B, Choudhary C, Crosetto N, et al. Flt3-dependent transformation by inactivating c-Cbl mutations in AML. Blood 2007;110(3):1004–12.
59. Caligiuri MA, Briesewitz R, Yu J, et al. Novel c-CBL and CBL-b ubiquitin ligase mutations in human acute myeloid leukemia. Blood 2007;110(3):1022–4.
60. Abbas S, Rotmans G, Lowenberg B, et al. Exon 8 splice site mutations in the gene encoding the E3-ligase CBL are associated with core binding factor acute myeloid leukemias. Haematologica 2008;93(10):1595–7.
61. Ko M, Huang Y, Jankowska AM, et al. Impaired hydroxylation of 5-methylcytosine in myeloid cancers with mutant TET2. Nature 2010;468(7325):839–43.
62. Tahiliani M, Koh KP, Shen Y, et al. Conversion of 5-methylcytosine to 5-hydroxymethylcytosine in mammalian DNA by MLL partner TET1. Science 2009;324(5929):930–5.
63. Ito S, D'Alessio AC, Taranova OV, et al. Role of Tet proteins in 5mC to 5hmC conversion, ES-cell self-renewal and inner cell mass specification. Nature 2010;466(7310):1129–33.
64. Bracken AP, Helin K. Polycomb group proteins: navigators of lineage pathways led astray in cancer. Nat Rev Cancer 2009;9(11):773–84.
65. Simon JA, Lange CA. Roles of the EZH2 histone methyltransferase in cancer epigenetics. Mutat Res 2008;647(1–2):21–9.
66. Cao R, Wang L, Wang H, et al. Role of histone H3 lysine 27 methylation in Polycomb-group silencing. Science 2002;298(5595):1039–43.
67. Czermin B, Melfi R, McCabe D, et al. Drosophila enhancer of Zeste/ESC complexes have a histone H3 methyltransferase activity that marks chromosomal Polycomb sites. Cell 2002;111(2):185–96.
68. Muller J, Hart CM, Francis NJ, et al. Histone methyltransferase activity of a Drosophila Polycomb group repressor complex. Cell 2002;111(2):197–208.
69. Kuzmichev A, Nishioka K, Erdjument-Bromage H, et al. Histone methyltransferase activity associated with a human multiprotein complex containing the Enhancer of Zeste protein. Genes Dev 2002;16(22):2893–905.
70. Guglielmelli P, Biamonte F, Score J, et al. EZH2 mutational status predicts poor survival in myelofibrosis. Blood 2011;118(19):5227–34.
71. Brecqueville M, Rey J, Bertucci F, et al. Mutation analysis of ASXL1, CBL, DNMT3A, IDH1, IDH2, JAK2, MPL, NF1, SF3B1, SUZ12, and TET2 in myeloproliferative neoplasms. Genes Chromosomes Cancer 2012;51(8):743–55.
72. Zhang J, Ding L, Holmfeldt L, et al. The genetic basis of early T-cell precursor acute lymphoblastic leukaemia. Nature 2012;481(7380):157–63.
73. van Haaften G, Dalgliesh GL, Davies H, et al. Somatic mutations of the histone H3K27 demethylase gene UTX in human cancer. Nat Genet 2009;41(5):521–3.

74. Ley TJ, Ding L, Walter MJ, et al. DNMT3A mutations in acute myeloid leukemia. N Engl J Med 2010;363(25):2424–33.
75. Walter MJ, Ding L, Shen D, et al. Recurrent DNMT3A mutations in patients with myelodysplastic syndromes. Leukemia 2011;25(7):1153–8.
76. Luedi PP, Hartemink AJ, Jirtle RL. Genome-wide prediction of imprinted murine genes. Genome Res 2005;15(6):875–84.
77. Lo HS, Wang Z, Hu Y, et al. Allelic variation in gene expression is common in the human genome. Genome Res 2003;13(8):1855–62.
78. Gimelbrant A, Hutchinson JN, Thompson BR, et al. Widespread monoallelic expression on human autosomes. Science 2007;318(5853):1136–40.
79. Kralovics R, Teo SS, Buser AS, et al. Altered gene expression in myeloprolifera- tive disorders correlates with activation of signaling by the V617F mutation of Jak2. Blood 2005;106(10):3374–6.
80. de Nooij-van Dalen AG, van Buuren-van Seggelen VH, Mulder A, et al. Isolation and molecular characterization of spontaneous mutants of lymphoblastoid cells with extended loss of heterozygosity. Mutat Res 1997;374(1):51–62.
81. Gupta PK, Sahota A, Boyadjiev SA, et al. High frequency in vivo loss of heterozy- gosity is primarily a consequence of mitotic recombination. Cancer Res 1997; 57(6):1188–93.
82. Hickson ID. RecQ helicases: caretakers of the genome. Nat Rev Cancer 2003; 3(3):169–78.
83. Lohman TM, Bjornson KP. Mechanisms of helicase-catalyzed DNA unwinding. Annu Rev Biochem 1996;65:169–214.
84. Villani G, Tanguy Le Gac N. Interactions of DNA helicases with damaged DNA: possible biological consequences. J Biol Chem 2000;275(43):33185–8.
85. Kralovics R. Genetic complexity of myeloproliferative neoplasms. Leukemia 2008; 22(10):1841–8.
86. Kruglyak L. The use of a genetic map of biallelic markers in linkage studies. Nat Genet 1997;17(1):21–4.

Genotype-Phenotype Interactions in the Myeloproliferative Neoplasms

Anna L. Godfrey, MRCP, FRCPath, Anthony R. Green, PhD, FRCPath*

KEYWORDS

- Myeloproliferative neoplasms • JAK2 • MPL • Hematopoiesis

KEY POINTS

- *JAK2V617F*-positive polycythemia vera (PV) and essential thrombocythemia (ET) share certain clinical characteristics and may be distinguished by factors that include *JAK2V617F* homozygosity and disease-specific differences in *JAK2*-related signaling.
- *JAK2* exon 12–mutated PV is characterized by a specific phenotype of isolated and marked erythrocytosis, which may reflect increased signaling strength through JAK2.
- *MPL* mutations, found in ET and primary myelofibrosis (PMF), do not define distinct subsets of these diseases but show certain clinical associations that vary with the specific mutation.
- Mutations in TET2, other epigenetic regulators, and other regulators of cytokine signaling are not specific to the classic myeloproliferative neoplasms (MPNs) but may influence prognosis and play roles in hematopoietic stem cell (HSC) dysregulation and progression to accelerated or blast-phase disease.

INTRODUCTION

The MPNs comprise a set of clonal HSC disorders, characterized by the overproduction of 1 or more mature myeloid cell types. The 3 classic Philadelphia-negative MPNs, which are discussed in this review, are PV, ET, and PMF. Although these disorders share certain clinical features—including bone marrow hypercellularity, frequent splenomegaly, and risks of thrombosis, hemorrhage, and transformation to acute myeloid leukemia (AML)—they also show important phenotypic differences. In PV, bone marrow panmyelosis is associated with increased numbers of red blood cells and, in some patients, neutrophilia and/or thrombocytosis. In ET, there is thrombocytosis with a normal red cell mass. PMF is characterized by proliferation predominantly

Cambridge Institute for Medical Research and Department of Haematology, University of Cambridge; Department of Haematology, Addenbrooke's Hospital, Hills Road, Cambridge CB2 0XY, UK
* Corresponding author.
E-mail address: arg1000@cam.ac.uk

Hematol Oncol Clin N Am 26 (2012) 993–1015
http://dx.doi.org/10.1016/j.hoc.2012.07.003
0889-8588/12/$ – see front matter © 2012 Elsevier Inc. All rights reserved.

of bone marrow megakaryocytes and granulocytes, resulting in deposition of fibrous connective tissue, and often associated with peripheral blood leukoerythroblastosis, cytopenias, and constitutional symptoms.

Although a relationship between these disorders was originally suggested by Dameshek in 1951,[1] it was not until 2005 that a molecular basis for this was identified, in the form of an acquired activating mutation in *JAK2* (*JAK2V617F*).[2–5] With sensitive detection techniques, this mutation is detectable in more than 95% of patients with PV and in 50% to 60% of those with ET or PMF. These early studies demonstrated that expression of *JAK2V617F* in retroviral bone marrow transplantation models caused erythrocytosis,[2,4] confirming its relevance to human MPNs. Moreover, in human studies, *JAK2V617F* has been identified in the stem cell–enriched $CD34^+CD38^-CD90^+Lin^-$ compartment, common myeloid progenitors, granulocyte-monocyte precursors, and megakaryocyte-erythroid precursors[6] as well as natural killer cells, B cells, and T cells in some patients,[7–9] confirming its origin in an early hematopoietic progenitor. The activating effects of the mutation are thought to reflect disruption of the normal autoinhibitory function of the JH2 domain, within which *JAK2V617F* is found,[10,11] and have been shown to affect downstream pathways, including STATs (especially STAT5), phosphatidylinositol 3-kinase, and MAP kinase pathways in cell lines and animal models.[2,4,12,13] STAT5 activation seems particularly important for *JAK2V617F*-induced cytokine independence in vitro[14] and erythrocytosis in vivo[15,16] and is in itself sufficient to support formation of endogenous erythroid colonies,[17] a cardinal feature of PV.

The *JAK2V617F* mutation is particularly common in the classic MPNs, although it is also found in approximately half of patients with the uncommon myelodysplastic (MDS)/MPN, refractory anemia with ringed sideroblasts and marked thrombocytosis,[18] and at lower frequencies in AML, other myeloproliferative, and myelodysplastic disorders.[19,20] The reason for the myeloid bias in these diseases is unclear, given the role of *JAK2* downstream of numerous cytokine receptors,[21] but could reflect qualitative differences in the consequences of JAK2V617F in the context of different receptors. An important question however, given the high prevalence of *JAK2V617F* in MPNs, is how it can be associated with several diseases with distinct clinical phenotypes (PV, ET, and PMF)? Conversely, the development of MPNs in the absence of *JAK2V617F* must be explained and is likely to reflect the presence of other mutations in *JAK2V617F*-negative patients. This review discusses specific factors that may contribute to disease phenotype in MPNs. Discussed first are *JAK2*-mutated MPNs, particularly focusing on the factors determining the differences between *JAK2*-mutated PV and ET. Then the mutations found in *JAK2V617F*-negative MPNs, especially *MPL* mutations in ET and PMF, together with the other mutations identified in a broader range of myeloid malignancies are discussed.

JAK2-MUTATED MPNS

Relationships Between Genotype and Phenotype in JAK2V617F-positive PV and ET

In 2005, a study of more than 800 ET patients demonstrated that in comparison to *JAK2V617F*-negative patients, *JAK2V617F*-positive patients were older; showed higher hemoglobin levels, neutrophil counts, bone marrow erythropoiesis, and granulopoiesis; showed lower platelet counts, mean corpuscular volume, serum erythropoietin, and ferritin; and showed a higher rate of PV transformation.[22] Subsequent studies have confirmed many of these associations,[23–27] supporting the view that *JAK2V617F*-positive ET resembles a mild form of PV and that the 2 disorders form a phenotypic continuum.[22] Although patients with PV have hemoglobin levels above the normal range (**Fig. 1**), patients with *JAK2V617F*-positive ET show a rightward shift in the normal Gaussian curve, such that some patients have hemoglobin levels in the normal range but others overlap with PV. Recent studies have identified factors that may cause this curve to shift rightwards from ET to PV. As discussed later, these include homozygosity for *JAK2V617F* and disease-specific differences in the signaling consequences of the *JAK2V617F* mutation.

Studies of JAK2V617F allele burden and clinical phenotype

A homozygous *JAK2V617F* sequencing pattern (>50% mutant) in granulocyte DNA was originally identified in 25% to 30% of those with PV, 9% to 20% with PMF, and 0% to 3% with ET and is a result of mitotic recombination.[2–5] Several clinical studies then investigated how *JAK2V617F* gene dosage may influence clinical phenotype by analyzing the associations between *JAK2V617F* allele burden, typically measured in granulocyte DNA, and clinical parameters. Initially these studies utilised sequencing, allele-specific polymerase chain reaction (PCR) and/or restriction enzyme digestion to divide patients into "heterozygous" (<50% mutant allele) and "homozygous" (>50% mutant allele) groups. In PV, "homozygous" PV was associated with higher hemoglobin and white cell counts and lower platelet counts at diagnosis, increased pruritus, more splenomegaly, and more need for cytoreduction compared with "heterozygous" PV.[28,29] Subsequent studies analyzed the associations between mutant allele burden, a continuous variable measured by real-time quantitative PCR (qPCR), and clinical features in PV and ET[30] (**Tables 1** and **2**). There is some discordance between studies in the associations found. This probably reflects methodologic differences between the studies, including in the use of retrospective or prospective data collection; different diagnostic and inclusion criteria; variable use of peripheral blood, granulocyte, or bone marrow DNA to determine allele burden[39]; and technical aspects of the qPCR assay, such as the precise probes and standards used.[30] Higher

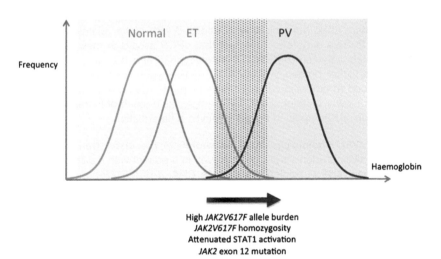

Fig. 1. Relationship between hemoglobin levels in normal individuals and those with *JAK2*-mutated ET and PV. Normal individuals show a gaussian distribution of hemoglobin levels (*green*). ET patients (*blue*) show a right shift from the normal curve but with the mean still in the normal range. Patients with PV show a further rightward shift, with hemoglobin levels above the normal range (*red*), which may reflect mechanisms such as *JAK2V617F* homozygosity, attenuated STAT1 signaling, or the presence of a *JAK2* exon 12 mutation. Hemoglobin levels in the midrange include patients with both ET and PV (*shaded*).

Table 1
Clinical parameters associated with *JAK2V617F* allele burden in polycythemia vera

	Association (References)	No Association (References)
Higher hemoglobin/hematocrit	9,31–34	35
Higher white cell/neutrophil count	9,31–33,35,36	
Lower platelet count	9,32,33,36	31,35
Lower mean corpuscular volume	31	
Lower serum ferritin	31	
Lower serum erythropoietin	31	
More splenomegaly	31–33,36	35
Increased pruritus	31,32,35	
Higher risk of thrombosis	31,37	32,33,35
Higher serum lactate dehydrogenase	31	
Higher leukocyte alkaline phosphatase and PRV-1 expression	31	
Higher risk of myelofibrotic transformation	32	

JAK2V617F allele burdens, however, have been reproducibly associated with higher hemoglobin levels, higher white cell counts, and lower platelet counts in PV, together with other features suggestive of more extreme PV (lower mean corpuscular volume, lower serum ferritin and erythropoietin levels, more splenomegaly, and more pruritus). These data are in keeping with the concept that a higher *JAK2V617F* allele burden promotes a PV-like rather than ET-like phenotype.

Higher *JAK2V617F* allele burdens in ET have been associated with some features in common with PV (higher white cell counts and more splenomegaly), but in contrast to PV, higher mutant allele burdens were associated with higher platelet counts (see **Tables 1** and **2**). This may reflect the fact that qPCR assays in these studies have not discriminated between *JAK2V617F* heterozygous and homozygous cells. It is possible that a higher burden of *JAK2V617F*-heterozygous cells is associated with more pronounced thrombocytosis but that a higher burden of homozygous-mutant cells results in a lower platelet count, for example, as a result of increased signaling strength through JAK2 impairing megakaryocytic differentiation.

Studies of JAK2V617F homozygosity in hematopoietic precursors from patients

A limitation of allele burden studies is that even in a patient with a *JAK2V617F* allele burden less than 50% in pooled granulocyte DNA, *JAK2V617F*-homozygous cells may still be present. To circumvent this issue, individual erythroid colonies from MPN patients have been genotyped to investigate the prevalence of homozygosity

Table 2
Clinical parameters associated with *JAK2V617F* allele burden in essential thrombocythemia

	Association (References)	No Association (References)
Higher white cell/neutrophil count	9,26,36	38
Higher platelet count	9,26	38
More splenomegaly	26,38	
Higher risk of thrombosis	26,37,38	

at the level of single precursors.[40] Although virtually all PV and ET patients produced both wild-type and mutant colonies, colonies with homozygosity for *JAK2V617F* were found in almost all of those with PV but none of 17 patients with ET. This contrasts to allele burden studies in which *JAK2V617F* burdens greater than 50% were identified in up to 55% of patients with PV by qPCR.[31,32,41] Subsequent studies have largely supported these observations from colony assays.[9,36] *JAK2V617F*-homozygous erythroid colonies have been reported, however, in a few patients with ET,[9,36,42] and granulocyte DNA *JAK2V617F* allele burdens over 50% have also been identified in 1% to 6% of ET patients.[9,26,37,43] Small homozygous clones can be identified in approximately half of ET patients when large numbers of colonies are grown in low erythropoietin conditions.[44] PV patients lacking *JAK2V617F*-homozygous colonies have also been reported.[9,36] Homozygosity for *JAK2V617F* in hematopoietic precursors is, therefore, preferentially associated with a clinical phenotype of PV rather than ET, but the association is not absolute and it has not been clear whether this relationship is causal. The authors have recently found that in PV, a higher proportion of homozygous colonies, relative to heterozygous colonies, is associated with higher hemoglobin levels, higher white cell counts, and lower platelet counts at the time of diagnosis but not at the time of colony assay.[44] These data support a causal role for *JAK2V617F* homozygosity in the development of a PV phenotype.

Little is known about the differential effects of *JAK2V617F* heterozygosity and homozygosity on hematopoietic cell function. The effect of *JAK2V617F* on expansion of hematopoietic progenitors has been assessed by measuring *JAK2V617F* allele burden in patient samples, either in immature and mature fractions isolated directly from bone marrow or blood or in CD34$^+$ cells and their progeny before and after a period of liquid culture. The observation that *JAK2V617F* allele burden may increase from more immature to mature fractions has suggested that any selective advantage of *JAK2V617F* may predominantly affect more mature cell types, although some in vitro culture methods have given conflicting results.[8,9,36,45] A more recent study of MPN bone marrow progenitor fractions also distinguished between heterozygous and homozygous *JAK2V617F* compartments and demonstrated that *JAK2V617F*-homozygous clones expanded from the HSC-enriched compartment to the differentiated erythroid and granulocytic compartments, at the expense of wild-type cells and in some cases *JAK2V617F*-heterozygous cells.[46] The effect of *JAK2V617F* homozygosity on erythroid cell growth has also been studied in cultures of erythroid colonies from patient samples, in which lowering the erythropoietin concentration had the most inhibitory effect on wild-type cells, a lesser effect on *JAK2V617F*-heterozygous cells, and least inhibition of *JAK2V617F*-homozygous cells.[9] There is, therefore, evidence that *JAK2V617F* exerts its selective effect preferentially in the later stages of at least some hematopoietic lineages, rather than at the HSC level, and moreover that this late advantage may be greatest for *JAK2V617F*-homozygous cells, especially in low erythropoietin conditions. This late expansion, together with the selective effects of relative erythropoietin deficiency in vivo, may help explain the observation that some patients with clear clinical PV seem to harbor small *JAK2V617F*-homozygous subclones, as assessed by erythroid colony assays.[40] Nonetheless, it remains unclear to what extent these effects of *JAK2V617F* homozygosity contribute to the clinical differences between PV and ET.

Mouse models of JAK2V617F-positive MPNs

Mouse models of *JAK2V617F*, which are reviewed comprehensively by Li and colleagues elsewhere,[47] have provided additional insights into the factors influencing phenotype. Where a murine *JAK2V617F* gene has been introduced into bone marrow cells that are transplanted into irradiated mice, the phenotype has varied at least in part with genetic background,[48] supporting the concept that constitutional genetic differences may alter the nature of the myeloproliferative phenotype between individuals. Nonetheless, these models with high, dysregulated *JAK2V617F* expression levels generally showed phenotypes resembling PV, with erythrocytosis, leukocytosis, and normal or near-normal platelet counts.[12,48–50] The effect of *JAK2V617F* gene dosage has been examined further in transgenic models. In one model derived from a mutated murine *Jak2* gene, mice with lower transgene expression levels developed variable erythrocytosis, leukocytosis, and thrombocytosis, whereas higher levels were associated with more severe leukocytosis, thrombocytosis, anemia, and bone marrow fibrosis.[51] In contrast, a transgenic model using human *JAK2V617F* showed erythrocytosis, leukocytosis, and thrombocytosis, all of which were more marked in mice with higher transgene copy numbers.[52] In a third model, human *JAK2V617F* was expressed at variable levels, depending on whether a *MxCre* or *VavCre* system was used.[53] Mice with lower *JAK2V617F* expression levels mice showed marked thrombocytosis, mild neutrophilia, and normal hemoglobin, reminiscent of human ET, whereas higher expression levels were associated with erythrocytosis, neutrophilia, and thrombocytosis, resembling human PV. The concept that increasing dosage may contribute to the differences between PV and ET is also supported by the observation that in one retroviral bone marrow transplantation model, secondary recipients of bone marrow with lower *JAK2V617F* expression levels showed a transient thrombocytosis that was not seen in recipients of marrow with higher expression levels.[50] Overall, these studies support the concept that *JAK2V617F* dosage can affect phenotype, although dysregulated *JAK2V617F* expression makes interpretation of these effects difficult.

In view of the likely significance of appropriate levels and patterns of *JAK2V617F* expression in determining phenotype, several groups have developed knock-in models in which *JAK2V617F* is expressed at physiologic levels under the normal regulatory elements of the mouse *Jak2* gene. Three knock-in models, all of which utilized a murine mutant *Jak2* gene, resembled PV with erythrocytosis, leukocytosis, splenomegaly, and variable thrombocytosis.[54–56] In one of these studies, mice homozygous for *Jak2V617F* were also generated but showed no further increase in hemoglobin levels.[56] In contrast, a fourth model, which carried a human mutant *JAK2* gene, showed thrombocytosis with minimal erythrocytosis, similar to the mild phenotypes seen in human ET,[57] with a proportion of mice transforming to a PV-like or MF-like disease. The phenotypic variation between these models may reflect technical issues associated with the different targeting strategies or inherent differences in the mutant human and mouse proteins.

In summary, mouse models indicate that *JAK2V617F* gene dosage and genetic background may influence disease phenotype, but the mechanisms responsible for the variable phenotypes seen between the heterozygous knock-in models remain unclear.

Different signaling consequences of JAK2V617F in PV and ET

Although there is evidence that the gene dosage of *JAK2V617F*, in particular homozygosity, may influence disease phenotype, there are differences in *JAK2V617F*-dependent signaling between PV and ET patients, which precede the acquisition of *JAK2V617F* homozygosity. Although expression arrays were previously used to investigate the consequences of *JAK2V617F* on gene expression, these studies generally compared peripheral blood leukocytes from MPN patients with normal individuals[58,59] and are, therefore, complicated by the effects of interindividual variation in gene expression and cellular heterogeneity within samples containing variable mixtures of normal and mutant cells. To circumvent these issues, a recent study analyzed differences in gene expression between clonally derived erythroid cells from patients with PV and ET.[60] For each patient, a *JAK2V617F*-heterozygous cell pool was compared with a corresponding wild-type cell sample from the same patient, thus controlling for interindividual variation in gene expression. A notable difference between PV and ET was that in ET, *JAK2V617F*-heterozygous cells showed strong up-regulation of genes related to interferon-γ (IFN-γ) signaling compared with wild-type cells, whereas PV mutant cells showed minimal up-regulation of this pathway. Levels of phosphorylated STAT1, the major downstream mediator of IFN-γ receptor signaling, were increased in mutant erythroblasts from ET patients compared with wild-type cells, consistent with the known role of JAK2 downstream of the IFN-γ receptor.[61] In contrast, PV patients showed no STAT1 activation in mutant cells, suggesting that *JAK2V617F*-induced STAT1 activation is attenuated or absent in patients with PV. Moreover, in K562 cells and CD34$^+$ cells from MPN patients, expression of a constitutively active STAT1 mutant caused increased megakaryocytic and reduced erythroid differentiation, whereas a dominant negative form of STAT1 had the opposite effect, indicating that these signaling differences could account for aspects of the PV and ET phenotypes.

This study[60] demonstrated that there are qualitative differences in signaling in *JAK2V617F*-heterozygous erythroid cells between PV and ET. The molecular mechanism for these differences remains unclear and could be due to either constitutional or acquired factors. It is also unclear whether differences in STAT1 signaling contribute to phenotype in PV and ET solely through direct effects on erythroid and megakaryocytic differentiation and whether these effects interact with *JAK2V617F* homozygosity.

JAK2 Exon 12 Mutations in PV

Mutations in exon 12 of *JAK2* were first identified in PV patients negative for *JAK2V617F* in 2007 and revealed a distinct subtype of PV.[62] Compared with PV patients with *JAK2V617F*, these patients were younger and had higher hemoglobin concentrations, lower white cell and platelet counts, and isolated bone marrow erythroid hyperplasia without granulocytic or megakaryocytic morphologic abnormalities. At least 20 different exon 12 mutations have been reported (**Table 3**) and, in contrast to *JAK2V617F* in PV, these are usually heterozygous, with homozygosity described in only a handful of patients[63–65,72] and in one case confirmed due to mitotic recombination.[65] The clinical features associated with exon 12 mutations were summarized in a recent series of 106 patients: 64% presented with isolated erythrocytosis, with 15% having additional leukocytosis, 12% additional thrombocytosis, and 9% both, with no significant differences between the different exon 12 mutations.[77] This study also confirmed the clinical associations described in the original report[62] and demonstrated that PV patients with *JAK2V617F* and exon 12 mutations exhibit a similar incidence of thrombosis, myelofibrosis, acute leukemia, and death.[77] The prevalence of these mutations in patients with erythrocytosis varies, depending on whether patients meeting criteria for PV or idiopathic erythrocytosis (absolute erythrocytosis in the absence of secondary causes and not fulfilling criteria for PV) are included.[64,71,72] In one study of 114 patients with PV, all had either *JAK2V617F* (either in granulocyte DNA or erythroid colonies) or an exon 12 mutation,[79] suggesting that almost all patients with true PV carry an activating mutation in *JAK2*. In another series of 58 patients, however, with idiopathic erythrocytosis and low serum erythropoietin,

Table 3
JAK2 exon 12 mutations described in case reports and case series in the literature[a]

Type	Mutation	Approximate Number of Patients	References
K539L-type	F537-K539delinsL	12	62–68
	K539L	6	62,64,69,70
	H538QK539L	4	62,64
	H538-K539delinsL	4	63,65,69,71
	H538-K539del	1	64
	H538DK539LI540S	1	64
E543del-type	N542-E543del	35	62–66,68–74
	E543-D544del	14	63–65,72,73
	R451-E543delinsK	8	63,71,75,76
	I540-E543delinsMK	4	63,65,75
	I540-E543delinsKK	1	68
	E543del	1	77
Duplications	V536-I546dup11	1	63
	V536-F547dup	1	64
	F537-F547dup	1	67
	F537-I546dup10+F547L	1	63
	547insL+I540-F547dup8	1	78
	F547V	1	77
Others	I540-N542delinsS	1	78
	D544-L545del	1	64

[a] Patients in a recent large case series with non-novel mutations are not included because many had been previously reported.[77]

27% were found to have a *JAK2* exon 12 mutation, highlighting that other mechanisms can cause isolated erythrocytosis.[72]

Similarly to *JAK2V617F*, exon 12 mutations have activating effects on the kinase: in Ba/F3 cells, the mutations can confer cytokine independence, with constitutively increased levels of activated JAK2, STAT5, and ERK1/2 in the absence of erythropoietin.[62] Use of the *JAK2K539L* allele in this assay resulted in more marked phosphorylation of JAK2 and ERK1/2 than the *V617F* allele, and the use of *JAK2K539L* in a retroviral murine bone marrow transplantation model caused more erythrocytosis but less marked leukocytosis and thrombocytosis than *V617F*, with expansion of erythroid and granulocytic but not megakaryocytic bone marrow compartments.[62] These findings suggest that the activating effect of exon 12 mutations may be stronger than *V617F* and that this activation is specifically associated with a more pronounced PV phenotype.

JAK2 exon 12 mutations, therefore, promote a phenotype characterized by an isolated and marked erythrocytosis, suggestive of a further rightward shift of the hemoglobin curve, depicted in **Fig. 1**. Consistent with this, exon 12 mutations have never been reported in ET. It remains unclear why the effects of *JAK2* exon 12 mutations should be more selective for erythroid progenitors than *JAK2V617F*. The phenotype may partly reflect the stronger activating effects of these mutations, particularly because certain aspects (higher hemoglobin and lower platelet counts) have also been associated with higher mutant allele burdens in *JAK2V617F*-positive PV. Conversely, *JAK2V617F*-positive PV is frequently associated with bone marrow panmyelosis, peripheral blood neutrophilia, and sometimes thrombocytosis. It is unclear why these features are less frequent with exon 12 mutations, but this may reflect qualitative differences in the signaling consequences of the 2 types of mutation.

JAK2V617F and Accelerated-Phase Disease: Myelofibrosis and Acute Myeloid Leukemia

Although *JAK2V617F* is also found in 50% to 60% of those with PMF, the additional factors determining the phenotype of this clinically heterogeneous disorder are less clear. It is likely that additional acquired mutations are important: most of the other mutations identified in MPNs are more common in PMF than in PV or ET and frequently coexist with *JAK2V617F* (discussed later). Moreover, the spectrum of genetic lesions in PMF shows increasing overlap both with secondary AML and with poor prognostic subgroups of other myeloid malignancies. These observations, together with fact that transformations of ET and PV to secondary myelofibrosis are well recognized, support the concept that PMF represents an accelerated phase of disease. Consistent with this idea, patients diagnosed with PMF may show prior evidence of an undiagnosed chronic-phase MPN.[80]

The role of *JAK2V617F* in progression of chronic-phase MPNs to AML is particularly complex. In individuals in whom *JAK2V617F* is detectable in the leukemic blasts, the mutation may have contributed to disease evolution through causing increased DNA damage[81] together with an impaired apoptotic response to DNA damage.[82] Other patients with *JAK2V617F*-positive chronic MPNs may, however, develop *JAK2V617F*-negative AML.[83,84] This may reflect evolution within a shared pre-JAK2 founder clone or independent transformation of a clonally unrelated HSC.[84] Other mutations, such as in *TET2*, are likely to play a role in such transformations (discussed later).

JAK2 MUTATION–NEGATIVE MPNS
Mutations Specific to JAK2V617F-Negative ET and PMF: MPL Mutations

Mutations in the thrombopoietin receptor gene, *MPL*, were first reported in *JAK2V617F*-negative myelofibrosis in 2006.[85] Several acquired mutations in *MPL* exon 10 have been reported in PMF and ET, of which the most common are *W515L* and *W515K* (**Table 4**). The *S505N* mutation was originally identified in patients with familial ET[91,92] and has also been confirmed to occur as an acquired change in ET and PMF.[86,87] Several other mutations have been reported outside exon 10, but it is unclear whether these are acquired or have functional significance.[71,87,94]

MPL mutations have been found in 4% to 9% of patients with PMF and 1% to 11% of those with ET,[86,88,89,95,96] depending on the sensitivity of the screening technique, but have not been identified in PV or other myeloid disorders.[88] When high-sensitivity assays are used for both *MPL* and *JAK2V617F* mutations, *MPL* mutations have been found in 15% to 24% of *JAK2V617F*-negative ET and PMF,[89,93] and, therefore, account for a significant proportion of *JAK2V617F*-negative MPNs. Homozygosity has been reported for most of the individual *MPL* mutations, either on the basis of

Table 4		
MPL exon 10 mutations described in essential thrombocythemia and myelofibrosis		
Mutation	**Selected References**	**Notes**
W515L	85–90	
W515K	86–90	2 different base substitutions[86]
W515A	87,89,90	
W515R	89,90	
S505N	86,87,89	Germline mutations in familial ET[91,92]
V501A	93	Coexisted with *W515L*
S505C	93	Coexisted with *W515L*

mutant allele burden estimations in granulocyte DNA[88,90,95,96] or sequencing of individual hematopoietic colonies,[42,86,89] and is likely to result from mitotic recombination.[94] Homozygosity is more common in PMF or post-MF AML compared with ET[90] and is found significantly more frequently with W515K (50%–80% of patients) than W515L (0–17% of patients) in both ET and PMF.[86,90,95,96] Other patients have compound mutations,[89,93,96] which may occur in the same subclone on the same or different chromosomes.[89,93] Depending on the screening assays used, 3% to 30% of patients with MPL mutations have also been found to carry JAK2V617F.[86,88,89,95,96] In some of these patients, analyses of hematopoietic colonies have demonstrated that the mutations are in different clones and, therefore, have either arisen independently or are the progeny of a shared founder clone.[97]

Like JAK2 mutations, the W515K, W515L, and S505N mutations have been shown to confer cytokine-independent growth when expressed in Ba/F3 cells, with activation of downstream targets, such as JAK2, STAT3, STAT5, AKT, and ERK.[85,87,91] The W515K and W515A mutants also induce myeloproliferative disorders in murine bone marrow transplantation models, but in contrast to the erythrocytosis observed with JAK2V617F, these are characterized by thrombocytosis, leukocytosis, extramedullary hematopoiesis, and megakaryocytic hyperplasia and reticulin fibrosis in spleen and bone marrow.[85,98] In vitro colony assays also confirm that the mutation preferentially exerts its effects in megakaryocytic precursors, because thrombopoietin-independent megakaryocyte colonies, but not erythropoietin-independent erythroid colonies, can be grown from patients with MPL mutations.[86,99]

In clinical studies, MPL-mutated patients show some clinical associations but do not form discrete subgroups within JAK2V617F-negative ET or PMF. Patients with MPL-mutated, as compared with MPL-negative, myelofibrosis are more often female, are older, show more severe anemia, and are more often transfusion dependent, with no difference in other hematological parameters or splenomegaly.[96] Patients with MPL-mutated ET, compared with JAK2V617F-positive ET, show lower hemoglobin levels, higher platelet counts, and higher serum erythropoietin levels, with reduced erythroid and granulocytic cellularity in bone marrow trephine biopsies.[86,95] Reduced hemoglobin levels are particularly associated with W515L mutations, whereas increased platelet counts are more associated with W515K mutations,[95] but these differences are unexplained at the molecular level. Among JAK2V617F-negative patients with ET, patients with MPL mutations are older and show less bone marrow cellularity and erythropoiesis compared with those without MPL mutations but without any differences in blood count parameters. MPL mutations in ET do not have prognostic significance in terms of thrombosis, major hemorrhage, myelofibrotic transformation, or survival.[86,95]

In summary, MPL-mutant disease in humans and mice is characterized by selective involvement of the megakaryocytic lineage, most likely as a result of the restricted expression of the thrombopoietin receptor, and this results in isolated thrombocytosis and/or myelofibrosis. By contrast, JAK2 is widely expressed and interacts with multiple cytokine receptors, as reflected by the additional involvement of erythroid and granulocytic lineages in JAK2-mutant disease.

Other Mutations in MPNs

Mutations in several other genes have been reported in MPNs. Of these, only TET2 mutations have been reproducibly identified in 5% or more of patients with PV or ET, with others more restricted to primary or secondary myelofibrosis and/or blast-phase MPNs as well as other chronic myeloid disorders, such as MDS and MDS/MPN overlap disorders. Many of these target genes, such as TET2, regulate chromatin structure, whereas others, such as *LNK* and *c-CBL*, may directly modulate transduction of cytokine signaling. The mechanisms by which these mutations act are reviewed elsewhere,[100,101] but their relevance to the MPN phenotype is discussed briefly in this article.

Mutations in TET2

TET2 mutations were first identified in patients with *JAK2V617F*-positive MPNs, in whom a high proportion of CD34[+] cells harbored the *JAK2* mutation, together with a group of MDS/AML patients with loss of heterozygosity at chromosome 4q24.[102] Other than *JAK2*, *TET2* is the most frequently mutated gene in patients with chronic-phase MPNs, including 10% to 16% of those with PV, 4% to 5% with ET, and 7% to 17% with myelofibrosis[102–104] as well as approximately 17% to 32% of those with blast-phase MPNs.[103,105,106] In MPNs, *TET2* mutations may be associated with older age and with lower hemoglobin levels but have no effects on survival, leukemic transformation, or thrombosis.[103] *TET2* mutations are also found in a spectrum of other myeloid disorders, such as MDS (14%); MDS/MPN, including chronic myelomonocytic leukemia (CMML) (20%–50%); and primary or secondary AML (12%–43%)[104,107–110] as well as some lymphomas.[111] They have been reported to be an adverse prognostic factor in CMML and some subtypes of AML.[104,109,112]

Mutations in *TET2* lead to reduced levels of genomic 5-hydroxymethylcytosine, which have been postulated as leading to reduced CpG demethylation and contributing to DNA hypermethylation, although CpG hypomethylation has been observed in MPN samples with *TET2* mutations.[113] Targeted inactivation of *TET2* in mice does not cause a phenotype resembling PV, ET, or PMF but rather a CMML-like disease with leukocytosis, neutrophilia, monocytosis, splenomegaly, and extramedullary hematopoiesis[111,114–116] and, in some cases, lymphoid abnormalities.[111] These mouse models also show increased numbers of stem cell–enriched Lin[–]Sca1[+]Kit[+] (LSK) cells, increased colony-forming progenitors, and increased HSC self-renewal.[111,114–116] Knockdown of *TET2* in cord blood CD34[+] cells also skews their differentiation toward the granulomonocytic lineage at the expense of lymphoid and erythroid lineages.[117] Together these studies indicate that *TET2* mutations are sufficient to cause myeloid malignancies, particularly with CMML-like phenotypes, but in isolation they do not cause classic MPN phenotypes. Their importance in chronic-phase MPNs, such as PV and ET, is likely through contributing to dysregulated HSC self-renewal, with other mutations (such as *JAK2V617F*) determining the relative expansion and differentiation of individual myeloid lineages.

TET2 mutations can coexist with *JAK2V617F* and can either precede or follow acquisition of *JAK2V617F*.[84,102,118] In at least 3 patients in whom a *JAK2V617F*-positive MPN preceded *JAK2V617F*-negative AML, *TET2* mutations were identified in the *JAK2V617F*-negative leukemic phase, and in 2 of these patients, the *TET2* mutation was also present in the chronic-phase disease, indicating that AML arose from a long-standing *JAK2V617F*-negative, *TET2*-mutated clone.[84,105] In other patients, *TET2* mutations were detected in the AML-phase but not chronic-phase samples.[106] *TET2* mutations may, therefore, arise either early in the development of chronic-phase MPNs or later in leukemic transformation.

Mutations in other epigenetic regulators: EZH2, ASXL1, IDH1, IDH2, and DNMT3A

EZH2 is a component of the polycomb repressive complex 2 (PRC2) and promotes transcriptional repression by catalyzing trimethylation of lysine 27 of histone H3 (H3K27) and recruiting DNA methyltransferases.[119] *EZH2* mutations have been identified in 6% to 13% of patients with myelofibrosis as well as 6% of those with MDS and 5% to 12% of CMML or MDS/MPN but are rare in chronic-phase PV (3%) and ET.[120–125] They may coexist with *JAK2V617F*, *ASXL1*, *TET2*, *c-CBL*, or *MPL* mutations.[121,122] Moreover, *EZH2* mutations seem to have phenotypic and prognostic significance in myelofibrosis, associated with higher white cell counts, larger spleen size at diagnosis, and reduced leukemia-free and overall survival in multivariable analyses.[121] Although *EZH2* mutations have been identified in secondary AML, in paired-sample studies they have most often also been found in the preceding chronic-phase MPN or MDS, suggesting that in spite of their association with reduced leukemia-free survival in myelofibrosis, they may be an early event rather than the trigger for transformation.[120,121]

ASXL1 forms part of a complex, first characterized in *Drosophila*, which removes monoubiquitin from histone H2A in nucleosomes.[126] Acquired mutations in *ASXL1* have been found in 13% to 30% of patients with myelofibrosis as well as 11% to 20% of patients with MDS, almost half of those with CMML, 5% with de novo AML, and up to 11% of secondary AML.[122,127–131] Mutations in patients with ET and PV are rare but have been reported.[132,133] *ASXL1* mutations do not have clear prognostic value in the MPNs[133] but are associated with poorer prognosis in MDS, CMML, and AML.[129–131]

Mutations in the isocitrate dehydrogenase 1 and 2 (*IDH1* and *IDH2*) genes were first identified in up to 23% of patients with AML, in which they confer an adverse prognosis,[134–137] and were subsequently found in 9% to 22% of patients with AML secondary to MPNs.[106,138,139] Mutations are less prevalent in chronic-phase disease, affecting 4% of patients with PMF and 1% to 2% of ET and PV,[139] 3% to 5% of MDS, and 10% to 15% of AML secondary to MDS[140,141] and are associated with inferior overall and leukemia-free survival in chronic-phase PMF and inferior overall survival in blast-phase PMF.[142] Unlike *EZH2* mutations, *IDH* mutations present in secondary AML are often absent from chronic-phase MPN samples and, therefore, may have a more direct role in transformation.[143] These mutations not only impair the capacity of IDH1 and IDH2 to catalyze conversion of isocitrate to α-ketoglutarate but also create a neomorphic catalytic function that converts α-ketoglutarate to 2-hydroxyglutarate.[144,145] Increased 2-hydroxyglutarate levels have been suggested to impair conversion of 5-methylcytosine to 5-hydroxymethylcytosine by TET2, resulting in reduced DNA demethylation.[146]

Lastly, inactivating mutations in the methyltransferase gene, *DNMT3A*, were identified in 22% of patients with de novo AML[147] and 2% to 8% of those with MDS,[148,149] conferring a worse prognosis in both groups. In MPNs, *DNMT3A* mutations were identified in 7% of patients with PV, 7% to 15% with PMF, and 14% with AML secondary to MPNs but not in ET.[150,151] These studies were too small to assess phenotypic or prognostic significance of the mutations.

In summary, mutations in epigenetic regulators are not specific for MPNs and are more common in PMF and secondary AML, compared with ET and PV, in keeping with the concept that PMF is a more genetically complex disease than ET and PV.

Mutations in other cytokine signaling regulators: LNK and c-CBL

LNK regulates thrombopoietin-dependent and erythropoietin-dependent JAK-STAT signaling by binding directly to JAK2 and cytokine receptors.[152,153] Overexpression of *LNK* suppresses both erythroid and megakaryocytic differentiation and attenuates thrombopoietin-induced or erythropoietin-induced STAT5 and MAPK pathway activation.[154,155] *LNK*-deficient mice show marked thrombocytosis and leukocytosis, splenomegaly with megakaryocytic hyperplasia, increased erythroid progenitors and fibrosis,[154–156] and increased LSK cells with enhanced repopulation ability.[152,157]

Consistent with the importance of activated JAK-STAT signaling in *JAK2*-mutated and *MPL*-mutated MPNs, *LNK* mutations are also fairly specific to MPNs, but, in keeping with its regulatory role in multiple hematopoietic lineages, they are not associated with a single phenotype. Mutations have been found in ET, myelofibrosis, *JAK2*-negative idiopathic erythrocytosis, and blast-phase MPNs, with a prevalence of approximately 6% in chronic-phase *JAK2V617F*-negative MPNs and 13% in blast-phase MPNs in small cohorts.[158–160] In some blast-phase patients, the mutation was absent in preceding chronic-phase samples, consistent with a role in disease progression.[160]

The CBL proteins are E3 ubiquitin ligases, which bind receptor tyrosine kinases after cytokine-induced stimulation and monoubiquitinate the receptors at multiple sites, triggering internalization, degradation, and termination of signaling.[161,162] In contrast to *LNK*, they regulate not only JAK-STAT signaling but also other cytokine receptors that are important in hematopoiesis, such as Flt3.[163,164] Consistent with this, *c-CBL* mutations have not been associated with chronic-phase PV or ET but have been found in approximately 6% of patients with myelofibrosis and in other myeloid malignancies, including primary and secondary AML, MDS, CMML, and other MDS/MPN syndromes, such as atypical CML.[163–168] Acquisition of *c-CBL* mutations has been associated temporally with transformation from ET to myelofibrosis[165] and from *JAK2V617F*-positive myelofibrosis to *JAK2V617F*-negative AML.[84] These data are in keeping with a main role for *c-CBL* mutations in disease progression within the MPNs.

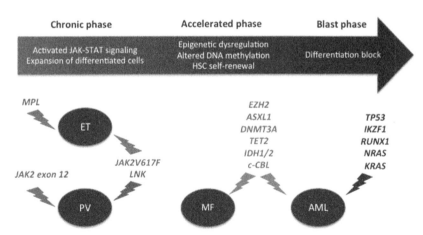

Fig. 2. Model for interactions between phenotype and genotype in PV, ET, and accelerated and blast-phase MPNs. Chronic-phase disease is characterized by mutations that activate JAK-STAT signaling pathways and lead to expansion of differentiated cells. Some of these mutations are phenotype-specific, such as *MPL* mutations in ET and *JAK2* exon 12 mutations in PV. *JAK2V617F* and *LNK* mutations are not phenotype-specific and presumably depend on other factors, such as gene dosage for JAK2V617F or constitutional factors, to determine the precise phenotype. Accelerated-phase disease may carry any of these mutations but is also characterized by increasing genetic complexity, with more frequent mutations in genes regulating DNA methylation (*TET2* and *IDH1/2*), other epigenetic mechanisms (*EZH2*, *ASXL1*, and *DNMT3A*), or other pathways in HSC self-renewal (*c-CBL*). Additional mutations that further promote HSC self-renewal and differentiation block may contribute to blast-phase transformation. Many of the mutations depicted have been identified in patients at each disease stage, highlighting the need for a greater understanding of how cooperation between mutations may account for HSC dysfunction and disease progression.

Other mutations implicated in leukemic progression
Mutations in various other genes have been implicated in leukemic progression of MPNs, including *TP53, IKZF1, RUNX1, NRAS,* and *KRAS*[84,101,169] but are not to be discussed further.

SUMMARY

Considering the different phenotypes and phases within the MPNs (**Fig. 2**), ET seems likely to represent the least genetically complex disorder, characterized by expansion of differentiated cells predominantly within the megakaryocytic lineage. *JAK2* exon 12–mutated PV has some similarities to ET, with expansion of differentiated cells principally within a single lineage, but the pronounced erythrocytosis may reflect stronger JAK2 signaling. *JAK2V617F*-positive PV frequently involves all 3 myeloid lineages, perhaps reflecting additional lesions, high levels of *JAK2V617F* homozygosity, and/ or genetic modifiers. Several lines of evidence are consistent with the concept of myelofibrosis as an accelerated phase, with frequent mutations in epigenetic regulators and other genes involved in HSC self-renewal. Lastly, blast-phase MPNs are characterized by a spectrum of mutations that are likely to further promote HSC self-renewal and also a block in differentiation.

REFERENCES

1. Dameshek W. Some speculations on the myeloproliferative syndromes. Blood 1951;6(4):372–5.
2. James C, Ugo V, Le Couedic JP, et al. A unique clonal JAK2 mutation leading to constitutive signalling causes polycythaemia vera. Nature 2005;434(7037):1144–8.
3. Baxter EJ, Scott LM, Campbell PJ, et al. Acquired mutation of the tyrosine kinase JAK2 in human myeloproliferative disorders. Lancet 2005;365(9464): 1054–61.
4. Levine RL, Wadleigh M, Cools J, et al. Activating mutation in the tyrosine kinase JAK2 in polycythemia vera, essential thrombocythemia, and myeloid metaplasia with myelofibrosis. Cancer Cell 2005;7(4):387–97.
5. Kralovics R, Passamonti F, Buser AS, et al. A gain-of-function mutation of JAK2 in myeloproliferative disorders. N Engl J Med 2005;352(17):1779–90.
6. Jamieson CH, Gotlib J, Durocher JA, et al. The JAK2 V617F mutation occurs in hematopoietic stem cells in polycythemia vera and predisposes toward erythroid differentiation. Proc Natl Acad Sci U S A 2006;103(16):6224–9.
7. Delhommeau F, Dupont S, Tonetti C, et al. Evidence that the JAK2 G1849T (V617F) mutation occurs in a lymphomyeloid progenitor in polycythemia vera and idiopathic myelofibrosis. Blood 2007;109(1):71–7.
8. Ishii T, Bruno E, Hoffman R, et al. Involvement of various hematopoietic-cell lineages by the JAK2V617F mutation in polycythemia vera. Blood 2006;108(9):3128–34.
9. Dupont S, Masse A, James C, et al. The JAK2 V617F mutation triggers erythropoietin hypersensitivity and terminal erythroid amplification in primary cells from patients with polycythemia vera. Blood 2007;110(3):1013–21.
10. Saharinen P, Silvennoinen O. The pseudokinase domain is required for suppression of basal activity of Jak2 and Jak3 tyrosine kinases and for cytokine-inducible activation of signal transduction. J Biol Chem 2002;277(49):47954–63.
11. Sanz A, Ungureanu D, Pekkala T, et al. Analysis of Jak2 catalytic function by peptide microarrays: the role of the JH2 domain and V617F mutation. PLoS One 2011;6(4):e18522.

12. Zaleskas VM, Krause DS, Lazarides K, et al. Molecular pathogenesis and therapy of polycythemia induced in mice by JAK2 V617F. PLoS One 2006;1:e18.

13. Kamishimoto J, Tago K, Kasahara T, et al. Akt activation through the phosphorylation of erythropoietin receptor at tyrosine 479 is required for myeloproliferative disorder-associated JAK2 V617F mutant-induced cellular transformation. Cell Signal 2011;23(5):849–56.

14. Funakoshi-Tago M, Tago K, Abe M, et al. STAT5 activation is critical for the transformation mediated by myeloproliferative disorder-associated JAK2 V617F mutant. J Biol Chem 2010;285(8):5296–307.

15. Yan D, Hutchison RE, Mohi G. Critical requirement for Stat5 in a mouse model of polycythemia vera. Blood 2011;119(15):3539–49.

16. Walz C, Ahmed W, Lazarides K, et al. Essential role for Stat5a/b in myeloproliferative neoplasms induced by BCR-ABL1 and JAK2(V617F) in mice. Blood 2012;119(15):3550–60.

17. Garcon L, Rivat C, James C, et al. Constitutive activation of STAT5 and Bcl-xL overexpression can induce endogenous erythroid colony formation in human primary cells. Blood 2006;108(5):1551–4.

18. Wardrop D, Steensma DP. Is refractory anaemia with ring sideroblasts and thrombocytosis (RARS-T) a necessary or useful diagnostic category? Br J Haematol 2009;144(6):809–17.

19. Levine RL, Loriaux M, Huntly BJ, et al. The JAK2V617F activating mutation occurs in chronic myelomonocytic leukemia and acute myeloid leukemia, but not in acute lymphoblastic leukemia or chronic lymphocytic leukemia. Blood 2005;106(10):3377–9.

20. Jones AV, Kreil S, Zoi K, et al. Widespread occurrence of the JAK2 V617F mutation in chronic myeloproliferative disorders. Blood 2005;106(6):2162–8.

21. Rane SG, Reddy EP. Janus kinases: components of multiple signaling pathways. Oncogene 2000;19(49):5662–79.

22. Campbell PJ, Scott LM, Buck G, et al. Definition of subtypes of essential thrombocythaemia and relation to polycythaemia vera based on JAK2 V617F mutation status: a prospective study. Lancet 2005;366(9501):1945–53.

23. Antonioli E, Guglielmelli P, Pancrazzi A, et al. Clinical implications of the JAK2 V617F mutation in essential thrombocythemia. Leukemia 2005;19(10):1847–9.

24. Wolanskyj AP, Lasho TL, Schwager SM, et al. JAK2 mutation in essential thrombocythaemia: clinical associations and long-term prognostic relevance. Br J Haematol 2005;131(2):208–13.

25. Cheung B, Radia D, Pantelidis P, et al. The presence of the JAK2 V617F mutation is associated with a higher haemoglobin and increased risk of thrombosis in essential thrombocythaemia. Br J Haematol 2006;132(2):244–5.

26. Kittur J, Knudson RA, Lasho TL, et al. Clinical correlates of JAK2V617F allele burden in essential thrombocythemia. Cancer 2007;109(11):2279–84.

27. Dahabreh IJ, Zoi K, Giannouli S, et al. Is JAK2 V617F mutation more than a diagnostic index? A meta-analysis of clinical outcomes in essential thrombocythemia. Leuk Res 2009;33(1):67–73.

28. Tefferi A, Lasho TL, Schwager SM, et al. The clinical phenotype of wild-type, heterozygous, and homozygous JAK2V617F in polycythemia vera. Cancer 2006;106(3):631–5.

29. Vannucchi AM, Antonioli E, Guglielmelli P, et al. Clinical profile of homozygous JAK2 617V>F mutation in patients with polycythemia vera or essential thrombocythemia. Blood 2007;110(3):840–6.

30. Vannucchi AM, Antonioli E, Guglielmelli P, et al. Clinical correlates of JAK2V617F presence or allele burden in myeloproliferative neoplasms: a critical reappraisal. Leukemia 2008;22(7):1299–307.
31. Vannucchi AM, Antonioli E, Guglielmelli P, et al. Prospective identification of high-risk polycythemia vera patients based on JAK2V617F allele burden. Leukemia 2007;21(9):1952–9.
32. Passamonti F, Rumi E, Pietra D, et al. A prospective study of 338 patients with polycythemia vera: the impact of JAK2 (V617F) allele burden and leukocytosis on fibrotic or leukemic disease transformation and vascular complications. Leukemia 2010;24(9):1574–9.
33. Silver RT, Vandris K, Wang YL, et al. JAK2(V617F) allele burden in polycythemia vera correlates with grade of myelofibrosis, but is not substantially affected by therapy. Leuk Res 2011;35(2):177–82.
34. Lippert E, Boissinot M, Kralovics R, et al. The JAK2-V617F mutation is frequently present at diagnosis in patients with essential thrombocythemia and polycythemia vera. Blood 2006;108(6):1865–7.
35. Tefferi A, Strand JJ, Lasho TL, et al. Bone marrow JAK2V617F allele burden and clinical correlates in polycythemia vera. Leukemia 2007;21(9):2074–5.
36. Moliterno AR, Williams DM, Rogers O, et al. Phenotypic variability within the JAK2 V617F-positive MPD: roles of progenitor cell and neutrophil allele burdens. Exp Hematol 2008;36(11):1480–6.
37. Carobbio A, Finazzi G, Antonioli E, et al. JAK2V617F allele burden and thrombosis: a direct comparison in essential thrombocythemia and polycythemia vera. Exp Hematol 2009;37(9):1016–21.
38. Antonioli E, Guglielmelli P, Poli G, et al. Influence of JAK2V617F allele burden on phenotype in essential thrombocythemia. Haematologica 2008;93(1):41–8.
39. Larsen TS, Pallisgaard N, Moller MB, et al. Quantitative assessment of the JAK2 V617F allele burden: equivalent levels in peripheral blood and bone marrow. Leukemia 2008;22(1):194–5.
40. Scott LM, Scott MA, Campbell PJ, et al. Progenitors homozygous for the V617F mutation occur in most patients with polycythemia vera, but not essential thrombocythemia. Blood 2006;108(7):2435–7.
41. Larsen TS, Pallisgaard N, Moller MB, et al. The JAK2 V617F allele burden in essential thrombocythemia, polycythemia vera and primary myelofibrosis– impact on disease phenotype. Eur J Haematol 2007;79(6):508–15.
42. Pardanani A, Lasho TL, Finke C, et al. Extending Jak2V617F and MplW515 mutation analysis to single hematopoietic colonies and B and T lymphocytes. Stem Cells 2007;25(9):2358–62.
43. Stein BL, Williams DM, Wang NY, et al. Sex differences in the JAK2 V617F allele burden in chronic myeloproliferative disorders. Haematologica 2010;95(7):1090–7.
44. Godfrey AL, Chen E, Pagano F, et al. JAK2V617F-homozygosity arises commonly and recurrently in PV and ET, but PV is characterized by expansion of a dominant homozygous subclone. Blood 2012. [Epub ahead of print].
45. Gaikwad A, Nussenzveig R, Liu E, et al. In vitro expansion of erythroid progenitors from polycythemia vera patients leads to decrease in JAK2 V617F allele. Exp Hematol 2007;35(4):587–95.
46. Anand S, Stedham F, Beer P, et al. Effects of the JAK2 mutation on the hematopoietic stem and progenitor compartment in human myeloproliferative neoplasms. Blood 2011;118(1):177–81.

47. Li J, Kent DG, Chen E, et al. Mouse models of myeloproliferative neoplasms: JAK of all grades. Dis Model Mech 2011;4(3):311–7.
48. Wernig G, Mercher T, Okabe R, et al. Expression of Jak2V617F causes a polycythemia vera-like disease with associated myelofibrosis in a murine bone marrow transplant model. Blood 2006;107(11):4274–81.
49. Bumm TG, Elsea C, Corbin AS, et al. Characterization of murine JAK2V617F-positive myeloproliferative disease. Cancer Res 2006;66(23):11156–65.
50. Lacout C, Pisani DF, Tulliez M, et al. JAK2V617F expression in murine hematopoietic cells leads to MPD mimicking human PV with secondary myelofibrosis. Blood 2006;108(5):1652–60.
51. Shide K, Shimoda HK, Kumano T, et al. Development of ET, primary myelofibrosis and PV in mice expressing JAK2 V617F. Leukemia 2008;22(1):87–95.
52. Xing S, Wanting TH, Zhao W, et al. Transgenic expression of JAK2V617F causes myeloproliferative disorders in mice. Blood 2008;111(10):5109–17.
53. Tiedt R, Hao-Shen H, Sobas MA, et al. Ratio of mutant JAK2-V617F to wild-type Jak2 determines the MPD phenotypes in transgenic mice. Blood 2008;111(8):3931–40.
54. Mullally A, Lane SW, Ball B, et al. Physiological Jak2V617F expression causes a lethal myeloproliferative neoplasm with differential effects on hematopoietic stem and progenitor cells. Cancer Cell 2010;17(6):584–96.
55. Marty C, Lacout C, Martin A, et al. Myeloproliferative neoplasm induced by constitutive expression of JAK2V617F in knock-in mice. Blood 2010;116(5):783–7.
56. Akada H, Yan D, Zou H, et al. Conditional expression of heterozygous or homozygous Jak2V617F from its endogenous promoter induces a polycythemia vera-like disease. Blood 2010;115(17):3589–97.
57. Li J, Spensberger D, Ahn JS, et al. JAK2 V617F impairs hematopoietic stem cell function in a conditional knock-in mouse model of JAK2 V617F-positive essential thrombocythemia. Blood 2010;116(9):1528–38.
58. Kralovics R, Teo SS, Buser AS, et al. Altered gene expression in myeloproliferative disorders correlates with activation of signaling by the V617F mutation of Jak2. Blood 2005;106(10):3374–6.
59. Pellagatti A, Vetrie D, Langford CF, et al. Gene expression profiling in polycythemia vera using cDNA microarray technology. Cancer Res 2003;63(14):3940–4.
60. Chen E, Beer PA, Godfrey AL, et al. Distinct clinical phenotypes associated with JAK2V617F reflect differential STAT1 signaling. Cancer Cell 2010;18(5):524–35.
61. Platanias LC. Mechanisms of type-I- and type-II-interferon-mediated signalling. Nat Rev Immunol 2005;5(5):375–86.
62. Scott LM, Tong W, Levine RL, et al. JAK2 exon 12 mutations in polycythemia vera and idiopathic erythrocytosis. N Engl J Med 2007;356(5):459–68.
63. Pietra D, Li S, Brisci A, et al. Somatic mutations of JAK2 exon 12 in patients with JAK2 (V617F)-negative myeloproliferative disorders. Blood 2008;111(3):1686–9.
64. Schnittger S, Bacher U, Haferlach C, et al. Detection of JAK2 exon 12 mutations in 15 patients with JAK2V617F negative polycythemia vera. Haematologica 2009;94(3):414–8.
65. Li S, Kralovics R, De Libero G, et al. Clonal heterogeneity in polycythemia vera patients with JAK2 exon12 and JAK2-V617F mutations. Blood 2008;111(7):3863–6.
66. Pardanani A, Lasho TL, Finke C, et al. Prevalence and clinicopathologic correlates of JAK2 exon 12 mutations in JAK2V617F-negative polycythemia vera. Leukemia 2007;21(9):1960–3.

67. Siemiatkowska A, Bieniaszewska M, Hellmann A, et al. JAK2 and MPL gene mutations in V617F-negative myeloproliferative neoplasms. Leuk Res 2010; 34(3):387–9.

68. Yeh YM, Chen YL, Cheng HY, et al. High percentage of JAK2 exon 12 mutation in Asian patients with polycythemia vera. Am J Clin Pathol 2010;134(2):266–70.

69. Martinez-Aviles L, Besses C, Alvarez-Larran A, et al. JAK2 exon 12 mutations in polycythemia vera or idiopathic erythrocytosis. Haematologica 2007;92(12): 1717–8.

70. Kouroupi E, Zoi K, Parquet N, et al. Mutations in exon 12 of JAK2 are mainly found in JAK2 V617F-negative polycythaemia vera patients. Br J Haematol 2008;142(4):676–9.

71. Williams DM, Kim AH, Rogers O, et al. Phenotypic variations and new mutations in JAK2 V617F-negative polycythemia vera, erythrocytosis, and idiopathic myelofibrosis. Exp Hematol 2007;35(11):1641–6.

72. Percy MJ, Scott LM, Erber WN, et al. The frequency of JAK2 exon 12 mutations in idiopathic erythrocytosis patients with low serum erythropoietin levels. Haematologica 2007;92(12):1607–14.

73. Ormazabal C, Hurtado C, Aranaz P, et al. Low frequency of JAK2 exon 12 mutations in classic and atypical CMPDs. Leuk Res 2008;32(9):1485–7.

74. Albiero E, Madeo D, Ruggeri M, et al. Loss of the JAK2 intramolecular auto-inhibition mechanism is predicted by structural modelling of a novel exon 12 insertion mutation in a case of idiopathic erythrocytosis. Br J Haematol 2008; 142(6):986–90.

75. Butcher CM, Hahn U, To LB, et al. Two novel JAK2 exon 12 mutations in JAK2V617F-negative polycythaemia vera patients. Leukemia 2008;22(4):870–3.

76. Colaizzo D, Amitrano L, Tiscia GL, et al. A new JAK2 gene mutation in patients with polycythemia vera and splanchnic vein thrombosis. Blood 2007;110(7): 2768–9.

77. Passamonti F, Elena C, Schnittger S, et al. Molecular and clinical features of the myeloproliferative neoplasm associated with JAK2 exon 12 mutations. Blood 2011;117(10):2813–6.

78. Bernardi M, Ruggeri M, Albiero E, et al. Isolated erythrocytosis in V617F negative patients with JAK2 exon 12 mutations: report of a new mutation. Am J Hematol 2009;84(4):258–60.

79. Scott LM, Beer PA, Bench AJ, et al. Prevalance of JAK2 V617F and exon 12 mutations in polycythaemia vera. Br J Haematol 2007;139(3):511–2.

80. Beer PA, Erber WN, Campbell PJ, et al. How I treat essential thrombocythemia. Blood 2011;117(5):1472–82.

81. Plo I, Nakatake M, Malivert L, et al. JAK2 stimulates homologous recombination and genetic instability: potential implication in the heterogeneity of myeloproliferative disorders. Blood 2008;112(4):1402–12.

82. Zhao R, Follows GA, Beer PA, et al. Inhibition of the Bcl-xL deamidation pathway in myeloproliferative disorders. N Engl J Med 2008;359(26):2778–89.

83. Campbell PJ, Baxter EJ, Beer PA, et al. Mutation of JAK2 in the myeloproliferative disorders: timing, clonality studies, cytogenetic associations, and role in leukemic transformation. Blood 2006;108(10):3548–55.

84. Beer PA, Delhommeau F, LeCouedic JP, et al. Two routes to leukemic transformation after a JAK2 mutation-positive myeloproliferative neoplasm. Blood 2010; 115(14):2891–900.

85. Pikman Y, Lee BH, Mercher T, et al. MPLW515L is a novel somatic activating mutation in myelofibrosis with myeloid metaplasia. PLoS Med 2006;3(7):e270.

86. Beer PA, Campbell PJ, Scott LM, et al. MPL mutations in myeloproliferative disorders: analysis of the PT-1 cohort. Blood 2008;112(1):141–9.
87. Chaligne R, Tonetti C, Besancenot R, et al. New mutations of MPL in primitive myelofibrosis: only the MPL W515 mutations promote a G1/S-phase transition. Leukemia 2008;22(8):1557–66.
88. Pardanani AD, Levine RL, Lasho T, et al. MPL515 mutations in myeloproliferative and other myeloid disorders: a study of 1182 patients. Blood 2006;108(10): 3472–6.
89. Boyd EM, Bench AJ, Goday-Fernandez A, et al. Clinical utility of routine MPL exon 10 analysis in the diagnosis of essential thrombocythaemia and primary myelofibrosis. Br J Haematol 2010;149(2):250–7.
90. Schnittger S, Bacher U, Haferlach C, et al. Characterization of 35 new cases with four different MPLW515 mutations and essential thrombocytosis or primary myelofibrosis. Haematologica 2009;94(1):141–4.
91. Ding J, Komatsu H, Wakita A, et al. Familial essential thrombocythemia associated with a dominant-positive activating mutation of the c-MPL gene, which encodes for the receptor for thrombopoietin. Blood 2004;103(11):4198–200.
92. Teofili L, Giona F, Martini M, et al. Markers of myeloproliferative diseases in childhood polycythemia vera and essential thrombocythemia. J Clin Oncol 2007; 25(9):1048–53.
93. Pietra D, Brisci A, Rumi E, et al. Deep sequencing reveals double mutations in cis of MPL exon 10 in myeloproliferative neoplasms. Haematologica 2011;96(4): 607–11.
94. Kawamata N, Ogawa S, Yamamoto G, et al. Genetic profiling of myeloproliferative disorders by single-nucleotide polymorphism oligonucleotide microarray. Exp Hematol 2008;36(11):1471–9.
95. Vannucchi AM, Antonioli E, Guglielmelli P, et al. Characteristics and clinical correlates of MPL 515W>L/K mutation in essential thrombocythemia. Blood 2008;112(3):844–7.
96. Guglielmelli P, Pancrazzi A, Bergamaschi G, et al. Anaemia characterises patients with myelofibrosis harbouring Mpl mutation. Br J Haematol 2007; 137(3):244–7.
97. Beer PA, Jones AV, Bench AJ, et al. Clonal diversity in the myeloproliferative neoplasms: independent origins of genetically distinct clones. Br J Haematol 2009;144(6):904–8.
98. Pecquet C, Staerk J, Chaligne R, et al. Induction of myeloproliferative disorder and myelofibrosis by thrombopoietin receptor W515 mutants is mediated by cytosolic tyrosine 112 of the receptor. Blood 2010;115(5):1037–48.
99. Chaligne R, James C, Tonetti C, et al. Evidence for MPL W515L/K mutations in hematopoietic stem cells in primitive myelofibrosis. Blood 2007;110(10): 3735–43.
100. Tefferi A. Novel mutations and their functional and clinical relevance in myeloproliferative neoplasms: JAK2, MPL, TET2, ASXL1, CBL, IDH and IKZF1. Leukemia 2010;24(6):1128–38.
101. Vainchenker W, Delhommeau F, Constantinescu SN, et al. New mutations and pathogenesis of myeloproliferative neoplasms. Blood 2011;118(7):1723–35.
102. Delhommeau F, Dupont S, Della Valle V, et al. Mutation in TET2 in myeloid cancers. N Engl J Med 2009;360(22):2289–301.
103. Tefferi A, Pardanani A, Lim KH, et al. TET2 mutations and their clinical correlates in polycythemia vera, essential thrombocythemia and myelofibrosis. Leukemia 2009;23(5):905–11.

104. Abdel-Wahab O, Mullally A, Hedvat C, et al. Genetic characterization of TET1, TET2, and TET3 alterations in myeloid malignancies. Blood 2009;114(1): 144–7.

105. Couronne L, Lippert E, Andrieux J, et al. Analyses of TET2 mutations in post-myeloproliferative neoplasm acute myeloid leukemias. Leukemia 2010;24(1): 201–3.

106. Abdel-Wahab O, Manshouri T, Patel J, et al. Genetic analysis of transforming events that convert chronic myeloproliferative neoplasms to leukemias. Cancer Res 2010;70(2):447–52.

107. Tefferi A, Lim KH, Abdel-Wahab O, et al. Detection of mutant TET2 in myeloid malignancies other than myeloproliferative neoplasms: CMML, MDS, MDS/MPN and AML. Leukemia 2009;23(7):1343–5.

108. Jankowska AM, Szpurka H, Tiu RV, et al. Loss of heterozygosity 4q24 and TET2 mutations associated with myelodysplastic/myeloproliferative neoplasms. Blood 2009;113(25):6403–10.

109. Kosmider O, Gelsi-Boyer V, Ciudad M, et al. TET2 gene mutation is a frequent and adverse event in chronic myelomonocytic leukemia. Haematologica 2009; 94(12):1676–81.

110. Nibourel O, Kosmider O, Cheok M, et al. Incidence and prognostic value of TET2 alterations in de novo acute myeloid leukemia achieving complete remission. Blood 2010;116(7):1132–5.

111. Quivoron C, Couronne L, Della Valle V, et al. TET2 inactivation results in pleiotropic hematopoietic abnormalities in mouse and is a recurrent event during human lymphomagenesis. Cancer cell 2011;20(1):25–38.

112. Chou WC, Chou SC, Liu CY, et al. TET2 mutation is an unfavorable prognostic factor in acute myeloid leukemia patients with intermediate-risk cytogenetics. Blood 2011;118(14):3803–10.

113. Ko M, Huang Y, Jankowska AM, et al. Impaired hydroxylation of 5-methylcytosine in myeloid cancers with mutant TET2. Nature 2010;468(7325):839–43.

114. Ko M, Bandukwala HS, An J, et al. Ten-Eleven-Translocation 2 (TET2) negatively regulates homeostasis and differentiation of hematopoietic stem cells in mice. Proc Natl Acad Sci U S A 2011;108(35):14566–71.

115. Li Z, Cai X, Cai CL, et al. Deletion of Tet2 in mice leads to dysregulated hematopoietic stem cells and subsequent development of myeloid malignancies. Blood 2011;118(17):4509–18.

116. Moran-Crusio K, Reavie L, Shih A, et al. Tet2 loss leads to increased hematopoietic stem cell self-renewal and myeloid transformation. Cancer Cell 2011;20(1): 11–24.

117. Pronier E, Almire C, Mokrani H, et al. Inhibition of TET2-mediated conversion of 5-methylcytosine to 5-hydroxymethylcytosine disturbs erythroid and granulomonocytic differentiation of human hematopoietic progenitors. Blood 2011;118(9): 2551–5.

118. Schaub FX, Looser R, Li S, et al. Clonal analysis of TET2 and JAK2 mutations suggests that TET2 can be a late event in the progression of myeloproliferative neoplasms. Blood 2010;115(10):2003–7.

119. Vire E, Brenner C, Deplus R, et al. The Polycomb group protein EZH2 directly controls DNA methylation. Nature 2006;439(7078):871–4.

120. Ernst T, Chase AJ, Score J, et al. Inactivating mutations of the histone methyltransferase gene EZH2 in myeloid disorders. Nat Genet 2010;42(8):722–6.

121. Guglielmelli P, Biamonte F, Score J, et al. EZH2 mutational status predicts poor survival in myelofibrosis. Blood 2011;118(19):5227–34.

122. Abdel-Wahab O, Pardanani A, Patel J, et al. Concomitant analysis of EZH2 and ASXL1 mutations in myelofibrosis, chronic myelomonocytic leukemia and blast-phase myeloproliferative neoplasms. Leukemia 2011;25(7):1200–2.
123. Nikoloski G, Langemeijer SM, Kuiper RP, et al. Somatic mutations of the histone methyltransferase gene EZH2 in myelodysplastic syndromes. Nat Genet 2010; 42(8):665–7.
124. Jankowska AM, Makishima H, Tiu RV, et al. Mutational spectrum analysis of chronic myelomonocytic leukemia includes genes associated with epigenetic regulation: UTX, EZH2, and DNMT3A. Blood 2011;118(14):3932–41.
125. Makishima H, Jankowska AM, Tiu RV, et al. Novel homo- and hemizygous mutations in EZH2 in myeloid malignancies. Leukemia 2010;24(10):1799–804.
126. Scheuermann JC, de Ayala Alonso AG, Oktaba K, et al. Histone H2A deubiquitinase activity of the polycomb repressive complex PR-DUB. Nature 2010; 465(7295):243–7.
127. Carbuccia N, Murati A, Trouplin V, et al. Mutations of ASXL1 gene in myeloproliferative neoplasms. Leukemia 2009;23(11):2183–6.
128. Gelsi-Boyer V, Trouplin V, Adelaide J, et al. Mutations of polycomb-associated gene ASXL1 in myelodysplastic syndromes and chronic myelomonocytic leukaemia. Br J Haematol 2009;145(6):788–800.
129. Gelsi-Boyer V, Trouplin V, Roquain J, et al. ASXL1 mutation is associated with poor prognosis and acute transformation in chronic myelomonocytic leukaemia. Br J Haematol 2010;151(4):365–75.
130. Thol F, Friesen I, Damm F, et al. Prognostic significance of ASXL1 mutations in patients with myelodysplastic syndromes. J Clin Oncol 2011;29(18):2499–506.
131. Pratcorona M, Abbas S, Sanders M, et al. Acquired mutations in ASXL1 in acute myeloid leukemia: prevalence and prognostic value. Haematologica 2012;97(3): 388–92.
132. Martinez-Aviles L, Besses C, Alvarez-Larran A, et al. TET2, ASXL1, IDH1, IDH2, and c-CBL genes in JAK2- and MPL-negative myeloproliferative neoplasms. Ann Hematol 2012;91(4):533–41.
133. Stein BL, Williams DM, O'Keefe C, et al. Disruption of the ASXL1 gene is frequent in primary, post-essential thrombocytosis and post-polycythemia vera myelofibrosis, but not essential thrombocytosis or polycythemia vera: analysis of molecular genetics and clinical phenotypes. Haematologica 2011;96(10): 1462–9.
134. Mardis ER, Ding L, Dooling DJ, et al. Recurring mutations found by sequencing an acute myeloid leukemia genome. N Engl J Med 2009;361(11):1058–66.
135. Paschka P, Schlenk RF, Gaidzik VI, et al. IDH1 and IDH2 mutations are frequent genetic alterations in acute myeloid leukemia and confer adverse prognosis in cytogenetically normal acute myeloid leukemia with NPM1 mutation without FLT3 internal tandem duplication. J Clin Oncol 2010;28(22):3636–43.
136. Schnittger S, Haferlach C, Ulke M, et al. IDH1 mutations are detected in 6.6% of 1414 AML patients and are associated with intermediate risk karyotype and unfavorable prognosis in adults younger than 60 years and unmutated NPM1 status. Blood 2010;116(25):5486–96.
137. Ward PS, Patel J, Wise DR, et al. The common feature of leukemia-associated IDH1 and IDH2 mutations is a neomorphic enzyme activity converting alpha-ketoglutarate to 2-hydroxyglutarate. Cancer Cell 2010;17(3):225–34.
138. Pardanani A, Lasho TL, Finke CM, et al. IDH1 and IDH2 mutation analysis in chronic- and blast-phase myeloproliferative neoplasms. Leukemia 2010;24(6): 1146–51.

139. Tefferi A, Lasho TL, Abdel-Wahab O, et al. IDH1 and IDH2 mutation studies in 1473 patients with chronic-, fibrotic- or blast-phase essential thrombocythemia, polycythemia vera or myelofibrosis. Leukemia 2010;24(7):1302–9.

140. Thol F, Weissinger EM, Krauter J, et al. IDH1 mutations in patients with myelodysplastic syndromes are associated with an unfavorable prognosis. Haematologica 2010;95(10):1668–74.

141. Kosmider O, Gelsi-Boyer V, Slama L, et al. Mutations of IDH1 and IDH2 genes in early and accelerated phases of myelodysplastic syndromes and MDS/myeloproliferative neoplasms. Leukemia 2010;24(5):1094–6.

142. Tefferi A, Jimma T, Sulai NH, et al. IDH mutations in primary myelofibrosis predict leukemic transformation and shortened survival: clinical evidence for leukemogenic collaboration with JAK2V617F. Leukemia 2012;26(3):475–80.

143. Green A, Beer P. Somatic mutations of IDH1 and IDH2 in the leukemic transformation of myeloproliferative neoplasms. N Engl J Med 2010;362(4):369–70.

144. Dang L, White DW, Gross S, et al. Cancer-associated IDH1 mutations produce 2-hydroxyglutarate. Nature 2009;462(7274):739–44.

145. Zhao S, Lin Y, Xu W, et al. Glioma-derived mutations in IDH1 dominantly inhibit IDH1 catalytic activity and induce HIF-1alpha. Science 2009;324(5924):261–5.

146. Figueroa ME, Abdel-Wahab O, Lu C, et al. Leukemic IDH1 and IDH2 mutations result in a hypermethylation phenotype, disrupt TET2 function, and impair hematopoietic differentiation. Cancer Cell 2010;18(6):553–67.

147. Ley TJ, Ding L, Walter MJ, et al. DNMT3A mutations in acute myeloid leukemia. N Engl J Med 2010;363(25):2424–33.

148. Walter MJ, Ding L, Shen D, et al. Recurrent DNMT3A mutations in patients with myelodysplastic syndromes. Leukemia 2011;25(7):1153–8.

149. Thol F, Winschel C, Ludeking A, et al. Rare occurrence of DNMT3A mutations in myelodysplastic syndromes. Haematologica 2011;96(12):1870–3.

150. Stegelmann F, Bullinger L, Schlenk RF, et al. DNMT3A mutations in myeloproliferative neoplasms. Leukemia 2011;25(7):1217–9.

151. Abdel-Wahab O, Pardanani A, Rampal R, et al. DNMT3A mutational analysis in primary myelofibrosis, chronic myelomonocytic leukemia and advanced phases of myeloproliferative neoplasms. Leukemia 2011;25(7):1219–20.

152. Bersenev A, Wu C, Balcerek J, et al. Lnk controls mouse hematopoietic stem cell self-renewal and quiescence through direct interactions with JAK2. J Clin Invest 2008;118(8):2832–44.

153. Gery S, Gueller S, Chumakova K, et al. Adaptor protein Lnk negatively regulates the mutant MPL, MPLW515L associated with myeloproliferative disorders. Blood 2007;110(9):3360–4.

154. Tong W, Lodish HF. Lnk inhibits Tpo-mpl signaling and Tpo-mediated megakaryocytopoiesis. J Exp Med 2004;200(5):569–80.

155. Tong W, Zhang J, Lodish HF. Lnk inhibits erythropoiesis and Epo-dependent JAK2 activation and downstream signaling pathways. Blood 2005;105(12):4604–12.

156. Velazquez L, Cheng AM, Fleming HE, et al. Cytokine signaling and hematopoietic homeostasis are disrupted in Lnk-deficient mice. J Exp Med 2002;195(12):1599–611.

157. Takaki S, Morita H, Tezuka Y, et al. Enhanced hematopoiesis by hematopoietic progenitor cells lacking intracellular adaptor protein, Lnk. J Exp Med 2002;195(2):151–60.

158. Oh ST, Simonds EF, Jones C, et al. Novel mutations in the inhibitory adaptor protein LNK drive JAK-STAT signaling in patients with myeloproliferative neoplasms. Blood 2010;116(6):988–92.

159. Lasho TL, Pardanani A, Tefferi A. LNK mutations in JAK2 mutation-negative erythrocytosis. N Engl J Med 2010;363(12):1189–90.
160. Pardanani A, Lasho T, Finke C, et al. LNK mutation studies in blast-phase myeloproliferative neoplasms, and in chronic-phase disease with TET2, IDH, JAK2 or MPL mutations. Leukemia 2010;24(10):1713–8.
161. Ogawa S, Sanada M, Shih LY, et al. Gain-of-function c-CBL mutations associated with uniparental disomy of 11q in myeloid neoplasms. Cell Cycle 2010; 9(6):1051–6.
162. Bacher U, Haferlach C, Schnittger S, et al. Mutations of the TET2 and CBL genes: novel molecular markers in myeloid malignancies. Ann Hematol 2010; 89(7):643–52.
163. Sargin B, Choudhary C, Crosetto N, et al. Flt3-dependent transformation by inactivating c-Cbl mutations in AML. Blood 2007;110(3):1004–12.
164. Caligiuri MA, Briesewitz R, Yu J, et al. Novel c-CBL and CBL-b ubiquitin ligase mutations in human acute myeloid leukemia. Blood 2007;110(3):1022–4.
165. Grand FH, Hidalgo-Curtis CE, Ernst T, et al. Frequent CBL mutations associated with 11q acquired uniparental disomy in myeloproliferative neoplasms. Blood 2009;113(24):6182–92.
166. Sanada M, Suzuki T, Shih LY, et al. Gain-of-function of mutated C-CBL tumour suppressor in myeloid neoplasms. Nature 2009;460(7257):904–8.
167. Makishima H, Cazzolli H, Szpurka H, et al. Mutations of e3 ubiquitin ligase cbl family members constitute a novel common pathogenic lesion in myeloid malignancies. J Clin Oncol 2009;27(36):6109–16.
168. Kohlmann A, Grossmann V, Klein HU, et al. Next-generation sequencing technology reveals a characteristic pattern of molecular mutations in 72.8% of chronic myelomonocytic leukemia by detecting frequent alterations in TET2, CBL, RAS, and RUNX1. J Clin Oncol 2010;28(24):3858–65.
169. Beer PA, Ortmann CA, Stegelmann F, et al. Molecular mechanisms associated with leukemic transformation of MPL-mutant myeloproliferative neoplasms. Haematologica 2010;95(12):2153–6.

Disordered Signaling in Myeloproliferative Neoplasms

Shubha Anand, PhD[a], Brian J.P. Huntly, MRCP, FRCPath, PhD[a,b,c],*

KEYWORDS

- Myeloproliferative neoplasms • JAK2 • Erythropoietin-receptor • MPL • Signaling

KEY POINTS

- Human myeloproliferative neoplasms (MPN) are defined by abnormal signaling patterns, which are central to the development of these diseases.
- The studies conducted so far suggest that multiple signaling pathways are upregulated, with many linked to specific recurrent mutations.
- Although the data suggest the induction of common signaling pathways, emerging evidence also suggests that specific signaling pathways or combinations of signaling abnormalities may dictate the phenotypic differences among MPN subtypes.
- Further delineating these signaling pathways and how they might differ from homeostatic signaling pathways in normal hematopoietic stem and progenitor populations will greatly inform knowledge of MPN and allow clinicians to more safely target signaling for therapeutic gain.

Human chronic myeloproliferative neoplasms (MPN) were first named and classed together by Dameshek in 1951.[1] These include polycythemia vera (PV), essential thrombocythemia (ET), and primary myelofibrosis (PMF). The MPN arise in long-term hematopoietic stem cells and are characterized by overproduction of one or more myeloid lineage.[2,3] In addition, although these disorders are associated with full terminal differentiation, they have a variable propensity to progress either to a myelofibrotic (MF) phase (for PV and ET) or to acute myeloid leukemia. These characteristics allow the use of MPN as a model system to examine the consequences of oncogene activation on normal myeloid ontogeny before this is distorted by further mutations that block differentiation. In addition, they also provide important in vivo model systems to probe the multistep progression to acute myeloid leukemia. It has long been recognized that MPN are associated with altered responsiveness to

[a] Department of Haematology, Cambridge Institute of Medical Research, University of Cambridge, Hills Road, Cambridge CB2 0XY, UK; [b] Cambridge University Hospitals, NHS Foundation Trust, Department of Haematology, Addenbrooke's Hospital, Hills Road, Cambridge CB2 0QQ, UK; [c] Wellcome trust/MRC Cambridge Stem Cell Institute, Cambridge Institute of Medical Research, University of Cambridge, Hills Road, Cambridge CB2 0XY, UK
* Corresponding author. Department of Haematology, Cambridge Institute of Medical Research, University of Cambridge, Cambridge CB2 0XY, UK.
E-mail address: bjph2@cam.ac.uk

Hematol Oncol Clin N Am 26 (2012) 1017–1035
http://dx.doi.org/10.1016/j.hoc.2012.07.004   **hemonc.theclinics.com**
0889-8588/12/$ – see front matter © 2012 Elsevier Inc. All rights reserved.

cytokines and abnormal activation of signaling pathways, and molecular mechanism was recently added to this observation with the identification of recurrent mutations in critical signaling intermediates, such as JAK2. This article outlines what is currently known about signaling abnormalities in MPN and places these findings in the context of the pathogenesis of the disease and the implications for therapy.

INITIAL CLUES ABOUT ALTERED SIGNALING PATHWAYS IN MPN

In 1974, Prchal and Axelrad[4] demonstrated the seminal finding that bone marrow (BM) cells from patients with PV could form colony-forming units–erythroid in vitro without the addition of erythropoietin (EPO). These colonies were therefore called endogenous erythroid colonies (EECs). Because overproduction of red blood cells in PV is also associated with reduced EPO levels, it was proposed that EECs were generated by progenitors either hypersensitive to EPO or whose growth was EPO-independent. This observation was confirmed by culturing BM or peripheral blood (PB) progenitor cells in vitro in the presence of neutralizing antibodies to EPO or EPO-R and by replating analysis in methylcellulose media.[5–9] Correa and coworkers[10] went on to develop serum-free culture medium to study the growth of PV progenitors in vitro and found that erythroid progenitors were also hypersensitive to other cytokines including insulin-like growth factor-1, but not to EPO. Other groups demonstrated hypersensitivity of erythroid progenitors to several cytokines involved in myeloid development, including interleukin (IL)-3, granulocyte-macrophage colony–stimulating factor (GM-CSF), and stem cell factor in patients with PV compared with normal control subjects.[11–13] By contrast, they did not observe any difference in response when PV progenitors were stimulated with cytokines with more pleiotrophic effects, including IL-4, IL-6, granulocyte colony–stimulating factor (G-CSF), and macrophage colony–stimulating factor (M-CSF). It was therefore concluded that erythroid or myeloid progenitor cells from patients with PV were hypersensitive to the predominant cytokines that instructed their proliferation and differentiation. Further experiments were performed to assess number, affinity, and internalization of I^{125}-labeled EPO and IL-3 receptors in erythroid progenitors from patients with PV and normal control subjects and excluded differences as an explanation for altered cytokine sensitivity.[14,15] Furthermore, no mutations were detected in the EPO receptor gene in patients with PV.[16,17]

MUTATIONS ASSOCIATED WITH ACTIVATED SIGNALING IN PATIENTS WITH MPN

Although the previously mentioned studies demonstrated abnormal signaling in patients with MPN, the molecular basis for these findings was not elucidated for a further two decades. In contrast, over the last 7 years several mutations have been described that provide a framework for the understanding of activated signaling in MPN.

JAK2 V617F Mutation

In 2005, several groups identified a somatic mutation (G-to-T substitution at position 1849) in the tyrosine kinase JAK2 in patients with MPN. This mutation occurs in most patients with PV (95%–99%), and in a significant proportion of patients with ET (50%–70%) and patients with IMF (40%–50%).[18–21] The mutation results in the substitution of valine to phenylalanine at codon 617 (V617F). JAK2 is a member of the Janus family of cytoplasmic tyrosine kinases, which also includes JAK1, JAK3, and TYK2. JAK kinases contain two homologous kinase domains: a catalytically active JH1 domain and what was until recently thought to be an inactive JH2 domain (**Fig. 1**). The V617F mutation alters the JH2 domain, which contains a similar amino acid sequence to JH1 and is also called the pseudokinase domain.[22,23] The JH2 domain was already

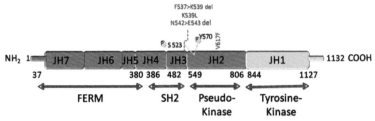

Fig. 1. The structure of Janus kinase 2 (JAK2). The different functional domains include the amino terminal FERM domain and SH2 domain and the carboxy terminal pseudokinase (JH2) and kinase domain (JH1), listed below the figure. The location of the JAK2V617F mutation in the pseudokinase domain and some of the exon 12 mutations are shown in red. Also shown are the two residues Ser523 and Tyr570, which are phosphorylated by JH2 domain to inhibit the kinase activity of JH1. The V617F mutation inhibits the kinase activity of the JH2 domain and blocks the phosphorylation of these two residues, thereby constitutively activating the kinase.

known to play a negative auto regulatory role in switching off the kinase activity of JAK2, because its deletion results in constitutive activation of the kinase.[24,25] However, Ungureanu and colleagues[26] have recently demonstrated that the JH2 pesudokinase domain also possesses catalytic activity and that it is this activity that regulates the JAK2 JH1 kinase activity. This occurs through auto-phosphorylation at two negative regulatory sites, one of which (Tyr570) had been previously shown to regulate response to cytokines.[24,25]

JAK2 is associated with the cytoplasmic tails of many cytokine receptors, including the type I cytokine receptors for EPO, TPO, G-CSF, GM-CSF, and IL-3, which are involved in myeloid or erythroid differentiation.[27] In particular, JAK2 is the only kinase specifically associated with EPO-R and MPL (TPO-R) and is also involved, by its N terminal FERM domain, in facilitating the transport of the receptor-JAK complex to the cell surface.[28,29] When a specific cytokine binds its cognate-receptor it induces receptor dimerization or oligomerization. JAK family members are preassembled on the receptor in the endoplasmic reticulum and ligand binding induces their transphosphorylation. The fully activated JAKs subsequently phosphorylate specific tyrosine residues on the receptor, which act as docking sites for STAT (signal transducers and activators of transcription) proteins and other SH2 domain-containing adaptor proteins (**Fig. 2**). The STAT proteins are, in turn, themselves phosphorylated inducing their dimerization and translocation to the nucleus, where they activate the transcription of target genes, many of which are involved in cell proliferation.[30,31] In addition to STAT proteins, JAK kinases can also activate other signaling pathways by binding SH2-containing adaptor proteins. These include RAS, mitogen-activated protein kinase-extracellular signal-related kinase (MAPK-ERK), protein kinase B (PKB or AKT), and phospholipase-B pathways.[31] The MPN V617F mutation is thought to abrogate the catalytic activity of the JH2 domain, thereby increasing the basal activity of JAK2.[26] In support of this notion, expression of JAK2 V617F in murine hematopoietic cells leads to cytokine hypersensitivity and cytokine-independent growth similar to EECs grown from patients with PV. Constitutive phosphorylation of JAK2 in the absence of ligand is also observed.[19–21,32] Cytokine-independent growth seems most effective if the cells also express homodimeric type 1 cytokine receptors, such as EPO-R, MPL, or G-CSF-R. This is hardly surprising, in that these are receptors that are differentially expressed on cells of the erythroid, megakaryocytic, and granulocytic lineages, the lineages preferentially amplified in MPNs.[33,34]

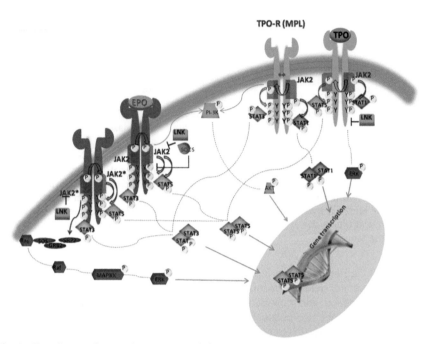

Fig. 2. Signaling pathways downstream of the EPO and TPO-R. JAK2 (*purple*) is associated with EPO-R and MPL receptors. The mutant JAK2 (JAK2*) and TPO-R (*red stars*) activate the signal transduction pathway in the absence of ligand. JAK2 phosphorylates specific tyrosine residues on the receptor, which act as docking sites for STAT proteins. STAT proteins are also phosphorylated by JAK2, mediating their dimerization and translocation to the nucleus, where they activate a specific gene expression program. In addition, other SH2-containing adaptor proteins are phosporylated, which in turn activate other pathways including the RAS, mitogen-activated protein kinase–extracellular signal-related kinase (MAPK-ERK), and PI-3K -AKT pathway. All pathways promote survival, proliferation, and differentiation of committed myeloid progenitors, ultimately through alterations in gene expression programs. The negative regulators SOCS1 and SOCS3 compete with STAT proteins to bind to the JAK2 catalytic domain resulting in abrogation of downstream signaling. Whether SOCS proteins can inhibit mutant JAK2 signaling is unclear. LNK negatively regulate signaling through the MPL and EPO receptors by reducing the duration of their response to cytokine stimulation. For further explanation, please see text.

JAK2 Exon 12 Mutations

Approximately 5% of patients with PV and almost half of patients with ET and MF do not harbor the JAK2 V617F mutation. Therefore, further studies were undertaken to identify complementing alleles that might be mutated in these patients. Scott and colleagues[35] analyzed JAK2V617F-negative patients with PV for mutations in all *JAK* kinase family members and their downstream mediators STAT5A and B. They found four novel mutations in exon 12 of *JAK2*. Of the initial 10 patients analyzed, six had mutations that either involved deletion or substitution affecting lysine at codon 539 (**Table 1**). The remaining four had N542-E543 deletion. Erythroid colonies could be grown from these patients in vitro in the absence of EPO, with all colonies heterozygous for the exon 12 mutation. However, unlike V617F, which can occur in the homozygous state, no colonies homozygous for exon 12 mutations were found. More recently, a large number of other JAK2 exon 12 mutations have been identified.[36] Structurally, all of the mutations are present

Table 1
Mutations predicted to alter canonical signaling in MPN

	Function	Disease	Mutation	Frequency	References
JAK2	Tyrosine kinase	PV, ET, MF	V617F	PV (95%) ET, MF	[18–21]
		PV	K539L	(~50%)	
		PV	F537-K539delinsL	Exon 12 mutations:	[35,36]
		PV	N542-E543del	PV (5%)	
MPL	Thrombopoietin receptor	ET, MF	W515L	ET (4%)	[41,42,45–48]
			W515K	MF (11%)	
			W515N		
			W515A		
LNK (SH2B3)	Adaptor protein; negative regulator of signaling	ET, MF	DEL mutant (loss of PH&SH2 domains) E208Q Other *LNK* mutations outside of PH&SH2 domains	ET (<5%) MF (<5%)	[56–60]
CBL	Adaptor protein; E3 ubiquitin ligase; negative regulator of signaling	MF	Missense mutations in RING finger domain leading to loss of ubiquitin ligase activity Other *CBL* mutations in Proline rich domain no loss of ubiquitin ligase activity	MF (6%)	[69,70]
SOCS3	E3 ubiquitin ligase; negative regulator of signaling	PV	SH2 mutant F136L	PV (2.4% in a Japanese cohort)	[72]

upstream of the JH2 pseudokinase domain (see **Fig. 1**), and are thought to modify the conformation of this domain, leading to an increased basal activity of JAK2. Unlike JAK2V617F, exon 12 mutations have not been found in patients with ET or PMF. Expression of mutant K539L JAK2 in murine Ba/F3 cells expressing the EPO-R led to factor-independent growth. However, no growth was observed in the absence of EPO-R, indicating that these mutants also required the presence of homodimeric type-1 cytokine receptors to manifest their effect. In addition, in a murine retroviral BM transplantation (BMT) assay model of MPN overexpressing the K539L JAK2 exon 12 mutant, the resultant myeloproliferative phenotype was distinct from V617F, suggesting that different mutations in the same kinase can lead to distinct clinical phenotypes, presumably through subtle differences in signaling.[35]

MPL Mutations

Several laboratories working on Tpo signaling had previously reported that overexpression of Tpo causes myelofibrosis in mice.[37–40] In support of abnormal TPO-MPL signaling in MPN pathogenesis, gain-of-function somatic mutations in JAK2V617F-negative patients with PMF and ET have since been identified in *MPL*. No mutations have been documented in patients with PV.[41] The first mutation reported was substitution of tryptophan to leucine at position 515 (W515L).[42] The tryptophan is located in the cytoplasmic membrane proximal region of the receptor and is involved in repression of the receptor in the absence of ligand[43] and the transforming activity of the mutant receptor is also dependent on its cell surface localization.[44] Similarly to JAK2 mutants, expression of mutant MPL receptor leads to cytokine independent growth and hypersensitivity to Tpo in cell lines in vitro[42] and mouse BM engineered to overexpress the mutant receptor generated myelofibrosis with marked thrombocytosis in recipient mice after transplantation. Subsequently, other mutations targeting the same amino acid have been identified (see **Table 1**).[45–48]

LNK Mutations

LNK proteins have no intrinsic catalytic activity or transcriptional domain, but demonstrate the ability to integrate signaling events within the cell. Lnk belongs to the PSM family of adaptor proteins (proline-rich, pleckstrin homology [PH] domain and Src homology 2 [SH2] domain-containing partner of the insulin receptor) and has been demonstrated to negatively regulate signaling through the MPL and EPO receptors by reducing the duration of their response to cytokine stimulation.[49–51] On cytokine stimulation, LNK binds by its SH2 domain to phosphorylated JAK2, leading to attenuation of signaling.[49,50,52] LNK can also bind MPL by its SH2 domain and was found to be colocalized with MPL to the plasma membrane in transfected cell lines.[53] As might be expected, LNK levels were found to be high in CD34+ cells from patients with MPN and LNK expression was induced in vitro on overexpression of mutant JAK2. However, mutant JAK2 and MPL seem equally sensitive to negative regulation by LNK compared with their wild-type (WT) counterparts.[54,55] LNK mutations have recently been identified in patients with ET and PMF that were negative for JAK2V617F, JAK2 exon 12, and MPLW515 mutations.[56] Both mutations were located in exon 2 of LNK. One of the mutations led to loss of PH and SH2 domains, whereas the other was a point mutation in the PH domain (see **Table 1**). More recently, around 14 LNK mutations have been detected in patients with MPN.[56–58] These mutations are not restricted to the PH or SH2 domains, have also been found to co-occur in JAK2V617F-positive patients,[59–61] and may facilitate progression of the MPN, as suggested by their lower incidence in chronic-phase MPN (<10% mutated) and increasing incidence in accelerated and blast phase MPN.[58,59] In vitro experiments in Ba/F3 MPL-expressing cells demonstrated that the SH2 domain LNK mutant could not inhibit TPO-dependent growth of these cells in contrast to WT LNK. The PH domain mutant was intermediate and partially retained its inhibitory effect. In addition, in BMT assays Lnk deficiency led to an accelerated onset of myeloproliferative disease induced by JAK2V617F, indicating that WT LNK inhibits oncogenic JAK2 activity.[62] LNK$^{-/-}$ mice exhibit a subtle MPN phenotype in the absence of mutant JAK2 expression, with an enlarged stem cell compartment suggestive of the fact that LNK plays a role in pathogenesis of MPN.[51,63]

CBL Mutations

CBL is the cellular homolog of the v-Cbl oncogene, which is the transforming gene of Casitas B lymphoma murine retrovirus. CBL proteins have a multidomain structure with a unique amino terminal tyrosine kinase binding domain, a linker region, and a RING finger domain. The C terminus of CBL contains tyrosine residues, which on phosphorylation interact with SH2 domain proteins. It also contains Proline rich regions, which interact with SH3 domain proteins.[64] The main role of CBL proteins is as negative regulators of signaling by different tyrosine kinases (receptor and non-receptor). The mechanism of action is by their RING finger domain, which is an E3 ubiquitin ligase that targets activated tyrosine kinases for degradation by ubiquitination.[65–67] CBL can also target cytokine receptors, including MPL, for degradation.[68] In classical MPNs, CBL mutations were first detected in JAK2 mutation–negative patients with PMF with an acquired uniparental disomy of the 11q region, in which the CBL gene lies. The mutations were missense mutations involving the RING finger and linker regions that abrogated ubiquitin ligase activity and led to autonomous growth of 32D/FLT3 cells in vitro.[69] More recently, mutations have also been detected in JAK2V617F-positive MPNs. These involved the proline-rich region of CBL and would be predicted not to affect the ubiquitination activity of CBL. However, in vitro these mutations do lead to factor-independent growth, although the mechanisms remain unclear. Interestingly, CBL mutations are more frequent in PMF compared with ET and PV,[70] and similarly to LNK mutations, acquisition of mutations in CBL may be late events in MPN, potentially heralding their transformation to acute myeloid leukemia.

Suppressors of Cytokine Signaling Alterations

Suppressors of cytokine signaling (SOCS) proteins were initially described as inhibitory regulators of the JAK-STAT signaling pathway. The SOCS family consists of eight intracellular proteins that exert their negative feedback through several mechanisms. Among the SOCS family members, SOCS1 and SOCS3 compete with STAT proteins to bind to the JAK2 catalytic domain resulting in abrogation of downstream signaling. They can also bind by their SH2 domains to phospho-tyrosines on activated cytokine receptors (eg, EPO-R), thus preventing JAK2 association with the receptor. SOCS proteins are also components of the ubiquitin E3 ligase family and target their binding partners, including activated JAKs, for ubiquitination and degradation.[71] SOCS3 germline mutation (F316L) has been detected in a small cohort of Japanese patients and in a patient with a heterozygous JAK2 exon 12 mutation. The mutation impairs the degradation of the SOCS-JAK complex after ubiquitination. However, because the SOCS3 mutation is a relatively rare event, its role in disease pathogenesis is unclear.[72] In addition, other mechanisms that impair SOCS expression have been described, including hypermethylation of CpG islands near the promoters of SOCS1 and SOCS-3 in patients with MPN.[73–76] Furthermore, functional studies into the role of SOCS proteins in the regulation of WT and mutant JAK2 are somewhat conflicting. In particular, one study suggests an inability of SOCS3 to negatively regulate mutant JAK2 and a stabilization of SOCS3 by JAK2-mediated phosphorylation.[77,78] However, these findings were not corroborated in another study,[79] highlighting the complex role of SOCS proteins in modulating abnormal signaling within patients with MPN.

STUDIES OF CANONICAL SIGNALING PATHWAY INDUCTION DOWNSTREAM OF MPN MUTATIONS

Studies to elucidate aberrant signaling pathways in MPN have been performed in a variety of in vitro and in vivo model systems, including cell line models, murine models, and in primary patient BM and fractionated cell populations. The data are summarized next for each of these separate systems.

In Vitro Studies of Activated Signaling Pathways in Cell Lines

Oncogenic signaling activation downstream of mutant JAK2 kinases has been extensively studied in factor-dependent murine cell lines, including Ba/F3, 32D, and FDCP (often cotransduced with the EPO-R) after transduction with retroviruses expressing the mutant kinases. Western blot analysis has uniformly demonstrated autophosphorylation of JAK2 along with constitutive activation of STAT5, PI3K (assessed by phosphorylation of AKT), and MAP kinase pathway (assessed by phosphorylation of ERK) in the absence of any cytokine stimulation.[19,20,34,35] Addition of EPO and IL-3 further stimulated these pathways.[19,20] A recent study comparing signaling pathways in Ba/F3-EPOR cells showed subtle differences in downstream signaling between the JAK2 V617F and exon 12 mutants. In this report, the PI3 kinase pathway was not activated by either the V617F or K539L mutant. The tyrosine phosphatase Shp2 and its adaptor Gab2 were differentially activated by the mutants and the JAK2V617F mutant was shown to have a higher catalytic activity for a synthetic STAT5 substrate compared with the K539L mutant in an in vitro kinase assay.[80] These differences in signaling might explain subtle phenotypic differences in the PV associated with the different mutants.

Similarly, when MPL mutant W515L was overexpressed in 32D cells constitutive activation of JAK2, STAT5, STAT3, MAP-K, and PI3K pathway was observed in vitro. The cells became hyperresponsive to TPO stimulation and TYK2 associated with the MPL receptor was also found to be activated on TPO addition.[42]

Murine Models of MPN and Signaling Pathways Activated In Vivo

The first murine models for MPN were generated in retroviral transduction and transplantation assays of murine progenitors overexpressing the JAK2 V617F mutant. These models exhibited subtly different MPN phenotypes depending on the strain of mice used for the study,[81–84] although the predominant phenotype was of erythrocytosis, similar to PV. Depending on the level of overexpression and genetic background, myelofibrosis and occasionally thrombocytosis were also observed. BM, splenocytes, and PB granulocytes from diseased mice were further assessed for activation of signaling pathways using Western blotting or intracellular detection of phosphorylated signaling intermediates by flow cytometry (phospho-flow).[81–84] Similarly to Ba/F3 cell lines overexpressing JAK2 V617F, JAK2, STAT5, and MAPK/ERK pathway activation was detected. However, the PI3K pathway was not found to be consistently activated.[84] Similarly, MPLW515L overexpression in murine BMT model results in marked thrombocytosis, leukocytosis, and a more severe phenotype than the JAK2 mutant model, with the features of the disease more closely resembling human ET and PMF.[42] Signaling intermediates were assessed in splenocytes, CD11b, and CD61+ myeloid cells from these mice. All cells showed constitutive phosphorylation of STAT5 and STAT3 (STAT3 > STAT5) and myeloid cells were hypersensitive to G-CSF and TPO.[85]

However, the in vitro and in vivo experiments described previously have all been performed in systems where MPN mutant proteins are overexpressed and this may render them less relevant to the human disease. To address this concern, several mouse models have been generated that express JAK2V617F from the endogenous murine Jak2 promoter[86–89] (and for a comprehensive review see[90]). All except one developed a PV phenotype, with this model, where human rather than mouse JAK2V617F was expressed under the control of murine JAK2 promoter, recapitulating an ET-like phenotype. Signaling pathways were examined in whole BM[82]; the LSK compartment[89]; and erythroblasts derived from BM, spleen, or liver of knock-in mice. The basal activation status of STAT5 and MAPK/ERK pathways was shown to be enhanced in JAK2V617F-positive cells.[82,87] Moreover, gene dosage of JAK2 was shown to directly affect downstream signaling as activation of STAT5 and MAPK/ERK pathways was increased in homozygous compared with heterozygous erythroblasts and AKT phosphorylation was only evident in the homozygous state.[86] In addition, differentiation-specific effects of signaling mutants were suggested. No significant difference in STAT5 phosphorylation was detected even after stimulation with cytokines (EPO+IL3) in the LSK cells, whereas downstream progenitors (MEPs) demonstrated obvious hypersensitivity to cytokines.[89]

In vivo modeling has also allowed the use of genetic strategies to dissect abnormal signaling activation in the pathogenesis of MPN. To determine if STAT pathway activation is necessary for JAK2V617F mediated transformation, two groups recently tested the ability of JAK2 V617F to generate MPN in the absence of STAT5. Yan and colleagues[91] abrogated the entire in vivo MPN phenotype and in vitro EEC formation on crossing Stat5 a/b deficient (−/−) mice with a JAK2V617F knock-in mouse model. However, restoration of one intact Stat5 allele (+/−) allowed re-establishment of the entire MPN phenotype.[91] Other critical pathways were assessed through use of specific inhibitors and dominant negative isoforms in vitro. Although chemical inhibition of the AKT pathway and expression of a dominant negative STAT3 isoform impaired EEC formation to a lesser degree than Stat5 loss, inhibition of the ERK pathway had no effect.[91] Similar centrality for the Stat5 pathway in development of the MPN phenotype was reported by Walz and colleagues[92] who retrovirally overexpressed JAK2V617F in BM from the same strain of Stat5a/b-deficient mice and transplanted the cells into lethally irradiated recipients. Similarly, no PV-like phenotype was evident; however, over time substantial myelofibrosis developed in the mice with activation of the MAPK/ERK signaling pathway. Differences in the development of myelofibrosis between the knock-in and retroviral model may represent different dosages of JAK2 V617F or the modulation of transplantation on disease phenotype, but taken together these studies demonstrate the importance of STAT5 to the pathogenesis of the MPN. Given the drive to develop STAT5-specific inhibitors, this observation also has clinical implications.[93,94] In contrast to the importance of Stat5, Src kinases, which can also be activated by EPO stimulation, seem to be redundant for the generation of the MPN phenotype associated with JAK2 V617F. In similar experiments retrovirally expressing JAK2 V617F in BM deficient for *Hck*, *Fgr*, or *Lyn*, no differences were found for the development of JAK2V617F-induced polycythemia.[84]

Signaling Abnormalities in MPN Patient Samples

Model systems cannot accurately reflect the cellular context or molecular complexity of human MPN. Therefore, studies of signaling abnormalities have also been performed in unfractionated and fractionated human patient material using Western blotting, immunohistochemistry, and phospho-flow. Mesa and colleagues[95] aimed to correlate the JAK2 mutant allele burden with the phosphorylation status of downstream signaling intermediates in the neutrophils of patients with MF. Using Western blotting analysis they demonstrated that STAT3 was preferentially activated in mutant JAK2 neutrophils compared with patients with WT JAK2. However, STAT5, MAPK/ERK, and AKT phosphorylation were not detected in most samples. Schwemmers and colleagues[96] also performed Western blot analysis from granulocytes of patients with ET and found constitutive activation of the PI3 kinase and MAPK/ERK pathways, irrespective of JAK2 mutation status. However, only JAK2 mutant and not mutation-negative patients strongly activated the STAT3 pathway. A larger analysis in BM biopsies of 114 patients with MPN and controls was performed by immunohistochemistry.[97] Patients with PV exhibited high STAT3 and STAT5 phosphorylation; patients with ET exhibited high STAT3 but lower STAT5 phosphorylation, whereas patients with PMF were low in STAT3 and STAT5. However, there was no correlation of STAT phosphorylation with JAK2 mutation status suggesting that aberrant STAT activation might be common to all MPNs irrespective of underlying mutations. Grimwade and colleagues[98] also examined BM trephines of patients with MPN using monoclonal antibodies to phospho-STAT5 and phospho-AKT. In contrast to the previous study they found all MPNs with a JAK2V617F mutation to demonstrate increased phosphorylation of STAT5 and AKT in more than 60% of megakaryocytes. MPNs with a JAK2 exon 12 or MPL mutation did not demonstrate this increase. It is likely that the discrepancies reported in these studies represent heterogeneity in the patient populations studied and technical differences between the modalities used to analyze signaling.

Our group set out to perform a systematic analysis of signaling pathways in two differentiation-specific compartments in the BM of patients with MPN.[99] CD34$^+$ cells represent a population enriched for hematopoietic stem and progenitor cells, whereas CD34$^-$ cells consist mainly of differentiating myeloid cells. To allow for systematic analysis of the small numbers of CD34$^+$ cells, we developed a phospho-flow cytometry assay to measure basal activation of signaling pathways in a limited number of MPN BM cells and compared these with the same phenotypic population in normal controls. Our studies revealed that only basal activation of the MAPK/ERK pathway was significantly increased in CD34$^+$ cells of patients with ET and patients with MF. However, in the more differentiated CD34$^-$ cells, STAT5 was activated in all MPNs compared with control subjects. When comparing specific disease phenotypes, patients with PV demonstrated higher levels of STAT5 activation compared with patients with ET and patients with MF showed higher STAT3 activation compared with patients with PV. However, we did not detect any MAPK/ERK and PI3K pathway activation in differentiated MPN cells. As previously, we found no correlation between JAK2 mutant allele burden and activation of signaling. Interestingly, certain signaling pathways (eg, ERK/MAPK and STAT3) actually seemed to be further activated in the JAK2-negative compared with JAK2-mutant patients with MPN. This might be caused by the presence of other signaling mutations in these cases and those different mutations or combinations of mutations may modulate signaling pathways in subtly different ways. We also assessed signaling after stimulation with EPO and were unable to increment signaling further in MPN CD34$^-$ or GPA$^+$ erythroid progenitor cells.[99] It might be that these cells are in a state of maximal signaling downstream of the EPO-R either from trace levels of endogenous cytokines or because of true cytokine independence. Further studies are required to differentiate between these possibilities.

A different approach, using downstream transcriptional correlates of signaling pathways, was adopted by Chen and colleagues[100] to identify signaling differences between ET and PV. They grew individual erythroid colonies from the PB of JAK2V617F-positive patients with PV and ET in methylcellulose supplemented with low concentrations of EPO. Colonies were pooled according to genotype (WT or mutant) and were then analyzed for differential gene expression by microarray. They found that ET JAK2 V617F colonies exhibited an interferon (IFN)-γ signaling signature, whereas patients with PV lacked this signature. In addition, this signature was associated with an increased level of phospho-STAT1 (as measured by both phospho-flow and immunoflourescence) in ET by comparison with patients with PV. The authors proposed that increased signaling by the IFN-γ pathway leads to megakaryopoiesis, whereas the absence of this signaling pathway in PV promotes erythropoiesis.

However, it remains to be determined if JAK2 WT patients with ET also have altered STAT1 signaling.[100]

NONCANONICAL JAK2 SIGNALING IN MPN: SIGNALING TO CHROMATIN

Initial evidence of JAK signaling to chromatin was first obtained in *Drosophila melanogaster*, where overactivation of the single JAK homolog Hopscotch (*hop*) was shown to disrupt heterochromatin gene silencing. This occurred through the dissociation of heterochromatin protein (HP) 1 from chromatin, leading to a reduction in H3 lysine9 dimethylation (H3K9me2), gene activation, and the development of hematopoietic tumors in *Drosophila* expressing a mutant *hop* (*hop*$^{Tum-l}$).[101] A recent study further demonstrated that JAK2 is present in the nucleus in human hematopoietic cells, where it directly phosphorylates histone H3 at tyrosine 41 (H3Y41ph). This phosphorylation prevents binding of HP1α to histone H3.[102] HP1α is known to repress the transcription of heterochromatin genes and its loss can lead to gene activation at specific loci.[103] Inhibition of mutant JAK2 signaling in the HEL cell line, using JAK2-specific inhibitors, led to increased binding of HP1α to chromatin without any effects on the levels of H3K9me3. One of the genes most downregulated by inhibition of JAK2 was the transcription factor *Imo2*, a gene critical for normal hematopoietic development. Downregulation of expression at this locus was associated with an increased binding of HP1α and a reciprocal decrease in phosphorylation of H3Y41 and H3K4me3 at the *Imo2* transcriptional start site. This led the authors to postulate that mutant JAK2 signaling may increase the expression of oncogenes, including but not limited to Imo2, leading to the development of the disease phenotype[102] (**Fig. 3**).

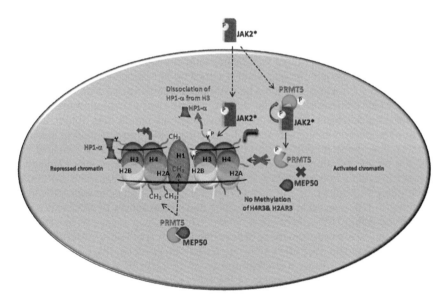

Fig. 3. Signaling to chromatin by mutant-JAK2. JAK2 is present in the nucleus in human hematopoietic cells, where it directly phosphorylates histone H3 (*orange*) at tyrosine 41 (H3Y41ph). This phosphorylation prevents binding of HP1α (*dark blue*) to histone H3. HP1α is known to repress the transcription of heterochromatin genes and its loss can lead to gene activation at specific loci. Mutant JAK2 (JAK2*) phosphorylates PRMT5 and disrupts its methylase activity and binding to MEP50, both of which have been predicted to lead to aberrant gene activation. For further explanation, please see text.

However, the consequences of H3Y41ph by WT-JAK2 for normal cell proliferation are not yet known.

Another potential epigenetic mechanism whereby mutant JAK2 can directly alter transcription is described by Liu and colleagues[104] who demonstrated an interaction between mutant JAK2 and the protein arginine methyltransferase 5 (PRMT5). PRMT5 mediates methylation of histone H4 arginine 3(H4R3me2), which in turn recruits the DNA methyltransferase DNMT3A to chromatin, with subsequent DNA methylation leading to gene silencing.[105] PRMT5 also binds to methylosome protein 50 (MEP50), forming a crucial component of the large 20S "methylosome" involved in methylating histones H2A, H3, and H4. Initial coimmunoprecipitation experiments in transfected cell lines demonstrated preferential binding of PRMT5 to mutant JAK2 by comparison with WT-JAK2, and these were confirmed with endogenous proteins in HEL cells. Phosphorylation of PRMT5 by JAK2 was found to disrupt its methylase activity and its binding to MEP50, both of which would be predicted to lead to aberrant gene activation (see **Fig. 3**).[104] In addition, knock-down of PRMT5 in human CD34$^+$ cells, resulted in an increase in erythroid colony formation in defined media.[104] However, the true contribution of PRMT5 to JAK2 mutant MPN pathogenesis is unclear, because phosphorylation of PRMT5 can occur in normal CD34$^+$ and cells from JAK2 WT and mutant patients with MPN. Moreover, mutations in other genes involved in epigenetic regulation have also been identified in MPNs. These include TET2, IDH1/2, EZH2, ASXL1, and DNMT3A. For an overview of the mutations in these genes and potential mechanisms for their effect on hematopoiesis, refer to articles elsewhere in this issue. Validation of these mechanisms and how dysregulation of epigenetic control may relate to alterations in "classical" signaling pathways remains to be seen.

ROLE OF THE MICROENVIRONMENT: SIGNALING INDUCTION BY SECRETED CYTOKINES IN MPN

The role of the microenvironment in MPN has long been appreciated. Indeed, myelofibrosis is a cell-nonautonomous, reactive condition in response to the secretion of proinflammatory cytokines, including hematopoietic cell-derived transforming growth factor-β1, which induces BM fibrosis, and stromal cell–derived osteoprotegerin, which promotes osteosclerosis.[106] Accumulating evidence also implicates autocrine/paracrine or microenvironmental secretion of cytokines in the dysregulation of signaling, facilitating the development of the MPN phenotype. In JAK2V617F patients with MPN, the proinflammatory cytokine tumor necrosis factor (TNF)-α was found to be increased in plasma from patients with MPN and to directly correlate with JAK2V617F allele burden.[107] Addition of JAK inhibitors to PB MNCs of patients with MPN led to a reduction in TNF-α levels in vitro, suggesting that kinase activity of JAK2 was essential for upregulating TNF-α. In addition, when colony-forming assays were performed on CD34$^+$ and MNCs in the presence of low concentrations of TNF-α, JAK2V617F cells demonstrated a proliferative advantage compared with WT cells. This observation was further confirmed by retroviral overexpression of JAK2V617F in a TNF-α null background, which led to an amelioration of the MPN phenotype. The authors therefore proposed that the acquisition of JAK2V617F not only leads to an increased production of TNF-α, but also provides the mutant cells with a proliferative advantage in limiting concentrations of the cytokine.[107] However, although these observations are interesting and noteworthy, it is still unclear how JAK2V617F upregulates TNF-α and how those cells become sensitized to the growth-promoting effects of TNF-α. Furthermore, other inflammatory cytokines, including oncostatin-M, have also been shown to be secreted by JAK2V617F myeloid cells, which then stimulated growth of fibroblasts and endothelial cells in BM and induced the production of angiogenic cytokines.[108] Finally, microenvironmental cues from BM stroma secreted cytokines including IL6, fibroblast growth factor, and chemokine C-X-C motif ligand 10/IFN-γ–inducible 10-kD protein (IP-10) have also been found to provide a survival advantage to JAK2V617F cells in vitro when tested in the presence of the JAK2 inhibitor atipro-mid.[109] Taken together, these studies indicate that humoral cytokines play an impor-tant role in disease development and might sustain the JAK2 mutant cells and potentially protect them from the effects of JAK inhibitors by stimulating prosurvival signaling through alternate pathways.

THERAPEUTIC IMPLICATIONS: INHIBITING SIGNALING IN MPN

The JAK-STAT and potentially other signaling pathways have emerged as attractive therapeutic targets because of the high incidence of JAK2 mutations in patients with MPN and the demonstration of activation of similar pathways even in patients who lack a JAK2 mutation. The clinical implications for disordered signaling in MPN and therapeutic experience with JAK2 selective inhibitors are not dealt with here but are covered in depth elsewhere in this issue.

SUMMARY

Human MPN are defined by abnormal signaling patterns and these signaling pathways are central to the development of these diseases. The studies conducted so far suggest that multiple signaling pathways are upregulated, with many linked to specific recurrent mutations. Although the data suggest the induction of common signaling pathways, emerging evidence also suggests that specific signaling pathways or combinations of signaling abnormalities may dictate the phenotypic differences among MPN subtypes. Further delineating these signaling pathways and how they might differ from homeostatic signaling pathways in normal hematopoietic stem and progenitor populations will greatly inform knowledge of MPN and allow clinicians to more safely target signaling for therapeutic gain.

REFERENCES

1. Dameshek W. Some speculations on the myeloproliferative syndromes. Blood 1951;6:372–5.
2. Campbell PJ, Green AR. The myeloproliferative disorders. N Engl J Med 2006; 355:2452–66.
3. Levine RL, Pardanani A, Tefferi A, et al. Role of JAK2 in the pathogenesis and therapy of myeloproliferative disorders. Nat Rev Cancer 2007;7:673–83.
4. Prchal JF, Axelrad AA. Letter: bone-marrow responses in polycythemia vera. N Engl J Med 1974;290:1382.
5. Casadevall N, Vainchenker W, Lacombe C, et al. Erythroid progenitors in poly-cythemia vera: demonstration of their hypersensitivity to erythropoietin using serum free cultures. Blood 1982;59:447–51.
6. Cashman J, Henkelman D, Humphries K, et al. Individual BFU-E in polycythemia vera produce both erythropoietin dependent and independent progeny. Blood 1983;61:876–84.
7. Eaves CJ, Eaves AC. Erythropoietin (Ep) dose-response curves for three classes of erythroid progenitors in normal human marrow and in patients with polycythemia vera. Blood 1978;52:1196–210.

8. Fisher MJ, Prchal JF, Prchal JT, et al. Anti-erythropoietin (EPO) receptor mono-clonal antibodies distinguish EPO-dependent and EPO-independent erythroid progenitors in polycythemia vera. Blood 1994;84:1982–91.

9. Zanjani ED, Lutton JD, Hoffman R, et al. Erythroid colony formation by polycy-themia vera bone marrow in vitro. Dependence on erythropoietin. J Clin Invest 1977;59:841–8.

10. Correa PN, Eskinazi D, Axelrad AA. Circulating erythroid progenitors in polycy-themia vera are hypersensitive to insulin-like growth factor-1 in vitro: studies in an improved serum-free medium. Blood 1994;83:99–112.

11. Dai CH, Krantz SB, Dessypris EN, et al. Polycythemia vera. II. Hypersensitivity of bone marrow erythroid, granulocyte-macrophage, and megakaryocyte progen-itor cells to interleukin-3 and granulocyte-macrophage colony-stimulating factor. Blood 1992;80:891–9.

12. Dai CH, Krantz SB, Green WF, et al. Polycythaemia vera. III. Burst-forming units-erythroid (BFU-E) response to stem cell factor and c-kit receptor expression. Br J Haematol 1994;86:12–21.

13. Dai CH, Krantz SB, Means RT Jr, et al. Polycythemia vera blood burst-forming units-erythroid are hypersensitive to interleukin-3. J Clin Invest 1991;87:391–6.

14. Emanuel PD, Eaves CJ, Broudy VC, et al. Familial and congenital polycythemia in three unrelated families. Blood 1992;79:3019–30.

15. Means RT Jr, Krantz SB, Sawyer ST, et al. Erythropoietin receptors in polycy-themia vera. J Clin Invest 1989;84:1340–4.

16. Hess G, Rose P, Gamm H, et al. Molecular analysis of the erythropoietin receptor system in patients with polycythaemia vera. Br J Haematol 1994;88:794–802.

17. Le Couedic JP, Mitjavila MT, Villeval JL, et al. Missense mutation of the erythro-poietin receptor is a rare event in human erythroid malignancies. Blood 1996;87: 1502–11.

18. Baxter EJ, Scott LM, Campbell PJ, et al. Acquired mutation of the tyrosine kinase JAK2 in human myeloproliferative disorders. Lancet 2005;365:1054–61.

19. James C, Ugo V, Le Couedic JP, et al. A unique clonal JAK2 mutation leading to constitutive signalling causes polycythaemia vera. Nature 2005;434:1144–8.

20. Kralovics R, Passamonti F, Buser AS, et al. A gain-of-function mutation of JAK2 in myeloproliferative disorders. N Engl J Med 2005;352:1779–90.

21. Levine RL, Wadleigh M, Cools J, et al. Activating mutation in the tyrosine kinase JAK2 in polycythemia vera, essential thrombocythemia, and myeloid metaplasia with myelofibrosis. Cancer Cell 2005;7:387–97.

22. Rane SG, Reddy EP. Janus kinases: components of multiple signaling path-ways. Oncogene 2000;19:5662–79.

23. Rane SG, Reddy EP. JAKs, STATs and Src kinases in hematopoiesis. Oncogene 2002;21:3334–58.

24. Feener EP, Rosario F, Dunn SL, et al. Tyrosine phosphorylation of Jak2 in the JH2 domain inhibits cytokine signaling. Mol Cell Biol 2004;24:4968–78.

25. Saharinen P, Silvennoinen O. The pseudokinase domain is required for suppression of basal activity of Jak2 and Jak3 tyrosine kinases and for cytokine-inducible activation of signal transduction. J Biol Chem 2002;277: 47954–63.

26. Ungureanu D, Wu J, Pekkala T, et al. The pseudokinase domain of JAK2 is a dual-specificity protein kinase that negatively regulates cytokine signaling. Nat Struct Mol Biol 2011;18:971–6.

27. Baker SJ, Rane SG, Reddy EP. Hematopoietic cytokine receptor signaling. Oncogene 2007;26:6724–37.

28. Huang LJ, Constantinescu SN, Lodish HF. The N-terminal domain of Janus kinase 2 is required for Golgi processing and cell surface expression of erythropoietin receptor. Mol Cell 2001;8:1327–38.

29. Royer Y, Staerk J, Costuleanu M, et al. Janus kinases affect thrombopoietin receptor cell surface localization and stability. J Biol Chem 2005;280:27251–61.

30. Darnell JE Jr, Kerr IM, Stark GR. Jak-STAT pathways and transcriptional activation in response to IFNs and other extracellular signaling proteins. Science 1994;264:1415–21.

31. Ihle JN. The Janus protein tyrosine kinases in hematopoietic cytokine signaling. Semin Immunol 1995;7:247–54.

32. Zhao R, Xing S, Li Z, et al. Identification of an acquired JAK2 mutation in polycythemia vera. J Biol Chem 2005;280:22788–92.

33. Lu X, Huang LJ, Lodish HF. Dimerization by a cytokine receptor is necessary for constitutive activation of JAK2V617F. J Biol Chem 2008;283:5258–66.

34. Lu X, Levine R, Tong W, et al. Expression of a homodimeric type I cytokine receptor is required for JAK2V617F-mediated transformation. Proc Natl Acad Sci U S A 2005;102:18962–7.

35. Scott LM, Tong W, Levine RL, et al. JAK2 exon 12 mutations in polycythemia vera and idiopathic erythrocytosis. N Engl J Med 2007;356:459–68.

36. Scott LM. The JAK2 exon 12 mutations: a comprehensive review. Am J Hematol 2011;86:668–76.

37. Villeval JL, Cohen-Solal K, Tulliez M, et al. High thrombopoietin production by hematopoietic cells induces a fatal myeloproliferative syndrome in mice. Blood 1997;90:4369–83.

38. Yan XQ, Lacey D, Fletcher F, et al. Chronic exposure to retroviral vector encoded MGDF (mpl-ligand) induces lineage-specific growth and differentiation of megakaryocytes in mice. Blood 1995;86:4025–33.

39. Yan XQ, Lacey D, Hill D, et al. A model of myelofibrosis and osteosclerosis in mice induced by overexpressing thrombopoietin (mpl ligand): reversal of disease by bone marrow transplantation. Blood 1996;88:402–9.

40. Yanagida M, Ide Y, Imai A, et al. The role of transforming growth factor-beta in PEG-rHuMGDF-induced reversible myelofibrosis in rats. Br J Haematol 1997; 99:739–45.

41. Pietra D, Brisci A, Rumi E, et al. Deep sequencing reveals double mutations in cis of MPL exon 10 in myeloproliferative neoplasms. Haematologica 2011;96:607–11.

42. Pikman Y, Lee BH, Mercher T, et al. MPLW515L is a novel somatic activating mutation in myelofibrosis with myeloid metaplasia. PLoS Med 2006;3:e270.

43. Staerk J, Lacout C, Sato T, et al. An amphipathic motif at the transmembrane-cytoplasmic junction prevents autonomous activation of the thrombopoietin receptor. Blood 2006;107:1864–71.

44. Marty C, Chaligne R, Lacout C, et al. Ligand-independent thrombopoietin mutant receptor requires cell surface localization for endogenous activity. J Biol Chem 2009;284:11781–91.

45. Beer PA, Campbell PJ, Scott LM, et al. MPL mutations in myeloproliferative disorders: analysis of the PT-1 cohort. Blood 2008;112:141–9.

46. Boyd EM, Bench AJ, Goday-Fernandez A, et al. Clinical utility of routine MPL exon 10 analysis in the diagnosis of essential thrombocythaemia and primary myelofibrosis. Br J Haematol 2010;149:250–7.

47. Chaligne R, Tonetti C, Besancenot R, et al. New mutations of MPL in primitive myelofibrosis: only the MPL W515 mutations promote a G1/S-phase transition. Leukemia 2008;22:1557–66.

48. Pardanani AD, Levine RL, Lasho T, et al. MPL515 mutations in myeloproliferative and other myeloid disorders: a study of 1182 patients. Blood 2006;108: 3472–6.

49. Tong W, Lodish HF. Lnk inhibits Tpo-mpl signaling and Tpo-mediated megakaryocytopoiesis. J Exp Med 2004;200:569–80.

50. Tong W, Zhang J, Lodish HF. Lnk inhibits erythropoiesis and Epo-dependent JAK2 activation and downstream signaling pathways. Blood 2005;105: 4604–12.

51. Velazquez L, Cheng AM, Fleming HE, et al. Cytokine signaling and hematopoietic homeostasis are disrupted in Lnk-deficient mice. J Exp Med 2002;195: 1599–611.

52. Bersenev A, Wu C, Balcerek J, et al. Lnk controls mouse hematopoietic stem cell self-renewal and quiescence through direct interactions with JAK2. J Clin Invest 2008;118:2832–44.

53. Gery S, Gueller S, Chumakova K, et al. Adaptor protein Lnk negatively regulates the mutant MPL, MPLW515L associated with myeloproliferative disorders. Blood 2007;110:3360–4.

54. Baran-Marszak F, Magdoud H, Desterke C, et al. Expression level and differential JAK2-V617F-binding of the adaptor protein Lnk regulates JAK2-mediated signals in myeloproliferative neoplasms. Blood 2010;116:5961–71.

55. Gery S, Cao Q, Gueller S, et al. Lnk inhibits myeloproliferative disorder-associated JAK2 mutant, JAK2V617F. J Leukoc Biol 2009;85:957–65.

56. Oh ST, Simonds EF, Jones C, et al. Novel mutations in the inhibitory adaptor protein LNK drive JAK-STAT signaling in patients with myeloproliferative neoplasms. Blood 2010;116:988–92.

57. Lasho TL, Pardanani A, Tefferi A. LNK mutations in JAK2 mutation-negative erythrocytosis. N Engl J Med 2010;363:1189–90.

58. Pardanani A, Lasho T, Finke C, et al. LNK mutation studies in blast-phase myeloproliferative neoplasms, and in chronic-phase disease with TET2, IDH, JAK2 or MPL mutations. Leukemia 2010;24:1713–8.

59. Ha JS, Jeon DS. Possible new LNK mutations in myeloproliferative neoplasms. Am J Hematol 2011;86:866–8.

60. Hurtado C, Erquiaga I, Aranaz P, et al. LNK can also be mutated outside PH and SH2 domains in myeloproliferative neoplasms with and without V617FJAK2 mutation. Leuk Res 2011;35:1537–9.

61. Lasho TL, Tefferi A, Finke C, et al. Clonal hierarchy and allelic mutation segregation in a myelofibrosis patient with two distinct LNK mutations. Leukemia 2011; 25:1056–8.

62. Bersenev A, Wu C, Balcerek J, et al. Lnk constrains myeloproliferative diseases in mice. J Clin Invest 2010;120:2058–69.

63. Takaki S, Morita H, Tezuka Y, et al. Enhanced hematopoiesis by hematopoietic progenitor cells lacking intracellular adaptor protein, Lnk. J Exp Med 2002; 195:151–60.

64. Kales SC, Ryan PE, Nau MM, et al. Cbl and human myeloid neoplasms: the Cbl oncogene comes of age. Cancer Res 2010;70:4789–94.

65. Joazeiro CA, Wing SS, Huang H, et al. The tyrosine kinase negative regulator c-Cbl as a RING-type, E2-dependent ubiquitin-protein ligase. Science 1999;286: 309–12.

66. Levkowitz G, Waterman H, Ettenberg SA, et al. Ubiquitin ligase activity and tyrosine phosphorylation underlie suppression of growth factor signaling by c-Cbl/ Sli-1. Mol Cell 1999;4:1029–40.

67. Yokouchi M, Kondo T, Houghton A, et al. Ligand-induced ubiquitination of the epidermal growth factor receptor involves the interaction of the c-Cbl RING finger and UbcH7. J Biol Chem 1999;274:31707–12.

68. Saur SJ, Sangkhae V, Geddis AE, et al. Ubiquitination and degradation of the thrombopoietin receptor c-Mpl. Blood 2010;115:1254–63.

69. Grand FH, Hidalgo-Curtis CE, Ernst T, et al. Frequent CBL mutations associated with 11q acquired uniparental disomy in myeloproliferative neoplasms. Blood 2009;113:6182–92.

70. Aranaz P, Hurtado C, Erquiaga I, et al. CBL mutations in myeloproliferative neoplasms are also found in its proline-rich domain and in patients with the V617FJAK2. Haematologica 2012;97(8):1234–41.

71. Dimitriou ID, Clemenza L, Scotter AJ, et al. Putting out the fire: coordinated suppression of the innate and adaptive immune systems by SOCS1 and SOCS3 proteins. Immunol Rev 2008;224:265–83.

72. Suessmuth Y, Elliott J, Percy MJ, et al. A new polycythaemia vera-associated SOCS3 SH2 mutant (SOCS3F136L) cannot regulate erythropoietin responses. Br J Haematol 2009;147:450–8.

73. Jost E, do ON, Dahl E, et al. Epigenetic alterations complement mutation of JAK2 tyrosine kinase in patients with BCR/ABL-negative myeloproliferative disorders. Leukemia 2007;21:505–10.

74. Teofili L, Martini M, Cenci T, et al. Epigenetic alteration of SOCS family members is a possible pathogenetic mechanism in JAK2 wild type myeloproliferative diseases. Int J Cancer 2008;123:1586–92.

75. Capello D, Deambrogi C, Rossi D, et al. Epigenetic inactivation of suppressors of cytokine signalling in Philadelphia-negative chronic myeloproliferative disorders. Br J Haematol 2008;141:504–11.

76. Chaligne R, Tonetti C, Besancenot R, et al. SOCS3 inhibits TPO-stimulated, but not spontaneous, megakaryocytic growth in primary myelofibrosis. Leukemia 2009;23:1186–90.

77. Elliott J, Suessmuth Y, Scott LM, et al. SOCS3 tyrosine phosphorylation as a potential bio-marker for myeloproliferative neoplasms associated with mutant JAK2 kinases. Haematologica 2009;94:576–80.

78. Hookham MB, Elliott J, Suessmuth Y, et al. The myeloproliferative disorder-associated JAK2 V617F mutant escapes negative regulation by suppressor of cytokine signaling 3. Blood 2007;109:4924–9.

79. Haan S, Wuller S, Kaczor J, et al. SOCS-mediated downregulation of mutant Jak2 (V617F, T875N and K539L) counteracts cytokine-independent signaling. Oncogene 2009;28:3069–80.

80. Zou H, Yan D, Mohi G. Differential biological activity of disease-associated JAK2 mutants. FEBS Lett 2011;585:1007–13.

81. Bumm TG, Elsea C, Corbin AS, et al. Characterization of murine JAK2V617F-positive myeloproliferative disease. Cancer Res 2006;66:11156–65.

82. Lacout C, Pisani DF, Tulliez M, et al. JAK2V617F expression in murine hematopoietic cells leads to MPD mimicking human PV with secondary myelofibrosis. Blood 2006;108:1652–60.

83. Wernig G, Mercher T, Okabe R, et al. Expression of Jak2V617F causes a polycythemia vera-like disease with associated myelofibrosis in a murine bone marrow transplant model. Blood 2006;107:4274–81.

84. Zaleskas VM, Krause DS, Lazarides K, et al. Molecular pathogenesis and therapy of polycythemia induced in mice by JAK2 V617F. PLoS One 2006; 1:e18.

85. Koppikar P, Abdel-Wahab O, Hedvat C, et al. Efficacy of the JAK2 inhibitor INCB16562 in a murine model of MPLW515L-induced thrombocytosis and myelofibrosis. Blood 2010;115:2919–27.

86. Akada H, Yan D, Zou H, et al. Conditional expression of heterozygous or homozygous Jak2V617F from its endogenous promoter induces a polycythemia vera-like disease. Blood 2010;115:3589–97.

87. Li J, Spensberger D, Ahn JS, et al. JAK2 V617F impairs hematopoietic stem cell function in a conditional knock-in mouse model of JAK2 V617F-positive essential thrombocythemia. Blood 2010;116:1528–38.

88. Marty C, Lacout C, Martin A, et al. Myeloproliferative neoplasm induced by constitutive expression of JAK2V617F in knock-in mice. Blood 2010;116:783–7.

89. Mullally A, Lane SW, Ball B, et al. Physiological Jak2V617F expression causes a lethal myeloproliferative neoplasm with differential effects on hematopoietic stem and progenitor cells. Cancer Cell 2010;17:584–96.

90. Li J, Kent DG, Chen E, et al. Mouse models of myeloproliferative neoplasms: JAK of all grades. Dis Model Mech 2011;4:311–7.

91. Yan D, Hutchison RE, Mohi G. Critical requirement for Stat5 in a mouse model of polycythemia vera. Blood 2012;119(15):3539–49.

92. Walz C, Ahmed W, Lazarides K, et al. Essential role for Stat5a/b in myeloproliferative neoplasms induced by BCR-ABL1 and Jak2V617F in mice. Blood 2012;119(15):3550–60.

93. Nelson EA, Walker SR, Weisberg E, et al. The STAT5 inhibitor pimozide decreases survival of chronic myelogenous leukemia cells resistant to kinase inhibitors. Blood 2011;117:3421–9.

94. Shah NP, Shannon K. Advancing the STATus of MPN pathogenesis. Blood 2012;119:3374–6.

95. Mesa RA, Tefferi A, Lasho TS, et al. Janus kinase 2 (V617F) mutation status, signal transducer and activator of transcription-3 phosphorylation and impaired neutrophil apoptosis in myelofibrosis with myeloid metaplasia. Leukemia 2006;20:1800–8.

96. Schwemmers S, Will B, Waller CF, et al. JAK2V617F-negative ET patients do not display constitutively active JAK/STAT signaling. Exp Hematol 2007;35:1695–703.

97. Teofili L, Martini M, Cenci T, et al. Different STAT-3 and STAT-5 phosphorylation discriminates among Ph-negative chronic myeloproliferative diseases and is independent of the V617F JAK-2 mutation. Blood 2007;110:354–9.

98. Grimwade LF, Happerfield L, Tristram C, et al. Phospho-STAT5 and phospho-Akt expression in chronic myeloproliferative neoplasms. Br J Haematol 2009;147:495–506.

99. Anand S, Stedham F, Gudgin E, et al. Increased basal intracellular signaling patterns do not correlate with JAK2 genotype in human myeloproliferative neoplasms. Blood 2011;118:1610–21.

100. Chen E, Beer PA, Godfrey AL, et al. Distinct clinical phenotypes associated with JAK2V617F reflect differential STAT1 signaling. Cancer Cell 2010;18:524–35.

101. Shi S, Calhoun HC, Xia F, et al. JAK signaling globally counteracts heterochromatic gene silencing. Nat Genet 2006;38:1071–6.

102. Dawson MA, Bannister AJ, Gottgens B, et al. JAK2 phosphorylates histone H3Y41 and excludes HP1alpha from chromatin. Nature 2009;461:819–22.

103. Panteleeva I, Boutillier S, See V, et al. HP1alpha guides neuronal fate by timing E2F-targeted genes silencing during terminal differentiation. EMBO J 2007;26:3616–28.

104. Liu F, Zhao X, Perna F, et al. JAK2V617F-mediated phosphorylation of PRMT5 downregulates its methyltransferase activity and promotes myeloproliferation. Cancer Cell 2011;19:283–94.
105. Zhao Q, Rank G, Tan YT, et al. PRMT5-mediated methylation of histone H4R3 recruits DNMT3A, coupling histone and DNA methylation in gene silencing. Nat Struct Mol Biol 2009;16:304–11.
106. Tefferi A. Pathogenesis of myelofibrosis with myeloid metaplasia. J Clin Oncol 2005;23:8520–30.
107. Fleischman AG, Aichberger KJ, Luty SB, et al. TNFalpha facilitates clonal expansion of JAK2V617F positive cells in myeloproliferative neoplasms. Blood 2011;118:6392–8.
108. Hoermann G, Cerny-Reiterer S, Herrmann H, et al. Identification of oncostatin M as a JAK2 V617F-dependent amplifier of cytokine production and bone marrow remodeling in myeloproliferative neoplasms. FASEB J 2012;26:894–906.
109. Manshouri T, Estrov Z, Quintas-Cardama A, et al. Bone marrow stroma-secreted cytokines protect JAK2(V617F)-mutated cells from the effects of a JAK2 inhibitor. Cancer Res 2011;71:3831–40.

Role of Germline Genetic Factors in MPN Pathogenesis

Ashot S. Harutyunyan, MD[a], Robert Kralovics, PhD[a,b,*]

KEYWORDS

- Myeloproliferative neoplasms • Hereditary predisposition • Familial clustering
- *JAK2* haplotype • Germline variants • Penetrance

KEY POINTS

- Myeloproliferative neoplasms (MPNs) are mainly driven by somatically acquired point mutations and chromosomal aberrations.
- Germline factors can predispose to the development of MPN, acquisition of somatic mutations, and chromosomal aberrations, as well as modify the clinical course of the disease.
- Familial clustering of MPN in 5% to 10% of cases, increased risk of the disease in relatives of patients with MPN, and the existence of biclonal MPN provide evidence of germline MPN susceptibility.
- Hereditary thrombocytosis and erythrocytosis have similar clinical symptoms as MPN; however, these disorders show distinct features, such as polyclonal hematopoiesis, single lineage involvement, and absence of disease progression.
- Germline mutations in *JAK2*, *MPL*, and *THPO* cause hereditary thrombocytosis, whereas germline mutations in *EPOR*, oxygen-sensing pathway genes, or genes affecting oxygen affinity of hemoglobin result in hereditary erythrocytosis.
- The common *JAK2* GGCC haplotype predisposes to the development of JAK2-postive MPN.
- A nonsynonymous germline variant in the *ERCC2* (*XPD*) gene increases the risk of leukemic transformation and the development of new primary tumors in patients with MPN.
- Rare germline variants in the regions of loss of heterozygosity can have an influence on MPN pathogenesis.
- The germline mutations responsible for the familial cases of MPN have not been identified so far.

INTRODUCTION

Myeloproliferative neoplasms (MPNs) are chronic hematological malignancies of clonal origin characterized by the predominant involvement of myeloid lineages, accumulation of terminally differentiated blood cells, and the tendency to transform to

[a] CeMM Research Center for Molecular Medicine of the Austrian Academy of Sciences, Lazarettgasse 14, BT25.3, Vienna 1090, Austria; [b] Department of Internal Medicine I, Division of Hematology and Blood Coagulation, Medical University of Vienna, Währinger Gurtel 18-20, Vienna 1090, Austria
* Corresponding author. CeMM Research Center for Molecular Medicine of the Austrian Academy of Sciences, Lazarettgasse 14, BT25.3, Vienna 1090, Austria.
E-mail address: robert.kralovics@cemm.oeaw.ac.at

Hematol Oncol Clin N Am 26 (2012) 1037–1051
http://dx.doi.org/10.1016/j.hoc.2012.07.005
0889-8588/12/$ – see front matter © 2012 Elsevier Inc. All rights reserved.

secondary acute myeloid leukemia (sAML). MPNs are a heterogeneous group of disorders and include 9 disease entities according to the 2008 World Health Organization classification.[1] The classic MPN or Ph-chromosome-negative MPN include polycythemia vera (PV), essential thrombocythemia (ET), and primary myelofibrosis (PMF). The MPN disease subtypes exhibit specific phenotypic features but share many clinical and molecular features.[2] MPNs are characterized by high numbers of differentiated cells of myeloid origin in peripheral blood, mainly red blood cells in PV or platelets in ET. Patients with PMF usually have a lower number of myeloid cells as a result of bone marrow fibrosis, and consequent extramedullary hematopoiesis often manifests with splenomegaly. PV and ET may progress into secondary myelofibrosis, which has a similar clinical presentation as PMF but a much higher rate of transformation to sAML.[3] Patients with MPN frequently have thrombotic or hemorrhagic complications; in some cases those complications are the first presentations of the disease.[2] Typically, MPNs are diseases of the elderly; the age of onset is around 50 to 60 years, although cases in younger ages are also observed, especially in the presence of familial history.[4] The life expectancy of patients with PV and ET is more than a decade. In PMF, the life expectancy is 3 to 5 years on average, whereas after the transformation to sAML, the median survival is a few months with no effective treatment available.[5] The treatment in MPN is directed toward controlling the symptoms and the progression of the disease; it proves to be enough in most cases.[6]

ROLE OF SOMATIC MUTATIONS IN MPN

Acquired genetic changes drive clonal progression in MPN, as in other cancers. Several recurrent chromosomal aberrations and point mutations have been identified in the pathogenesis of MPN, with variable frequency in PV, ET, and PMF. The most common somatic mutation in MPN is the V617F mutation in the Janus kinase 2 (JAK2) gene, observed in about 95% of patients with PV and 50% to 60% in ET and PMF.[7–10] The JAK2-V617F mutation is often associated with acquired uniparental disomy on the short arm of chromosome 9 (9pUPD), which makes the mutation homozygous particularly in PV and PMF.[9] Mutations in exon 12 of JAK2 are present in 1% to 3% of PV cases.[11,12] Somatic activating mutations in the thrombopoietin receptor gene (MPL) are detected in 1% to 5% of the cases of PMF and ET, predominantly in a mutually exclusive manner with JAK2 mutations.[13] Other mutations commonly found in patients with MPN are in TET2,[14–16] CBL,[17,18] EZH2,[19,20] and ASXL1,[21] with variable frequency in 3 MPN subtypes (**Fig. 1**). Another group of mutations are acquired during the disease progression and transformation to sAML, such as TP53,[22,23] RUNX1,[22,24,25] NPM1,[25,26] FLT3, IDH1, and IDH2.[27–29] Several recurrent

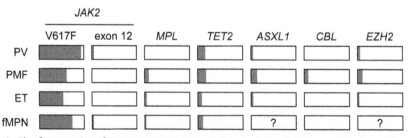

Fig. 1. The frequencies of common somatic mutations in 3 classic MPNs and in familial cases of MPN (fMPN). The red bars display the average frequency of the mutations obtained from multiple reports.

chromosomal aberrations have been described in patients with MPN. Deletions on chromosome 13q, 20q, 12p, uniparental disomies (UPDs) of 9p, 1p, 11q, 7q, trisomy of chromosome 8 and 9, and gains of chromosome 9p are often observed in the chronic phase of the disease,[25,30] whereas deletions of 5q, 7q, UPDs of 17p, and gains of chromosome 1q and 3q are mostly present in advanced disease and at leukemic transformation.[23,25,30,31] This remarkable diversity of somatic mutations and chromosomal aberrations in MPN contributes to the genetic complexity of the disease, similar to other forms of cancer. The variability in mutation frequencies in 3 subtypes of MPN partially explains the clinical differences among PV, ET, and PMF. However, a significant part of the phenotypic diversity is yet unexplained.

PREDISPOSITION TO MPN

Although MPNs are mainly driven by somatically acquired point mutations and chromosomal aberrations, germline factors have been shown to play a role in MPN pathogenesis. There are several lines of evidence that point out the importance of germline genetics in MPN. The phenotypic diversity of MPN (ie, the existence of 3 clinically different disease entities with similar mutational profile) is not properly explained by somatic defects and environmental factors. Thus, hereditary factors have been suggested to play a role in influencing the disease phenotype and resulting in the development of PV, ET, or PMF in the presence of the same mutations, most notably JAK2-V617F.[32,33] There have been some reports of the existence of biclonal MPN when 2 independent malignant clones develop in the same patient.[34–38] The probability of occurrence of such an event is extremely low, and the only explanation of that phenomenon could be the existence of hereditary predisposition in such patients. Surprisingly high number of patients with MPN have close relatives with MPN.[39,40] Common polymorphisms also have influence of predisposing to MPN, exemplified by the discovery of an MPN risk haplotype spanning JAK2 gene.[38,41,42]

GGCC HAPLOTYPE

In 2008, a study investigated the influence of germline single nucleotide polymorphisms (SNP) in several candidate genes on the clinical phenotype of the disease, particularly the difference between PV and ET.[32] They found that several SNPs in the region of the JAK2 gene are significantly different in PV compared with ET. Two other groups followed up this discovery and refined the association, showing that a common haplotype (46/1 or GGCC) in the JAK2 locus predisposes to JAK2-V617F-positive MPN.[41,42] The difference of haplotype frequency is caused by a different proportion of patients with PV and ET that carried the JAK2 mutation. In parallel, Olcaydu and colleagues (2009)[38] investigated the multiple acquisition of JAK2-V617F in MPN. Studying the patients who were V617F positive that were heterozygous for the common haplotype on JAK2, denoted as GGCC, the mutation was found to be gained significantly more often on one of the alleles. Following up on this finding, Olcaydu and colleagues[38] (2009) came to the same conclusion that the GGCC haplotype predisposes to V617F-postive MPN. Later it was demonstrated that the same haplotype also predisposes to the JAK2-exon12 mutation-positive MPN[43] and MPL-positive MPN.[44] Moreover, it was shown that the JAK2 haplotype is a susceptibility factor for ET and PMF independent of JAK2 status.[45,46]

Overall, the GGCC haplotype seems to be one of the major germline factors involved in the pathogenesis of MPN. The association of the haplotype with JAK2-V617F-positive MPN is one of the strongest reported so far, with an odds ratio around 2.5.[38,41,42] Most of the SNP associations for other diseases have odds ratios less than

1.5. In the era of genome-wide association studies, it is remarkable that *JAK2* haplotype association was found by other approaches, underlining its strong susceptibility. So far, no other common SNP has been reported to be associated with MPN. Although there might be more SNPs with high frequency in populations that predispose to MPN, it is highly unlikely that there will be another one of similar strength as the *JAK2* haplotype. The *JAK2* haplotype explains a major proportion of MPN heritability, which is more than 50% of the increased risk in the relatives of patients with MPN.[41] The population attributable risk percent has been estimated to be from 28%[41] to 46%.[42] Thus, the *JAK2* GGCC haplotype is the major common genetic susceptibility factor for MPN.

FAMILIAL CLUSTERING OF MPN

As soon as cellular and molecular markers became available to separate MPN from other hereditary conditions, such as familial erythrocytosis, several distinct pedigrees with true clonal MPN have been described.[47] Subsequent reports have shown frequent familial clustering of MPN, with an estimated 5% to 10% of MPN having familial history[40,48] and a several-fold increase of MPN risk in the relatives of patients with MPN.[39] Familial cases of MPN are defined as 2 or more cases among relatives.[40] However, it must be taken into account that 2 cases of sporadic MPN can also occur in a family by chance within populations of many millions of people.

So far, the causative germline mutations have only been found in a small proportion of familial MPN. For the rest of the families, the underlying genetic cause remains unknown. The germline mutations involved in familial MPN have to confer much higher risk than the GGCC haplotype, which increases the risk twofold to threefold. The estimated average penetrance level of MPN mutations is around 30%[49]; however, the penetrance varies significantly among individual families. Some reports have shown disease anticipation in familial MPN when in each following generation the age of onset of the disease is lower.[40,50] However, others have not confirmed this phenomenon.[39] Familial clustering of MPN is one of the most convincing evidences that germline factors play an important role in MPN pathogenesis.

CLINICAL AND GENETIC HETEROGENEITY IN FAMILIAL MPN

The MPN pedigree structures published to date show clear heterogeneity. Most of the families show the autosomal dominant pattern of inheritance,[40,47] although in some other cases autosomal recessive inheritance cannot be excluded.[39] The familial MPN in most cases display low penetrance[4,40,47]; however, there are pedigrees with high, almost complete penetrance. The age of onset in familial cases of MPN is lower than in sporadic MPN,[4,47] but there is evidence of variability.[40]

The MPN families also differ according to MPN subtype. There are families whereby all the affected members have the same subtype of the disease[4,40] (eg, ET, PV,[47] or PMF), whereas in other families the affected members have different diagnoses.[4,40] In addition, some families have an unusually high tendency to transform to sAML. This myriad of MPN family types points toward extreme genetic heterogeneity and supports the idea that there might be many different germline mutations that all cause MPN.

Perhaps the most intriguing variability in familial MPN cases is the somatic acquisition of *JAK2*, *MPL*, and *TET2* mutations in a subpopulation of familial cases.[4,49,51] This variability leads to the hypothesis that familial MPN may be comprised of 2 subgroups of fundamentally different diseases. The first group, true familial MPN, comprises the families whereby the underlying germline defect does not itself drive the disease but predisposes to the acquisition of oncogenic mutations, like JAK2-V617F. These pedigrees are predicted to have lower penetrance and a later age of onset because the disease initiation depends on the acquisition of a somatic mutation. There have been several familial linkage studies performed on families with MPN and most of the candidate genes frequently mutated somatically have been ruled out.[47] The second group, MPN-like disorders, is discussed later.

HEREDITARY ERYTHROCYTOSIS AND THROMBOCYTOSIS

In a proportion of pedigrees, the germline mutation itself is causing the disease. These MPN-like families have higher penetrance of the disease, an earlier age of onset, and do not carry somatic *JAK2* mutations. From another point of view, these families might not be considered true familial MPN but rather forms of hereditary thrombocytosis or erythrocytosis. It is important to differentiate true familial MPN from the cases of hereditary erythrocytosis and thrombocytosis, which can have clinical manifestations somewhat similar to PV and ET, respectively. There are several differences between these two disorders. Hereditary thrombocytosis and erythrocytosis are characterized by polyclonal hematopoiesis, involvement of single myeloid lineage, high penetrance, and absence of progression of the disease. By contrast, in patients with familial MPN, hematopoiesis is clonal, usually involves multiple lineages, and the disease frequently progresses to secondary myelofibrosis and sAML.[50,52] Progenitor cells from patients with familial MPN form spontaneous erythroid colonies, a feature absent in healthy people or hereditary erythrocytosis.[50,51,53]

In many cases of hereditary erythrocytosis and thrombocytosis, the underlying germline mutation is known. Mutations in oxygen-sensing pathway genes (*VHL*,[54] *EGLN1*,[55] and so forth) or genes affecting oxygen affinity of hemoglobin result in hereditary secondary erythrocytosis as a consequence of high erythropoietin levels.[50] *EPOR* truncating mutations cause primary familial and congenital polycythemia in which the erythrocytosis is primary as a result of the removal of inhibitory domain by the truncations and hypersensitivity to erythropoietin.[56] Hereditary thrombocytosis is caused by mutations in the thrombopoietin gene (*THPO*), which explains only a part of those cases.[57,58]

There is another group of families that have the MPN-like phenotype but also share some characteristics of hereditary thrombocytosis. These cases are caused by germline mutations in *MPL* and *JAK2* genes and are discussed in the following section.

GERMLINE MPL MUTATIONS

A germline mutation in the thrombopoietin receptor gene (*MPL*) has been found in familial cases of thrombocytosis.[59–62] The change is serine to asparagine (S505N), which is an activating mutation. Screening for germline *MPL* mutations in pediatric cases of thrombocytosis identified S505N mutation in several families.[63,64] It was also shown that there was a founder effect for the mutation. Although the patients have single lineage involvement and progenitors are not cytokine independent, the patients have some MPN-like properties, such as an increased risk of thrombotic events, splenomegaly, and progression of the disease to secondary myelofibrosis.[64] Recently, another germline MPL mutation, Y252H, has been shown to be associated with thrombocytosis.[61] Somatic MPL mutations (mostly W515) are found in some cases of ET and PMF.

GERMLINE JAK2 MUTATIONS

Recently, several groups identified germline mutations in the *JAK2* gene in familial cases of thrombocytosis.[65,66] The mutations, V617I and R564Q, are located in the pseudokinase domain, in the vicinity of the V617F mutation. The authors have also identified a family with hereditary thrombocytosis, previously diagnosed as ET, to carry the germline JAK2-H608N mutation.[67] All the families have a very similar phenotype, isolated thrombocytosis, absence of the somatic JAK2-V617F mutation, and high penetrance.[65,66] This type of disease can also be considered MPN-like because it does not possess true MPN characteristics.

OTHER FAMILIAL MYELOID DISORDERS

Malignant myeloid disorders other than MPN, such as myelodysplastic syndromes (MDS), juvenile myelomonocytic leukemia (JMML), and acute myeloid leukemia (AML), also show familial clustering. Several groups have studied those cases and identified germline mutations responsible for the development of the diseases. Inherited mutations in the CEBPA gene have been implicated in the development of AML,[68] whereas germline mutations in GATA2,[69] RUNX1,[70] TERC,[71] and TERT[72] predispose to the development of MDS. These mutations explain a part of the familial cases of MDS and AML; although for the remaining proportion of families, predisposing mutations are yet to be identified.

It has been shown that germline mutations in CBL cause developmental abnormalities and predispose to JMML.[73] Interestingly, CBL mutations are also acquired somatically in patients with JMML without familial history as well as in a wider spectrum of myeloid disorders, including MPN.[17,18] Similarly, somatic RUNX1 mutations are detected in several patients with MDS and secondary AML.[22,25,30] These facts illustrate the phenomenon of germline mutations in certain genes causing very specific neoplastic disorder, while the somatic mutations in the same gene are found in different related or even unrelated malignancies.

GGCC HAPLOTYPE IN FAMILIAL MPN: POPULATION (COMMON) AND FAMILIAL (RARE) SUSCEPTIBILITY

After the discovery of the MPN predisposition locus on JAK2, it was reasonable to consider the possibility that the JAK2 GGCC haplotype can contribute to the familial clustering of MPN. The authors investigated this issue in a large collection of MPN families and found that, although the GGCC haplotype is indeed a risk factor for developing JAK2-positive MPN in familial cases, the effect is similar to that observed in sporadic cases of MPN.[49] Thus, the GGCC haplotype cannot explain the familial clustering of MPN. Moreover, there is a difference of several orders of magnitude in the risk conferred by the familial predisposition loci (as yet unknown) and the GGCC haplotype.[49] Apparently, the GGCC haplotype only influences the acquisition of the JAK2 mutations (mainly V617F) and has an additive effect in the case of true familial MPN when there is an increased predisposition to the acquisition of somatic oncogenic mutations (**Fig. 2**).

GERMLINE FACTORS IN CLINICAL PICTURE: STAT1 PHOSPHORYLATION

The factors determining which subtype of MPN patients will develop while carrying the same somatic mutation has been a matter of study of many researchers. Recently, a report investigated the JAK-STAT pathway in single cells from patients with PV and ET both bearing heterozygous JAK2-V617F. They demonstrated that STAT1 phosphorylation is high in ET, whereas there are high levels of STAT5 phosphorylation in PV.[74] The authors attributed these differences to other unidentified somatic mutations. However, it is also likely that these differences have a germline basis. It is

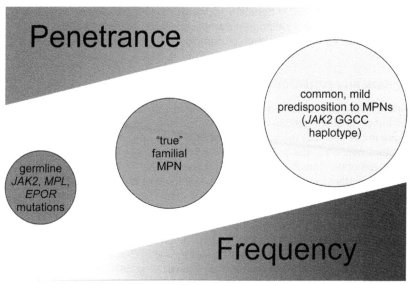

Fig. 2. Different types of germline predisposition in MPN and MPN-like disorders. The size of the circles corresponds to the respective frequency of the germline variants. The darker shade of the colors shows higher frequency and penetrance.

a matter of further investigation to find out which mechanism is responsible for the observed differences between PV and ET.

GERMLINE POLYMORPHISMS INFLUENCING CLINICAL COURSE OF MPNS

Germline factors in MPN can also impact the rate of disease complications in MPN. Recently, it has been found that a coding polymorphism in the *ERCC2* (*XPD*) gene increases the risk of transformation to sAML.[75] The patients with ET or PV who are homozygous for the risk variant had about a 5-fold higher risk of leukemic transformation than those with alternative genotypes. Moreover, the patients who were homozygous for the risk allele also had about a 4-fold higher risk of developing new primary nonmyeloid malignancies. ERCC2 is involved in the nucleotide excision repair pathway. It has been suggested that the risk genotype results in patients being more sensitive to DNA damage and developing sAML or nonmyeloid malignancies on long-term exposure to treatment.[75] This finding is more evidence that the variety of clinical manifestations in MPN might be partly caused by germline polymorphisms.

RARE GERMLINE ALLELES AND ACQUIRED CHROMOSOMAL ABERRATIONS

Germline mutations in the genome not only can predispose to the disease but also influence the clinical course of the disease. Every person carries multiple deleterious mutations in the genome, which do not have any effect in the heterozygous state. However, in MPN, patients acquire large-scale chromosomal abnormalities, which, in combination with germline deleterious variants, can alter the clinical phenotype of the patients. Particularly, deletions and UPDs can remove the wild-type allele. Recently, the authors have shown one such case when a patient with PV with chromosome 14q UPD developed anemia and later transformed to sAML.[76] The patient carried a germline heterozygous nonsense mutation in the Fanconi anemia complementation group M (*FANCM*) gene. After the somatically acquired UPD on 14q, the malignant clone cells became homozygous for the *FANCM* mutation and subsequently developed anemia (**Fig. 3**). This mechanism of MPN pathogenesis has not been thoroughly investigated and can yet provide an intriguing layer of complexity in the disease development and progression.

DISCUSSION AND FUTURE DIRECTIONS

Several studies have focused on the identification of germline genetic factors involved in MPN and the characterization of their precise role. Many exciting discoveries have emerged in the field, but there is still a long way to go. By now it is obvious that germline factors play an important role in MPN pathogenesis despite the fact that these diseases are driven mainly by acquired genetic lesions.

Germline factors predisposing to the development of MPN can be categorized in 2 groups: common, mild predisposition, which generally raises the incidence of the disease in the population, and rare, strong predisposition, which is responsible for the familial clustering of the disease. Consequently, these two groups of hereditary factors have a different frequency in the population and penetrance (**Fig. 4**).

A very strong common susceptibility factor, *JAK2* GGCC haplotype, has been shown have a 2- to 3-fold increased risk of developing JAK2-positive MPN. This is perhaps the strongest common predisposition factor in MPN. It is also one of the strongest SNP associations identified in any disease so far. There are definitely more SNPs that predispose to MPN; however, their effect is predicted to be much lower than the GGCC haplotype. It would be particularly interesting in JAK2-negative cases because the GGCC haplotype does not play a significant role in those. However, JAK2-negative cases are likely to be a rather heterogeneous group and might not have a common germline susceptibility factor.

There is much more work yet to be done in familial MPN. The familial case of MPN can be grouped into true familial MPN with low penetrance and driven by acquired somatic mutations and MPN-like disorders, which have high penetrance, are driven by the causative germline mutations, and mainly involve single lineage (cases of hereditary thrombocytosis and erythrocytosis). Considering only the true familial MPN, so far there is no germline mutation found. For MPN-like disorders, a few genes carrying germline mutations have been identified, most notably *MPL* and *JAK2* (**Table 1**). However, still most familial MPN-like disorders have no mutation found.

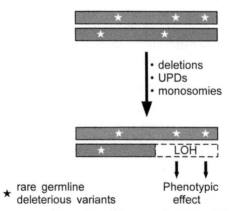

Fig. 3. Interaction between somatic and germline genetic factors. Alleles underlying germline recessive traits are made homozygous or hemizygous by somatic UPD, deletions, or monosomies, consequently influencing the clinical phenotype. White stars denote mutations.

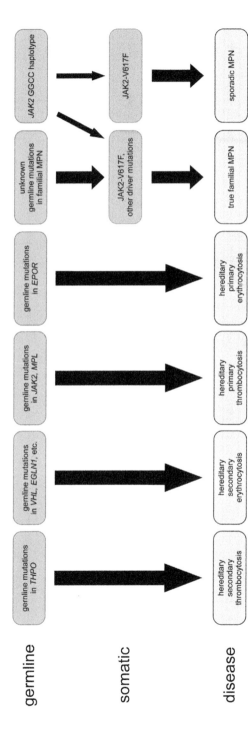

Fig. 4. Mechanisms of development of MPN and MPN-like disorders. Although MPN-like disorders are solely caused by germline mutations, in MPN germline variants predispose to acquisition of somatic mutations, which in turn drive the disease.

Table 1
Summary of identified germline mutations predisposing to MPN and MPN-related disorders

Gene	Germline Mutation	Disease	Inheritance	Clonality	Disease Progression	Lineage Involvement	Somatic Mutations
Unknown	Unknown	Familial MPN	Autosomal dominant with low penetrance	Clonal	Yes	Multilineage	Yes
JAK2	GGCC haplotype	Sporadic and familial MPN	Codominant	Clonal	Yes	Multilineage	Yes (JAK2)
	Missense mutations (V617I, H564Q, H608N)	Hereditary thrombocytosis/ET	Autosomal dominant	Polyclonal	No	Multilineage	No
MPL	Missense mutations (S505N, Y252H)	Hereditary thrombocytosis	Autosomal dominant	Polyclonal	No	Megakaryocytic	No
THPO	Splice site/missense/regulatory mutations	Hereditary thrombocytosis	Autosomal dominant	Polyclonal	No	Megakaryocytic	No
EPOR	Truncating mutations	Primary familial and congenital erythrocytosis	Autosomal dominant	Polyclonal	No	Erythroid	No
VHL	Loss-of-function mutations	Hereditary secondary erythrocytosis	Autosomal recessive	Polyclonal	No	Erythroid	No
HIF2a (EPAS1)	Missense mutations	Hereditary secondary erythrocytosis	Autosomal dominant	Polyclonal	No	Erythroid	No
EGLN1 (PHD2)	Loss-of-function mutations	Hereditary secondary erythrocytosis	Autosomal dominant	Polyclonal	No	Erythroid	No
HBB	High oxygen affinity variants	Hereditary secondary erythrocytosis	Autosomal dominant	Polyclonal	No	Erythroid	No
DPGM	Loss-of-function mutations	Hereditary secondary erythrocytosis	Autosomal dominant	Polyclonal	No	Erythroid	No

Both of those types of families, with *MPL* or *JAK2* mutations, are very homogenous, with early onset of the disease and thrombocytosis. The true familial MPNs look very heterogeneous at the first glance, but taking into account the evidence from MPN-like diseases, true familial MPN might consist of several homogeneous groups, each caused by a mutation in a different gene. On the other hand, quite often it is difficult to distinguish between hereditary thrombocytosis and ET if the germline mutation is unknown. Undoubtedly, the current technologies of second-generation sequencing will uncover many mutations in familial MPN and, in the process, some families previously diagnosed as true MPN will be reevaluated as MPN-like diseases.

Overall, it seems that true familial MPNs are diseases arising as a result of a very complex interaction between several factors. Germline mutations predispose the patients to acquire somatic mutations, whereas the GGCC haplotype and possibly other common SNPs enhance the risk of the disease. In addition, the various chromosomal aberrations interacting with germline deleterious provide another ground for the complexity. Because these diseases do not conform to classical Mendelian rules, the possibility of oligogenic inheritance cannot be ruled out.

The identification the causative mutations in familial MPN will not only help devise optimal treatment strategies for those cases but, in general, it will also enhance the understanding of MPN pathogenesis. The same genes mutated in the germline in familial MPN can be somatically mutated in other patients. *JAK2* and *MPL* are the best examples of that.

REFERENCES

1. Tefferi A, Vardiman JW. Classification and diagnosis of myeloproliferative neoplasms: the 2008 World Health Organization criteria and point-of-care diagnostic algorithms. Leukemia 2008;22:14.
2. Campbell PJ, Green AR. The myeloproliferative disorders. N Engl J Med 2006; 355:2452.
3. Dingli D, Schwager SM, Mesa RA, et al. Presence of unfavorable cytogenetic abnormalities is the strongest predictor of poor survival in secondary myelofibrosis. Cancer 2006;106:1985.
4. Bellanne-Chantelot C, Chaumarel I, Labopin M, et al. Genetic and clinical implications of the Val617Phe JAK2 mutation in 72 families with myeloproliferative disorders. Blood 2006;108:346.
5. Ostgard LS, Kjeldsen E, Holm MS, et al. Reasons for treating secondary AML as de novo AML. Eur J Haematol 2010;85:217.
6. Tefferi A, Vainchenker W. Myeloproliferative neoplasms: molecular pathophysiology, essential clinical understanding, and treatment strategies. J Clin Oncol 2011;29:573.
7. Baxter EJ, Scott LM, Campbell PJ, et al. Acquired mutation of the tyrosine kinase JAK2 in human myeloproliferative disorders. Lancet 2005;365:1054.
8. James C, Ugo V, Le Couedic JP, et al. A unique clonal JAK2 mutation leading to constitutive signalling causes polycythaemia vera. Nature 2005;434:1144.
9. Kralovics R, Passamonti F, Buser AS, et al. A gain-of-function mutation of JAK2 in myeloproliferative disorders. N Engl J Med 2005;352:1779.
10. Levine RL, Wadleigh M, Cools J, et al. Activating mutation in the tyrosine kinase JAK2 in polycythemia vera, essential thrombocythemia, and myeloid metaplasia with myelofibrosis. Cancer Cell 2005;7:387.
11. Pietra D, Li S, Brisci A, et al. Somatic mutations of JAK2 exon 12 in patients with JAK2 (V617F)-negative myeloproliferative disorders. Blood 2008;111:1686.

12. Scott LM, Tong W, Levine RL, et al. JAK2 exon 12 mutations in polycythemia vera and idiopathic erythrocytosis. N Engl J Med 2007;356:459.

13. Pikman Y, Lee BH, Mercher T, et al. MPLW515L is a novel somatic activating mutation in myelofibrosis with myeloid metaplasia. PLoS Med 2006;3:e270.

14. Delhommeau F, Dupont S, Della Valle V, et al. Mutation in TET2 in myeloid cancers. N Engl J Med 2009;360:2289.

15. Langemeijer SM, Kuiper RP, Berends M, et al. Acquired mutations in TET2 are common in myelodysplastic syndromes. Nat Genet 2009;41:838.

16. Tefferi A, Pardanani A, Lim KH, et al. TET2 mutations and their clinical correlates in polycythemia vera, essential thrombocythemia and myelofibrosis. Leukemia 2009;23:905.

17. Dunbar AJ, Gondek LP, O'Keefe CL, et al. 250K single nucleotide polymorphism array karyotyping identifies acquired uniparental disomy and homozygous mutations, including novel missense substitutions of c-Cbl, in myeloid malignancies. Cancer Res 2008;68:10349.

18. Sanada M, Suzuki T, Shih LY, et al. Gain-of-function of mutated C-CBL tumour suppressor in myeloid neoplasms. Nature 2009;460:904.

19. Ernst T, Chase AJ, Score J, et al. Inactivating mutations of the histone methyltransferase gene EZH2 in myeloid disorders. Nat Genet 2010;42:722.

20. Nikoloski G, Langemeijer SM, Kuiper RP, et al. Somatic mutations of the histone methyltransferase gene EZH2 in myelodysplastic syndromes. Nat Genet 2010; 42:665.

21. Carbuccia N, Murati A, Trouplin V, et al. Mutations of ASXL1 gene in myeloproliferative neoplasms. Leukemia 2009;23:2183.

22. Beer PA, Delhommeau F, LeCouedic JP, et al. Two routes to leukemic transformation after a JAK2 mutation-positive myeloproliferative neoplasm. Blood 2010;115:2891.

23. Harutyunyan A, Klampfl T, Cazzola M, et al. p53 lesions in leukemic transformation. N Engl J Med 2011;364:488.

24. Ding Y, Harada Y, Imagawa J, et al. AML1/RUNX1 point mutation possibly promotes leukemic transformation in myeloproliferative neoplasms. Blood 2009; 114:5201.

25. Klampfl T, Harutyunyan A, Berg T, et al. Genome integrity of myeloproliferative neoplasms in chronic phase and during disease progression. Blood 2011; 118:167.

26. Falini B, Mecucci C, Tiacci E, et al. Cytoplasmic nucleophosmin in acute myelogenous leukemia with a normal karyotype. N Engl J Med 2005;352:254.

27. Green A, Beer P. Somatic mutations of IDH1 and IDH2 in the leukemic transformation of myeloproliferative neoplasms. N Engl J Med 2010;362:369.

28. Pardanani A, Lasho TL, Finke CM, et al. IDH1 and IDH2 mutation analysis in chronic- and blast-phase myeloproliferative neoplasms. Leukemia 2010;24: 1146.

29. Tefferi A, Lasho TL, Abdel-Wahab O, et al. IDH1 and IDH2 mutation studies in 1473 patients with chronic-, fibrotic- or blast-phase essential thrombocythemia, polycythemia vera or myelofibrosis. Leukemia 2010;24:1302.

30. Thoennissen NH, Krug UO, Lee DH, et al. Prevalence and prognostic impact of allelic imbalances associated with leukemic transformation of Philadelphia chromosome-negative myeloproliferative neoplasms. Blood 2010;115:2882.

31. Rumi E, Harutyunyan A, Elena C, et al. Identification of genomic aberrations associated with disease transformation by means of high-resolution SNP array analysis in patients with myeloproliferative neoplasm. Am J Hematol 2011;86:974.

32. Pardanani A, Fridley BL, Lasho TL, et al. Host genetic variation contributes to phenotypic diversity in myeloproliferative disorders. Blood 2008;111:2785.

33. Wernig G, Gonneville JR, Crowley BJ, et al. The Jak2V617F oncogene associated with myeloproliferative diseases requires a functional FERM domain for transformation and for expression of the Myc and Pim proto-oncogenes. Blood 2008;111:3751.

34. Beer PA, Jones AV, Bench AJ, et al. Clonal diversity in the myeloproliferative neoplasms: independent origins of genetically distinct clones. Br J Haematol 2009;144:904.

35. Beer PA, Ortmann CA, Campbell PJ, et al. Independently acquired biallelic JAK2 mutations are present in a minority of patients with essential thrombocythemia. Blood 2010;116:1013.

36. Hussein K, Bock O, Theophile K, et al. Biclonal expansion and heterogeneous lineage involvement in a case of chronic myeloproliferative disease with concurrent MPLW515L/JAK2V617F mutation. Blood 2009;113:1391.

37. Kralovics R. Genetic complexity of myeloproliferative neoplasms. Leukemia 2008;22:1841.

38. Olcaydu D, Harutyunyan A, Jager R, et al. A common JAK2 haplotype confers susceptibility to myeloproliferative neoplasms. Nat Genet 2009;41:450.

39. Landgren O, Goldin LR, Kristinsson SY, et al. Increased risks of polycythemia vera, essential thrombocythemia, and myelofibrosis among 24,577 first-degree relatives of 11,039 patients with myeloproliferative neoplasms in Sweden. Blood 2008;112:2199.

40. Rumi E, Passamonti F, Della Porta MG, et al. Familial chronic myeloproliferative disorders: clinical phenotype and evidence of disease anticipation. J Clin Oncol 2007;25:5630.

41. Jones AV, Chase A, Silver RT, et al. JAK2 haplotype is a major risk factor for the development of myeloproliferative neoplasms. Nat Genet 2009;41:446.

42. Kilpivaara O, Mukherjee S, Schram AM, et al. A germline JAK2 SNP is associated with predisposition to the development of JAK2(V617F)-positive myeloproliferative neoplasms. Nat Genet 2009;41:455.

43. Olcaydu D, Skoda RC, Looser R, et al. The 'GGCC' haplotype of JAK2 confers susceptibility to JAK2 exon 12 mutation-positive polycythemia vera. Leukemia 2009;23:1924.

44. Jones AV, Campbell PJ, Beer PA, et al. The JAK2 46/1 haplotype predisposes to MPL-mutated myeloproliferative neoplasms. Blood 2010;115:4517.

45. Pardanani A, Lasho TL, Finke CM, et al. The JAK2 46/1 haplotype confers susceptibility to essential thrombocythemia regardless of JAK2V617F mutational status-clinical correlates in a study of 226 consecutive patients. Leukemia 2010;24:110.

46. Tefferi A, Lasho TL, Patnaik MM, et al. JAK2 germline genetic variation affects disease susceptibility in primary myelofibrosis regardless of V617F mutational status: nullizygosity for the JAK2 46/1 haplotype is associated with inferior survival. Leukemia 2010;24:105.

47. Kralovics R, Stockton DW, Prchal JT. Clonal hematopoiesis in familial polycythemia vera suggests the involvement of multiple mutational events in the early pathogenesis of the disease. Blood 2003;102:3793.

48. Rumi E. Familial chronic myeloproliferative disorders: the state of the art. Hematol Oncol 2008;26:131.

49. Olcaydu D, Rumi E, Harutyunyan A, et al. The role of the JAK2 GGCC haplotype and the TET2 gene in familial myeloproliferative neoplasms. Haematologica 2011;96:367.

50. Rumi E, Passamonti F, Picone C, et al. Disease anticipation in familial myelopro-liferative neoplasms. Blood 2008;112:2587.

51. Rumi E, Passamonti F, Pietra D, et al. JAK2 (V617F) as an acquired somatic muta-tion and a secondary genetic event associated with disease progression in familial myeloproliferative disorders. Cancer 2006;107:2206.

52. Skoda R. The genetic basis of myeloproliferative disorders. Hematology Am Soc Hematol Educ Program 2007;1–10.

53. Kralovics R, Skoda RC. Molecular pathogenesis of Philadelphia chromosome negative myeloproliferative disorders. Blood Rev 2005;19:1.

54. Ang SO, Chen H, Hirota K, et al. Disruption of oxygen homeostasis underlies congenital Chuvash polycythemia. Nat Genet 2002;32:614.

55. Albiero E, Ruggeri M, Fortuna S, et al. Analysis of the oxygen sensing pathway genes in familial chronic myeloproliferative neoplasms and identification of a novel EGLN1 germ-line mutation. Br J Haematol 2011;153:405.

56. de la Chapelle A, Traskelin AL, Juvonen E. Truncated erythropoietin receptor causes dominantly inherited benign human erythrocytosis. Proc Natl Acad Sci U S A 1993;90:4495.

57. Liu K, Kralovics R, Rudzki Z, et al. A de novo splice donor mutation in the throm-bopoietin gene causes hereditary thrombocythemia in a Polish family. Haemato-logica 2008;93:706.

58. Wiestner A, Schlemper RJ, van der Maas AP, et al. An activating splice donor mutation in the thrombopoietin gene causes hereditary thrombocythaemia. Nat Genet 1998;18:49.

59. Ding J, Komatsu H, Wakita A, et al. Familial essential thrombocythemia associ-ated with a dominant-positive activating mutation of the c-MPL gene, which encodes for the receptor for thrombopoietin. Blood 2004;103:4198.

60. El-Harith el HA, Roesl C, Ballmaier M, et al. Familial thrombocytosis caused by the novel germ-line mutation p.Pro106Leu in the MPL gene. Br J Haematol 2009;144:185.

61. Lambert MP, Jiang J, Batra V, et al. A novel mutation in MPL (Y252H) results in increased thrombopoietin sensitivity in essential thrombocythemia. Am J Hematol 2012;87:532.

62. Moliterno AR, Williams DM, Gutierrez-Alamillo LI, et al. Mpl Baltimore: a thrombo-poietin receptor polymorphism associated with thrombocytosis. Proc Natl Acad Sci U S A 2004;101:11444.

63. Teofili L, Giona F, Martini M, et al. Markers of myeloproliferative diseases in child-hood polycythemia vera and essential thrombocythemia. J Clin Oncol 2007;25: 1048.

64. Teofili L, Giona F, Torti L, et al. Hereditary thrombocytosis caused by MPLSer505-Asn is associated with a high thrombotic risk, splenomegaly and progression to bone marrow fibrosis. Haematologica 2010;95:65.

65. Etheridge L, Corbo LM, Kaushansky K, et al. A Novel activating JAK2 mutation, JAK2R564Q, causes familial essential thrombocytosis (fET) via mechanisms distinct from JAK2V617F. Blood (ASH Annual Meeting Abstracts) 2011; 118(21):123.

66. Mead AJ, Rugless MJ, Jacobsen SE, et al. Germline JAK2 mutation in a family with hereditary thrombocytosis. N Engl J Med 2012;366:967.

67. Rumi E, Harutyunyan A, Pietra D, et al. A novel germline JAK2 mutation in familial thrombocytosis. Haematologica 2012;97(s1):244.

68. Smith ML, Cavenagh JD, Lister TA, et al. Mutation of CEBPA in familial acute myeloid leukemia. N Engl J Med 2004;351:2403.

69. Hahn CN, Chong CE, Carmichael CL, et al. Heritable GATA2 mutations associated with familial myelodysplastic syndrome and acute myeloid leukemia. Nat Genet 2011;43:1012.

70. Song WJ, Sullivan MG, Legare RD, et al. Haploinsufficiency of CBFA2 causes familial thrombocytopenia with propensity to develop acute myelogenous leukaemia. Nat Genet 1999;23:166.

71. Yamaguchi H, Baerlocher GM, Lansdorp PM, et al. Mutations of the human telomerase RNA gene (TERC) in aplastic anemia and myelodysplastic syndrome. Blood 2003;102:916.

72. Kirwan M, Vulliamy T, Marrone A, et al. Defining the pathogenic role of telomerase mutations in myelodysplastic syndrome and acute myeloid leukemia. Hum Mutat 2009;30:1567.

73. Niemeyer CM, Kang MW, Shin DH, et al. Germline CBL mutations cause developmental abnormalities and predispose to juvenile myelomonocytic leukemia. Nat Genet 2010;42:794.

74. Chen E, Beer PA, Godfrey AL, et al. Distinct clinical phenotypes associated with JAK2V617F reflect differential STAT1 signaling. Cancer Cell 2010;18:524.

75. Hernandez-Boluda JC, Pereira A, Cervantes F, et al. A polymorphism in the XPD gene predisposes to leukemic transformation and new nonmyeloid malignancies in essential thrombocythemia and polycythemia vera. Blood 2012;119:5221.

76. Harutyunyan A, Gisslinger B, Klampfl T, et al. Rare germline variants in regions of loss of heterozygosity may influence clinical course of hematological malignancies. Leukemia 2011;25:1782.

Role of *TET2* and *ASXL1* Mutations in the Pathogenesis of Myeloproliferative Neoplasms

Omar Abdel-Wahab, MD[a,b], Ayalew Tefferi, MD[c],
Ross L. Levine, MD[a,b],*

KEYWORDS

• ASXL1 • TET2 • Myelofibrosis • Myeloproliferative neoplasms • JAK2

KEY POINTS

- Mutations in *TET2* are loss-of-function mutations present in 9% to 16% of patients with polycythemia vera (PV), 4% to 5% of patients with essential thrombocytosis (ET), and 7% to 17% of patients with primary myelofibrosis (PMF) or myelofibrosis arising from PV or ET.
- TET2 is a member of the TET family of α-ketoglutarate and Fe(II)-dependent dioxygenases, which oxidize 5-methylcytosine on DNA to produce 5-hydroxymethylcytosine followed by 5-formylcytosine and 5-carboxylcytosine. This enzymatic activity of TET2 is thought to facilitate demethylation of DNA.
- Additional sex combs like 1 (ASXL1) is the mammalian homologue of *Drosophila* ASXL, a protein known to affect both Trithorax group and Polycomb group gene function. Although several functions have been ascribed to ASXL1 in nonmammalian and nonhematopoietic cell contexts, the function of ASXL1 in mammalian hematopoietic cells is not yet fully delineated.
- Mutations in *ASXL1* are most common amongst MPN patients with PMF (13%–26%) or post-PV/ET MF (22%–38%) as compared with patients with PV (2%–5%) or ET (5%–10%).
- The clinical importance of *TET2* and *ASXL1* mutations amongst patients with MPNs is not yet clear. *ASXL1* mutations may confer worsened overall survival amongst patients with PMF/post-PV/ET MF, but this needs to be validated in larger, prospective studies.

Disclosures: The authors have no relationships to disclose.
[a] Human Oncology and Pathogenesis Program, Memorial Sloan-Kettering Cancer Center, 1275 York Avenue, New York, NY 10065, USA; [b] Leukemia Service, Department of Medicine, Memorial Sloan-Kettering Cancer Center, 1275 York Avenue, New York, NY 10065, USA; [c] Department of Hematology, Mayo Clinic, Rochester, MN, USA
* Corresponding author. Human Oncology and Pathogenesis Program, Memorial Sloan-Kettering Cancer Center, 1275 York Avenue, New York, NY.
E-mail address: leviner@mskcc.org

Hematol Oncol Clin N Am 26 (2012) 1053–1064
http://dx.doi.org/10.1016/j.hoc.2012.07.006
0889-8588/12/$ – see front matter © 2012 Elsevier Inc. All rights reserved.

hemonc.theclinics.com

EVIDENCE FOR MUTATIONS OUTSIDE OF THE JAK-STAT PATHWAY IN PATIENTS WITH MYELOPROLIFERATIVE NEOPLASMS

Myeloproliferative neoplasms (MPNs) are clonal disorders of hematopoiesis characterized by excess production of mature-appearing cells within the blood stream. The MPNs were initially grouped together by William Dameshek in 1951.[1] However, in 2005, the first biologic basis unifying the pathogenesis of the different MPNs was discovered when activating mutations in *JAK2* were identified in 95% of patients with polycythemia vera (PV), 55% to 60% of patients with essential thrombocytosis (ET), and 50% of patients with primary myelofibrosis (PMF).[2–5] This discovery was quickly followed by the discovery of additional mutations, resulting in activation of the JAK-STAT pathway in MPN patients, including exon 12 mutations in *JAK2*,[6] thrombopoietin receptor (*MPL*) mutations,[7] and loss-of-function mutations in *LNK*, a negative regulator of JAK-STAT signaling (**Table 1**).[8,9]

Although the discovery of mutations in *JAK2* and *MPL* provided seminal insight into MPN pathogenesis, several lines of evidence suggest that mutations in genes other than *JAK2* and *MPL* must be present in MPN patients. First was the question of how a single mutation in *JAK2*, which appeared to be sufficient for MPN pathogenesis from in vivo studies, could result in the development of 3 phenotypically different diseases. One attractive hypothesis to this question was that additional acquired or inherited genetic modifiers outside of *JAK2* or *MPL* could be present and modify the MPN phenotype. Secondly, clonal analysis of patients with *JAK2/MPL* mutations demonstrated the presence of *JAK2* wild-type endogenous erythroid colonies, clear evidence that an additional aberration responsible for erythropoietin-independent growth must be present.[10] Clonality analysis of patients with a cytogenetic abnormality in conjunction with the *JAK2V617F* mutation also revealed that some patients had cytogenetically abnormal clones with and without the *JAK2V617F* mutation.[11] Finally, several reports have shown that leukemic blasts of acute myeloid leukemia (AML) derived from a *JAK2V617F* MPN are frequently *JAK2* wild-type,[12,13] suggesting that the MPN and AML clones can arise from 2 different progenitor cells or that an ancestral clone bearing an abnormality preceding the *JAK2V617F* mutation can give rise to both the JAK2-positive MPN and the JAK2-negative AML. Thus, additional novel mutations in MPN pathogenesis have been speculated to exist since the discovery of mutations in *JAK2*.

Table 1
Frequency of somatic genetic mutations in patients with MPNs

MPN	Gene Mutation[a]					
	JAK2V617F	*JAK2* Exon 12	*MPL*	*LNK*	*TET2*	*ASXL1*[b]
Polycythemia vera (PV)	95%	3%–5%	NR	Present	9.8%–16%	2%–5%
Essential thrombocytosis (ET)	55%–60%	NR	3%–5%	3%–6%	4.4%–5%	5%–10%
Primary myelofibrosis (MF)	50%–60%	NR	8%–10%	3%–6%	7.7%–17%	13%–26%
Post-PV/ET MF	50%–60%	NR	NR	NR	14%	22%–38.5%

[a] NR, not reported.
[b] Several manuscripts used to delineate mutational frequency of *ASXL1* contain the controversial p.Gly646TrpfsX12 variant which has not definitively proven to be a somatic mutation.

DISCOVERY OF *TET2* MUTATIONS IN MPN PATIENTS

Mutations in *TET2* (Ten-Eleven-Translocation 2) were the first described recurrent somatic alterations in MPN patients in a gene not directly known to be involved in the JAK-STAT signaling pathway. *TET2* mutations were originally described by Delhommeau and colleagues[14] and Langemeijer and colleagues[15,16] in 2009 in patients with MPNs and myelodysplastic syndrome. Through careful examination of primary PV patient samples, Delhommeau and colleagues[14] noticed that most of *JAK2V617F* mutant PV patients ($\sim$85%) had expansion of CD34+CD38+—committed progenitor cells over CD34+CD38− multipotent progenitors in ex vivo liquid cultures. In contrast, a minority ($\sim$15%) of *JAK2V617F* mutant PV patients were characterized by relative expansion of the more immature multipotent progenitor cells (CD34+ CD38−). Hypothesizing that a novel genetic abnormality might be responsible for this immunophenotypic difference in these 2 patient subsets, the investigators performed single nucleotide polymorphism arrays (Affymetrix 500K) and comparative genomic hybridization array (aCGH) (Agilent 244K) on a small number of patient samples. They found that 3 of the 5 *JAK2V617F* mutant PV patients with expansion of CD34+CD38− cells had loss of heterozygosity at chromosomal locus 4q24. One of these 5 patients had a deletion of a 325 kB region of DNA at 4q24, the only gene present in this region being *TET2*. This deletion then led to sequencing of *TET2* in these patient samples and the identification of somatic *TET2* mutations in MPNs. Since then, sequencing of *TET2* has led to the identification of *TET2* mutations in every myeloid disorder.[15–21] Mutations in *TET2* have been found in all coding regions and can appear as missense, nonsense, or frameshift mutations. Mutations in *TET2* are less uncommonly biallelic (ie, involving both copies of *TET2*), consistent with mutations in *TET2* being haploinsufficient loss-of-function mutations in most patients.

BIOCHEMICAL FUNCTION OF TET2

TET2 is a member of the *TET* family of genes, the first member of which to be described was *TET1* (Ten-Eleven-Translocation 1). *TET1*, located on chromosome 10, was originally identified in cases of adult and pediatric AML as a translocation partner with *MLL* (located on chromosome 11).[22] Although *TET1* was the original gene member identified in hematologic malignancies, no sequence alterations in *TET1* or *TET3* have been identified to date.[17]

The function of *TET1* was first described in a landmark publication by Tahiliani and colleagues[23] in 2009. They pursued the identification of human enzymes that modify bases of nucleic acids as a means to understand how catalytic modifications of DNA bases affect the genetic code. As such, they undertook in silico approach to identify human homologues of the trypanosome proteins JBP1 and JBP2, which are known to oxidize the 5-methyl group of thymine.[24] Such enzymes were not previously known to exist in higher organisms. Surprisingly, they found that the *TET* family of genes was human homologues of these trypanosomal enzymes. Further characterization of *TET1* revealed that it is a 2-oxoglutarate- and Fe(II)—dependent dioxygenase that serves to oxidize the 5-methyl group of cytosine, leading to formation of 5-hydroxymethylcytosine (**Fig. 1**).

More recent work has identified that all 3 TET proteins are enzymes that can convert 5-methylcytosine (5mC) into 5-hydroxymethylcytosine (5hmC). Moreover, 2 groups have reported that TET proteins can further convert 5hmC into 5-formylcytosine (5fC) and 5-carboxylcytosine (5caC) in 2 successive oxidation reactions (see **Fig. 1**).

The discovery of these novel enzymatic activities by the TET proteins has provided insight into potential mechanisms by which 5mC is dynamically regulated as well as

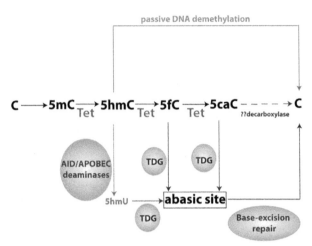

Fig. 1. Role of TET2 in DNA hydroxymethylation and DNA demethylation. The TET family of enzymes (TET1-3) are α-ketoglutarate and Fe(II)-dependent enzymes that hydroxylate the 5-methyl group on methylcytosine (5mC) to create 5-hydroxymethylcytosine (5hmC). TET family of enzymes then further oxidize 5hmC into 5-formylcytosine (5fC) and 5-carboxylcytosine (5caC). These activities of the TET family of enzymes may then promote demethylation of DNA in 4 potential pathways, which are being investigated further: (1) Because 5hmC is not recognized by maintenance DNA methyltransferases, 5hmC can result in DNA demethylation over time with DNA replication in a passive manner (*orange lines and text*); (2) 5fC and 5caC are excised by thymine DNA glycosylase (TDG) into an abasic site, which could then be regenerated into an unmodified cytosine by the base-excision repair pathway (BER) (*blue lines and text*); (3) 5hmC may also be converted by the activation-induced deaminase (AID)/APOBEC (apolipoprotein B mRNA editing enzyme complex) family of cytosine demethylases into 5-hydroxymethyluracil (5hmU), which may then be repaired through the action of DNA glycosylases and the BER pathway (*green text*); finally, there is a possibility that 5caC may be further decarboxylated by a yet undiscovered decarboxylase into unmodified cytosine (*purple text*).

demethylated in both active and passive processes. For instance, DNMT1 (DNA methyltransferase 1), the DNA methyltransferase responsible for maintaining DNA methylation, does not recognize 5hmC. Thus, conversion of 5mC into 5hmC may lead to replication-dependent passive demethylation of DNA (see **Fig. 1**). Furthermore, oxidized derivatives of 5hmC may serve in a replication-independent, active DNA demethylation process. Proof for this concept comes from the finding that thymine DNA glycosylase (TDG) can excise 5fC or 5caC in the context of CpG sites (TDG has minimal activity toward 5hmC). The resulting abasic site following TDG-excision can then be repaired by the base-excision repair (BER) pathway to generate unmethylated cytosines. There is also evidence that 5hmC can be actively deaminated into 5-hydroxymethyluracil (5hmU) by the activation-induced deaminase/apolipoprotein B mRNA editing enzyme complex. The resulting 5hmU could then be removed via the action of DNA glycosylases and the BER pathway. Finally, Ito and colleagues[25] proposed that 5mC might be converted to cytosine simply by iterative oxidation of 5hmC by TET enzymes followed by a single decarboxylation of 5caC to regenerate cytosine by a yet unidentified putative decarboxylase. Although no decarboxylase capable of removing the carboxyl group from 5caC has been identified, this latter mechanism of iterative 5mC oxidation followed by decarboxylation is attractive in its simplicity, and no DNA repair mechanism is required to effect DNA demethylation.

BIOLOGIC ROLE OF TET2 IN HEMATOPOIESIS

In parallel with the biochemical characterization of TET2's enzymatic function have been extensive functional studies of the biologic ramifications of TET2 loss. Initial evidence of the role of TET2 in hematopoiesis came from xenograft studies in the initial reports of TET2 mutations by Delhommeau and colleagues.[14,16] They noted that xenografting JAK2V617F-positive CD34+ cells from MPN subjects with (n = 2) and those without TET2 mutations (n = 3) into NOD-SCID mice revealed a more efficient engraftment of TET2 mutant cells over TET2 wild-type CD34+ cells. Moreover, the hematopoiesis was skewed toward increased frequency of myeloid progenitors over lymphoid progenitors in TET2 mutant patients.

More recently, independent reports of the phenotype of TET2 knockout mice have been published using at least 4 different targeting alleles (**Fig. 2**A). Conditional deletion of the first coding exon of TET2 by Moran-Crusio and colleagues[26] showed that TET2 loss leads to a progressive enlargement of the hematopoietic stem cell compartment and eventual myeloproliferation in vivo, including splenomegaly, monocytosis, and extramedullary hematopoiesis. In addition, TET2$^{+/-}$ mice displayed increased stem cell self-renewal and extramedullary hematopoiesis, demonstrating that TET2 haploinsufficiency contributes to hematopoietic transformation in vivo (see **Fig. 2**B). In a simultaneous publication, Quivoron and colleagues[27] also found a similar phenotype in a gene-trap TET2 knockout model and a conditional TET2 knockout, where the final coding exon of TET2 was floxed (see **Fig. 2**).

Just after the initial 2 TET2 knockout mouse models were published, 2 additional reports using different models of TET2 deletion were published.[28,29] All 4 publications revealed a similar effect of TET2 loss on increased hematopoietic stem cell self-renewal and development of an MPN resembling human chronic myelomonocytic leukemia. To date, there is no evidence that TET2 loss in vivo results in development of myelofibrosis in mice.[26]

Three of the 4 TET2 knockout mouse studies have revealed a clear linkage between loss of TET2 and decreased hmC in vivo.[27–29] The effect of TET2 loss on 5mC in patients however has yet to be clarified, and the genetic targets of TET2 loss are not yet well understood.

DISCOVERY OF ASXL1 MUTATIONS

Within the same year as discovery of TET2 mutations in myeloid cancers, mutations were identified in another putative epigenetic modifier in myeloid malignancies, Additional sex combs like 1 (ASXL1). Mutations in ASXL1 were originally identified based on aCGH studies of MDS samples.[30] Gelsi-Boyer and colleagues[30–32] performed Agilent 244K CGH arrays on patients with MDS and noticed deletions in one patient at 20q11. In this particular patient, the 20q deletions involved only 2 possible genes: ASXL1 and DNMT3B. Sequencing efforts of both genes followed and mutations in ASXL1 were found in 4 of 35 MDS patients (11%). Further sequencing of ASXL1 has delineated the frequency of ASXL1 mutations in MPNs and other myeloid disorders (see **Table 1**). From these studies, ASXL1 is most commonly mutated amongst MPN patients with PMF and post-PV/ET MF compared with PV or ET. This is in contrast to mutations in TET2, which appear to be somewhat evenly distributed in PV/ET compared with myelofibrosis (see **Table 1**).

BIOLOGIC ROLE OF ASXL1 IN HEMATOPOIESIS

ASXL1 is the human homologue of Drosophila Additional sex combs (Asx). Asx deletion results in a homeotic phenotype characteristic of Polycomb (PcG) and Trithorax

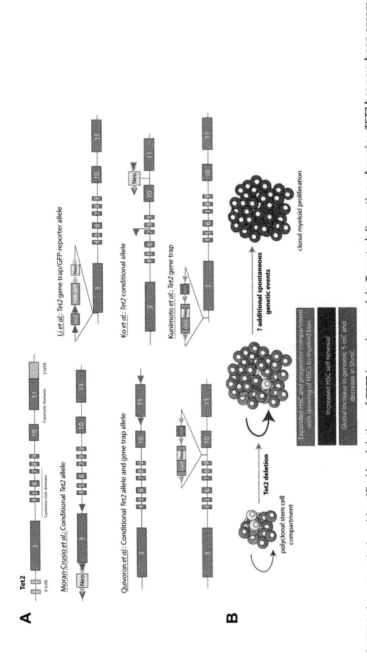

Fig. 2. The role of TET2 in hematopoiesis as identified by deletion of *TET2* in murine models. Targeted disruption of murine *TET2* has now been accomplished by deletion of *TET2* in murine models. Targeted disruption of murine *TET2* has now been accomplished using at least 6 different constructs each targeting *TET2* in a different location and manner (A). This includes conditional deletion of TET2 by targeting the first coding exon (as done by Moran-Crusio and colleagues[26]), the last coding exon encoding the enzymatic function of TET2 (as done by Quivoron and colleagues[27]), or the exons 8–10 (as done by Ko and colleagues[29]). Several groups have also studied mice with germline deletion of TET2 as accomplished by several different gene-trap constructs (A). Nearly all of these models have revealed that deletion of *TET2*, whether in a conditional, hematopoietic-specific manner or in the germline, results in expansion of the hematopoietic-stem progenitor compartment and increased hematopoietic stem cell self-renewal shortly after deletion (B). Overt myeloproliferation is also evident following TET2 deletion in vivo but with a latency of at least 3 to 6 months, suggesting the acquisition of additional collaborating events are required for disease initiation and progression in vivo.

group (TxG) gene deletions,[33] which led to the hypothesis that *Asx* has dual functions in silencing and activation of homeotic gene expression. In addition, functional studies in *Drosophila* suggest that *Asx* encodes a chromatin-associated protein with similarities to PcG proteins.[34] The mechanisms by which *ASXL1* mutations contribute to myeloid transformation have not been delineated. A series of in vitro studies in nonhematopoietic cells have suggested a variety of activities for ASXL1, including physical cooperativity with HP1a and LSD1 to repress retinoic acid-receptor activity and interaction with peroxisome proliferator—activated receptor gamma to suppress lipogenesis (**Fig. 3**).[35–37]

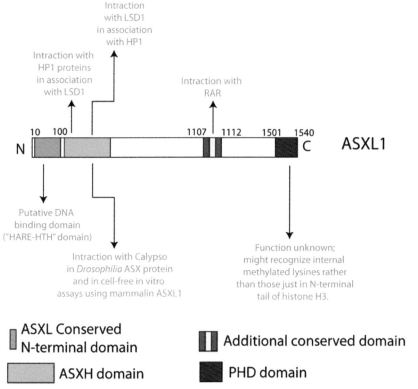

Fig. 3. Conserved domains of mammalian ASXL proteins and possible functions of ASXL1. ASXL1 contains a globular N-terminal domain that is conserved amongst ASX proteins and contains a potential DNA-binding motif based on homology with other proteins of known function. This domain has been referred to as a HARE-HTH domain (*H*B1, *A*SXL1, *r*estriction *e*ndonuclease *h*elix-turn *h*elix domain). Just distal to this domain is a domain that has been shown to bind Calypso (the mammalian homologue of BAP1) and serve as a deubiquitinase for histone H2A lysine 119. This activity has been shown in vivo in *Drosophila* and in cell-free assays using human ASXL1 purified protein. This same domain has also been suggested to bind to HP1 proteins and LSD1 (this activity has never been studied in a hematopoietic context). Distal to these domains lies a conserved domain, which has been suggested to physically interact with the retinoic acid receptor (another activity that has never been verified in hematopoietic cells). Finally, a plant homeo finger domain (PHD domain) lies at the extreme C-terminus of all ASXL proteins. The function of this PHD domain has not yet been identified.

All 3 *ASXL* family members are characterized by an amino-terminal homology domain and a C-terminal plant homeodomain (PHD domain) (see **Fig. 3**).[35,38,39] Recent bioinformatic analysis of the conserved domains of mammalian ASXL proteins has suggested that the N-terminal domain of *ASXL1* (amino acids 10–100) might represent a unique DNA binding motif, termed a HARE-HTH domain (*H*B1, *A*SXL1, *r*estriction *e*ndonuclease *h*elix-*t*urn *h*elix domain) (see **Fig. 3**).[40] In addition, based on comparative analysis with other PHD-domain containing proteins, the PHD domain of ASXL proteins appeared unique and was predicted to potentially recognize internal methylated lysines on histone H3 tails as opposed to lysines on the N-terminal tail of histone H3. Further functional investigations of these domains are needed to understand the role of these domains of ASXL1.

Drosophila Asx forms a complex with the chromatin deubiquitinase Calypso, which constitutes the Polycomb-repressive deubiquitinase (PR-DUB) complex. The PR-DUB complex removes monoubiquitin from histone H2A at lysine 119 (see **Fig. 3**). The mammalian homologue of Calypso, BAP1, directly associates with ASXL1, and the mammalian BAP1-ASXL1 complex was shown to possess deubiquitinase activity in vitro.[41]

The function of ASXL1 in hematopoiesis has not yet been fully delineated. A gene-trap hypomorphic mouse model of ASXL1 has been reported; however, this germline allele results in significant perinatal lethality. A small number of surviving mice were analyzed for an overt, short-latency hematopoietic phenotype. This model, created by Fisher and colleagues,[39] placed a PGK promoter-drive neomycin expression cassette into exon 5 of *ASXL1* interrupting the reading frame of *ASXL1* (this allele is referred to as *Asxl1*^{tm1BC}), which is predicted to lead to expression of a truncated protein lacking the nuclear interacting domains as well as the PHD domain. However, mice homozygous for this allele (*Asxl1*$^{tm1BC/tm1BC}$) did neither develop any overt hematologic malignancy in the first few months of age nor did they observe defects in the number of multipotent progenitors. The homozygous *Asxl1*$^{tm1BC/tm1BC}$ allele in this study was associated with approximately 75% perinatal lethality, and when the mice were backcrossed to a full C57BL/6J background, complete embryonic lethality was observed. Thus, further investigation of the function of ASXL1 in hematopoiesis using a conditional knockout model for postnatal and hematopoietic-specific deletion is of importance to the field.

CLINICAL IMPORTANCE OF *ASXL1* AND *TET2* MUTATIONS IN MPN PATIENTS

In contrast to the detailed clinical correlative studies of the effects of the *TET2* and *ASXL1* mutations on survival and response to therapy amongst patients with AML and MDS, comparatively fewer and smaller studies have been published thus far in MPN patients. Amongst patients with MPNs, *ASXL1* mutations are enriched amongst patients with more advanced age as well as in patients with PMF and post-PV/ET MF compared with PV or ET (see **Table 1**).[14,31,42] Brecqueville and colleagues[43] have recently reported that *ASXL1* mutant PMF patients have a significantly worsened overall survival compared with their wild-type counterparts. However, this was a modest study with 9 *ASXL1* mutant patients versus 35 wild-type patients and requires detailed study in much larger patient cohorts.

So far, few clear clinical associations or correlates have been identified for *TET2* mutant MPN patients compared with wild-type counterparts. *TET2* mutations cluster roughly equally amongst patients with classic MPNs (see **Table 1**).[16] The largest study of the clinical impact of *TET2* mutations on outcome amongst MPN patients was performed by Tefferi and colleagues[16,44] who did not identify an impact of

TET2 mutations on survival or leukemic transformation in a cohort of 89 PV patients and 60 PMF patients. *TET2* mutations were significantly associated with the development of hemoglobin less than 10 g/dL in patients with PMF.

From the current literature, neither mutations in *TET2* nor those in *ASXL1* appear to increase the risk of developing leukemic transformation in patients with chronic phase MPNs.[14,45] However, reports from 4 groups have identified that a substantial subset of MPN patients who transform to AML acquire *TET2* mutations in the leukemic state, whereas *TET2* mutations were not present in the MPN state.[12,13,18,45] In contrast, analysis of paired samples from the chronic and leukemic state has revealed that *ASXL1* mutations are not enriched in the leukemic state compared with the MPN phase of disease.[14] These data suggest that mutations in *ASXL1* may be critical for MPN initiation and may represent an early event in the clonal evolution of MPNs, in contrast for the more pleiotropic role of *TET2* mutations in MPN initiation and progression.

SUMMARY

The identification and characterization of mutations in *TET2* and *ASXL1* have provided important insights into the pathogenesis of MPNs and cancer biology in general. Mutations in *TET2* have been recently discovered to be important components in the dynamic regulation of DNA methylation and appear to be valuable biomarkers in prognostication of patients with normal karyotype AML.[46,47] Likewise, mutations in *ASXL1* predict for worsened outcome in MDS patients,[48] even in the absence of currently clinically used clinical outcome predictors. Despite these important insights, many unresolved questions regarding the biologic and clinical importance of these alterations still exist. For example, the prognostic importance of mutations in *TET2* and *ASXL1* in MPN patients is not clear. Given the relative rarity of these mutations in many chronic phase MPN patients, larger sequencing studies with comprehensive mutational data and pristine clinical annotation are urgently needed. Moreover, further functional studies to understand the effects of these alterations in combination with *JAK2* and *MPL* mutations are needed to better understand the biologic contribution of these alterations to MPN phenotype, outcome, and therapeutic response. Lastly, in vitro and in vivo studies in model systems and patient cohorts are needed to address the impact of mutations in epigenetic modifiers on the response to MPN therapies, including hydroxyurea, interferon, and JAK2-targeted therapy.

REFERENCES

1. Dameshek W. Some speculations on the myeloproliferative syndromes. Blood 1951;6(4):372–5.
2. Baxter EJ, Scott LM, Campbell PJ, et al. Acquired mutation of the tyrosine kinase JAK2 in human myeloproliferative disorders. Lancet 2005;365(9464):1054–61.
3. James C, Ugo V, Le Couedic JP, et al. A unique clonal JAK2 mutation leading to constitutive signalling causes polycythaemia vera. Nature 2005;434(7037): 1144–8.
4. Kralovics R, Passamonti F, Buser AS, et al. A gain-of-function mutation of JAK2 in myeloproliferative disorders. N Engl J Med 2005;352(17):1779–90.
5. Levine RL, Wadleigh M, Cools J, et al. Activating mutation in the tyrosine kinase JAK2 in polycythemia vera, essential thrombocythemia, and myeloid metaplasia with myelofibrosis. Cancer Cell 2005;7(4):387–97.
6. Scott LM, Tong W, Levine RL, et al. JAK2 exon 12 mutations in polycythemia vera and idiopathic erythrocytosis. N Engl J Med 2007;356(5):459–68.

7. Pikman Y, Lee BH, Mercher T, et al. MPLW515L is a novel somatic activating mutation in myelofibrosis with myeloid metaplasia. PLoS Med 2006;3(7):e270.

8. Pardanani A, Lasho T, Finke C, et al. LNK mutation studies in blast-phase myelo-proliferative neoplasms, and in chronic-phase disease with TET2, IDH, JAK2 or MPL mutations. Leukemia 2010;24(10):1713–8.

9. Oh ST, Simonds EF, Jones C, et al. Novel mutations in the inhibitory adaptor protein LNK drive JAK-STAT signaling in patients with myeloproliferative neoplasms. Blood 2010;116(6):988–92.

10. Kralovics R, Stockton DW, Prchal JT. Clonal hematopoiesis in familial polycy-themia vera suggests the involvement of multiple mutational events in the early pathogenesis of the disease. Blood 2003;102(10):3793–6.

11. Beer PA, Jones AV, Bench AJ, et al. Clonal diversity in the myeloproliferative neoplasms: independent origins of genetically distinct clones. Br J Haematol 2009;144(6):904–8.

12. Campbell PJ, Baxter EJ, Beer PA, et al. Mutation of JAK2 in the myeloproliferative disorders: timing, clonality studies, cytogenetic associations, and role in leukemic transformation. Blood 2006;108(10):3548–55.

13. Theocharides A, Boissinot M, Girodon F, et al. Leukemic blasts in transformed JAK2-V617F-positive myeloproliferative disorders are frequently negative for the JAK2-V617F mutation. Blood 2007;110(1):375–9.

14. Abdel-Wahab O, Manshouri T, Patel J, et al. Genetic analysis of transforming events that convert chronic myeloproliferative neoplasms to leukemias. Cancer Res 2010;70(2):447–52.

15. Langemeijer SM, Kuiper RP, Berends M, et al. Acquired mutations in TET2 are common in myelodysplastic syndromes. Nat Genet 2009;41(7):838–42.

16. Tefferi A, Pardanani A, Lim KH, et al. TET2 mutations and their clinical correlates in polycythemia vera, essential thrombocythemia and myelofibrosis. Leukemia 2009;23(5):905–11.

17. Abdel-Wahab O, Mullally A, Hedvat C, et al. Genetic characterization of TET1, TET2, and TET3 alterations in myeloid malignancies. Blood 2009;114(1):144–7.

18. Couronne L, Lippert E, Andrieux J, et al. Analyses of TET2 mutations in post-myeloproliferative neoplasm acute myeloid leukemias. Leukemia 2010;24(1):201–3.

19. Jankowska AM, Szpurka H, Tiu RV, et al. Loss of heterozygosity 4q24 and TET2 mutations associated with myelodysplastic/myeloproliferative neoplasms. Blood 2009;113(25):6403–10.

20. Tefferi A, Levine RL, Lim KH, et al. Frequent TET2 mutations in systemic masto-cytosis: clinical, KITD816V and FIP1L1-PDGFRA correlates. Leukemia 2009;23(5):900–4.

21. Tefferi A, Lim KH, Abdel-Wahab O, et al. Detection of mutant TET2 in myeloid malignancies other than myeloproliferative neoplasms: CMML, MDS, MDS/MPN and AML. Leukemia 2009;23(7):1343–5.

22. Lorsbach RB, Moore J, Mathew S, et al. TET1, a member of a novel protein family, is fused to MLL in acute myeloid leukemia containing the t(10;11)(q22;q23). Leukemia 2003;17(3):637–41.

23. Tahiliani M, Koh KP, Shen Y, et al. Conversion of 5-methylcytosine to 5-hydroxy-methylcytosine in mammalian DNA by MLL partner TET1. Science 2009;324(5929):930–5.

24. Iyer LM, Tahiliani M, Rao A, et al. Prediction of novel families of enzymes involved in oxidative and other complex modifications of bases in nucleic acids. Cell Cycle 2009;8(11):1698–710.

25. Ito S, Shen L, Dai Q, et al. Tet proteins can convert 5-methylcytosine to 5-formyl-cytosine and 5-carboxylcytosine. Science 2011;333(6047):13003.

26. Moran-Crusio K, Reavie L, Shih A, et al. Tet2 loss leads to increased hematopoi-etic stem cell self-renewal and myeloid transformation. Cancer Cell 2011;20(1):11–24.

27. Quivoron C, Couronne L, Della Valle V, et al. TET2 inactivation results in pleio-tropic hematopoietic abnormalities in mouse and is a recurrent event during human lymphomagenesis. Cancer Cell 2011;20(1):25–38.

28. Li Z, Cai X, Cai C, et al. Deletion of Tet2 in mice leads to dysregulated hemato-poietic stem cells and subsequent development of myeloid malignancies. Blood 2011;118(17):4509–18.

29. Ko M, Bandukwala HS, An J, et al. Ten-Eleven-Translocation 2 (TET2) negatively regulates homeostasis and differentiation of hematopoietic stem cells in mice. Proc Natl Acad Sci U S A 2011;108(35):14566–71.

30. Gelsi-Boyer V, Trouplin V, Adelaide J, et al. Mutations of polycomb-associated gene ASXL1 in myelodysplastic syndromes and chronic myelomonocytic leukaemia. Br J Haematol 2009;145(6):788–800.

31. Carbuccia N, Murati A, Trouplin V, et al. Mutations of ASXL1 gene in myeloprolif-erative neoplasms. Leukemia 2009;23(11):2183–6.

32. Carbuccia N, Trouplin V, Gelsi-Boyer V, et al. Mutual exclusion of ASXL1 and NPM1 mutations in a series of acute myeloid leukemias. Leukemia 2010;24(2):469–73.

33. Gaebler C, Stanzl-Tschegg S, Heinze G, et al. Fatigue strength of locking screws and prototypes used in small-diameter tibial nails: a biomechanical study. J Trauma 1999;47(2):379–84.

34. Sinclair DA, Milne TA, Hodgson JW, et al. The Additional sex combs gene of Drosophila encodes a chromatin protein that binds to shared and unique Polycomb group sites on polytene chromosomes. Development 1998;125(7):1207–16.

35. Cho YS, Kim EJ, Park UH, et al. Additional sex comb-like 1 (ASXL1), in cooper-ation with SRC-1, acts as a ligand-dependent coactivator for retinoic acid receptor. J Biol Chem 2006;281(26):17588–98.

36. Lee SW, Cho YS, Na JM, et al. ASXL1 represses retinoic acid receptor-mediated transcription through associating with HP1 and LSD1. J Biol Chem 2010;285(1):18–29.

37. Park UH, Yoon SK, Park T, et al. Additional sex comb-like (ASXL) proteins 1 and 2 play opposite roles in adipogenesis via reciprocal regulation of per-oxisome proliferator-activated receptor {gamma}. J Biol Chem 2011;286(2):1354–63.

38. Fisher CL, Lee I, Bloyer S, et al. Additional sex combs-like 1 belongs to the enhancer of trithorax and polycomb group and genetically interacts with Cbx2 in mice. Dev Biol 2010;337(1):9–15.

39. Fisher CL, Pineault N, Brookes C, et al. Loss-of-function Additional sex combs-like1 mutations disrupt hematopoiesis but do not cause severe myelodysplasia or leukemia. Blood 2010;115(1):38–46.

40. Aravind L, Iyer LM. The HARE-HTH and associated domains: novel modules in the coordination of epigenetic DNA and protein modifications. Cell Cycle 2012;11(1):119–31.

41. Scheuermann JC, de Ayala Alonso AG, Oktaba K, et al. Histone H2A deubiquiti-nase activity of the Polycomb repressive complex PR-DUB. Nature 2010;465(7295):243–7.

42. Abdel-Wahab O, Pardanani A, Patel J, et al. Concomitant analysis of EZH2 and ASXL1 mutations in myelofibrosis, chronic myelomonocytic leukemia and blast-phase myeloproliferative neoplasms. Leukemia 2011;25(7):1200–2.
43. Brecqueville M, Rey J, Bertucci F, et al. Mutation analysis of ASXL1, CBL, DNMT3A, IDH1, IDH2, JAK2, MPL, NF1, SF3B1, SUZ12, and TET2 in myeloproliferative neoplasms. Genes Chromosomes Cancer 2012;51(8):743–55.
44. Delhommeau F, Dupont S, Della Valle V, et al. Mutation in TET2 in myeloid cancers. N Engl J Med 2009;360(22):2289–301.
45. Beer PA, Delhommeau F, Lecouedic JP, et al. Two routes to leukemic transformation following a JAK2 mutation-positive myeloproliferative neoplasm. Blood 2010; 115(14):2891–900.
46. Metzeler KH, Becker H, Maharry K, et al. ASXL1 mutations identify a high-risk subgroup of older patients with primary cytogenetically normal AML within the ELN Favorable genetic category. Blood 2011;118(26):6920–9.
47. Patel JP, Gonen M, Figueroa ME, et al. Prognostic relevance of integrated genetic profiling in acute myeloid leukemia. N Engl J Med 2012;366(12):1079–89.
48. Bejar R, Stevenson K, Abdel-Wahab O, et al. Clinical effect of point mutations in myelodysplastic syndromes. N Engl J Med 2011;364(26):2496–506.

Myeloproliferative Neoplasm Animal Models

Ann Mullally, MD[a], Steven W. Lane, MD[b], Kristina Brumme, BA[a],
Benjamin L. Ebert, MD, PhD[a],*

KEYWORDS

- Myeloproliferative neoplasms • Preclinical murine models • BCR-ABL • JAK2V617F
- Hematopoietic stem cells • Bone marrow microenvironment • Myelofibrosis
- Oncogenes

KEY POINTS

- Retroviral transduction of *BCR-ABL* into murine bone marrow cells followed by transplantation into irradiated syngeneic mice established the field of myeloproliferative neoplasm (MPN) animal modeling.
- The effects of the *JAK2V617F* mutation in hematopoietic cells has been extensively modeled in vivo using retroviral, transgenic, knock-in, and xenograft murine models.
- The considerable phenotypic differences observed between broadly similar *JAK2V617F* murine models highlights the inherent variability in murine models that can occur as a result of multiple factors, such as promoter, oncogene expression level, murine versus human protein, and mouse strain.
- Mutant oncogenes found in human acute myelogenous leukemia (AML), such as *RAS* and *FLT3*, induce MPNs in mice, indicating that these genetic lesions are insufficient to cause AML and suggesting that additional cooperating genetic events are required for AML development.
- As the increasing genetic complexity of MPNs has become apparent, additional genetic models have been developed to investigate the functional effects and therapeutic susceptibilities of compound genetic lesions in MPNs.

INTRODUCTION

Animal models have been used extensively in the study of myeloproliferative neoplasms (MPNs) and have played a key role in advancing the biologic understanding of these diseases (**Boxes 1–3**). In general, these models have faithfully recapitulated human MPNs in mice, enabled detailed characterization of the effects of specific MPN-associated genetic abnormalities on the hematopoietic stem and progenitor

[a] Division of Hematology, Department of Medicine, Brigham and Women's Hospital, Harvard Medical School, Boston, MA 02115, USA; [b] Queensland Institute of Medical Research, Brisbane 4006, Australia
* Corresponding author. 1 Blackfan Circle, Karp Building 5.210, Boston, MA 02115.
E-mail address: bebert@partners.org

Hematol Oncol Clin N Am 26 (2012) 1065–1081
http://dx.doi.org/10.1016/j.hoc.2012.07.007   hemonc.theclinics.com
0889-8588/12/$ – see front matter © 2012 Elsevier Inc. All rights reserved.

Box 1
Retroviral bone marrow transplant murine MPN models

In the retroviral bone marrow transplantation (BMT) assay, bone marrow is harvested from donor mice that have been stimulated with 5-fluorouracil (5-FU). The 5-FU–stimulated bone marrow cells are then transduced ex vivo with a retroviral construct expressing the gene of interest. This results in stable but random integration of the transgene into the host cell genome. The transduced cells are then transplanted into irradiated syngeneic mice, where hematopoietic reconstitution is polyclonal. Transgene expression is generally high (nonphysiologic), and differences in the site of retroviral integration may result in variation in transgene expression level. Because retroviruses preferentially transduce mitotically active cells, quiescent long-term hematopoietic stem cells (LT-HSCs) are relatively resistant to retroviral integration.

---

cell (HSPC) compartment, and provided excellent in vivo models for testing novel MPN therapeutic agents. In this review, the authors focus primarily on murine models of the *JAK2V617F* mutation and on the insights these have provided, and also briefly outline the central role *BCR-ABL* models played in establishing and developing the field. Models of additional genetic lesions found in human MPNs are discussed, and genetic models that induce an MPN phenotype in mice are outlined. The authors describe the use of *JAK2V617F* models in the preclinical development of janus kinase 2 (JAK2) inhibitors and other MPN therapies. Studies of the bone marrow microenvironment that have been performed using MPN models are summarized, and some thoughts are provided as to how MPN animal models might be used in the future.

MPN MURINE MODELS
BCR-ABL

The faithful modeling of human MPNs in mice began in 1990 with the demonstration that retroviral transduction of *BCR-ABL* into murine bone marrow cells, followed by transplantation into irradiated syngeneic mice, recapitulated human chronic

---

Box 2
Genetically engineered murine MPN models

Genetically engineered murine models can be classified as transgenic or endogenous. Transgenic mice express the gene of interest under the control of ectopic promoter and enhancer elements. They are generated by pronuclear injection of the transgene into a single cell of a mouse embryo, in which it randomly integrates into the mouse genome. Knock-in mice express the gene of interest from their native promoters and thus represent endogenous genetically engineered mice. They are generated through the modification of embryonic stem (ES) cells using a DNA construct that contains sequences homologous to the target gene. The relevant mutation is thus introduced to the gene of interest under the control of its endogenous promoter via homologous recombination in ES cells. Conditional knock-in mice use site-specific recombinases, such as Cre, to control the timing and tissue-specificity of gene expression. Inducible transgenic and knock-in models use exogenous ligands (eg, doxycycline or interferon) to reversibly control the timing of target-gene expression. In general, transgenic models result in overexpression of the gene of interest through the use of exogenous promoters, whereas expression is at physiologic levels in knock-in models, in which the gene of interest is expressed from its endogenous promoter. Knock-out mice are genetically engineered mice, in which the gene of interest is inactivated by replacing it or disrupting it with an artificial piece of DNA. This is achieved in ES cells via homologous recombination. Because germline homozygous gene deletions can be embryonically lethal, conditional knock-out mice are often generated to circumvent this problem.

Box 3
Xenograft murine MPN models

In xenograft murine MPN models, human MPN CD34+ cells are transplanted and propagated in immunodeficient mice. To achieve engraftment, investigators have used NOD/SCID (nonobese diabetic/severe combined immunodeficiency) mice absolutely deficient in B and T cells and having impaired natural killer cell function.[1,2] Further impairment of the murine immune system has been achieved by depletion of natural killer cells using CD122 antibodies[3] or by crossing with a mouse strain deficient for the common gamma chain of the interleukin (IL)-2 receptor[4] (NSG mice). Although these models allow the study of primary human MPN cells in vivo, some aspects of the bone marrow microenvironment are not recapitulated because of the absence of immune cells and species incompatibility for some cytokines and cytokine receptors.

---

myelogenous leukemia (CML) in mice.[5,6] These groundbreaking experiments established the retroviral BMT assay and, with it, the ability to accurately model human hematologic malignancies in mice.

Retroviral

The retroviral *BCR-ABL* model has provided several important insights into the molecular pathophysiology of CML. These include the demonstration that BCR-ABL expression in vivo is sufficient to induce CML,[5,6] the identification of key *BCR-ABL* activated downstream signaling pathways in CML stem cells,[7] and the provision of an accurate preclinical model that continues to be used in the evaluation of novel CML therapeutics.[8]

Transgenic

Several *BCR-ABL* transgenic models have been developed and used primarily to investigate the kinetics and therapeutic susceptibilities of CML-propagating stem cells. Here, we discuss 2 models that have been particularly informative in this regard. Perez-Caro and colleagues[9] generated transgenic mice that expressed BCR-ABL under the control of the *Sca-1* promoter, thus restricting transgene expression to the Sca-1–positive cell population, which includes HSCs. The mice developed a CML-like disease characterized by neutrophilia and hepatosplenomegaly as a result of extramedullary hematopoiesis, with most animals progressing to blast crisis. A subset of mice developed additional solid tumors, indicating that *Sca-1*–driven BCR-ABL expression is not restricted to hematopoietic cells. The course of the CML-like disease was not modified by treatment with imatinib, suggesting that the HSC compartment in CML is insensitive to ABL kinase inhibition.

Koschmieder and colleagues[10] developed an inducible *BCR-ABL* transgenic model in which the tetracycline transactivator protein was placed under the control of the murine stem cell leukemia (*SCL*) gene 3′ enhancer, and double transgenic *SCL*–tetracycline transactivator protein/*BCR-ABL* mice were generated. With tetracycline withdrawal, BCR-ABL expression was induced in the HSPC compartment. These mice developed a CML-like disease that is reversible and reinducible, suggesting that sustained BCR-ABL expression is required for the development of a CML disease phenotype.[10] The CML-initiating cell population was found to be present in the lineage^low^Sca1+Kit^high^ (LSK) compartment,[11] and more recently, this population has been further refined and shown to be present solely in the most immature LT-HSC compartment.[12,13] *BCR-ABL*–positive LT-HSCs outcompete normal LT-HSCs and aberrantly mobilize to the spleen in this model.[12,13] Finally, CML-propagating stem cells have been found to be resistant to treatment with imatinib alone,[11] whereas the combination of imatinib with histone deacetylase inhibitors seems to mitigate some of this resistance, in this *BCR-ABL*–inducible murine model.[14]

Xenograft

Xenograft models of chronic-phase CML have been problematic in that most SCID-repopulating cells are *BCR-ABL* negative,[15] a finding thought to relate, at least in part, to the presence of a reservoir of normal HSCs in chronic-phase CML. These findings suggest that *BCR-ABL*–positive SCID-repopulating cells (SRCs) from chronic-phase CML do not have a proliferative advantage over wild-type SRCs. A major caveat of these experiments is the incompatibilities between cytokine receptors on human cells and cytokines produced by a murine microenvironment. Transplanting *BCR-ABL*–positive cells taken from long-term culture-initiating cell assays results in more durable leukemic cell engraftment in NOD/SCID mice,[16] as does the transplantation of cells from patients with CML in accelerated or blast phase.[17]

JAK2V617F

JAK2V617F is the most common molecular abnormality in *BCR-ABL*–negative MPNs, and it has been extensively studied in vivo using retroviral, transgenic, knock-in, and xenograft murine models. In general, these models reliably recapitulate the clinical features of human MPNs in mice (**Figs. 1** and **2**, **Table 1**), and they have helped advance the biologic understanding of *JAK2V617F*-mediated MPNs in humans.

Retroviral

Immediately following the discovery of the *JAK2V617F* mutation, retroviral models were generated to assess the phenotypic effects of JAK2V167F in vivo.[18–22] Mice transplanted with JAK2V617F expressing donor bone marrow developed striking polycythemia after a short latency with a high degree of penetrance. Leukocytosis,

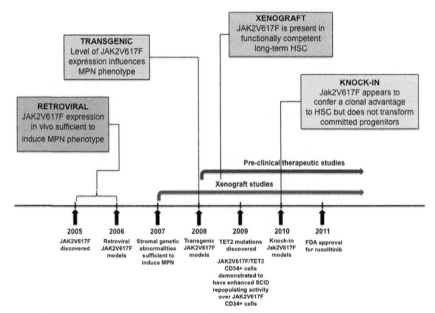

Fig. 1. Timeline for development of *JAK2V617F* murine models. FDA, Food and Drug Administration.

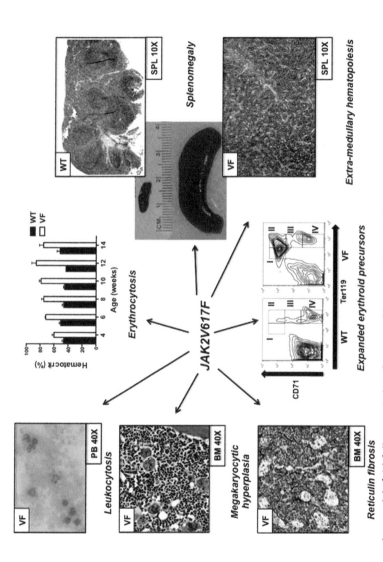

Fig. 2. JAK2V617F murine models faithfully recapitulate features of human MPN. MPN features common to most retroviral and genetic *JAK2V617F* models. WT, wild-type; VF, JAK2V617F; PB, peripheral blood; BM, bone marrow; SPL, spleen. (*Data from* Mullally A, Lane SW, Ball B, et al. Physiologic Jak2V617F expression causes a lethal myeloproliferative neoplasm with differential effects on hematopoietic stem and progenitor cells. Cancer Cell 2010;17(6):584–96.)

Table 1
Jak2V617F knock-in murine MPN models

First Author	JAK2 Origin	Strain	Type	VF:WT Expression	Homozygotes	Phenotype	Myelofibrosis
Akada[26]	Mouse	129Sv/C57Bl/6	Conditional	<1:1	Yes	PV-like	Yes
Marty[27]	Mouse	129Sv/C57Bl/6	Constitutive	~1:1	No	PV-like	Yes
Mullally[28,31]	Mouse	129Sv/C57Bl/6	Conditional	<1:1	No	PV-like	Yes, with BMT
Li[29]	Human	129Sv/C57Bl/6	Conditional	~1:1	No	ET-like	No

splenomegaly resulting from extramedullary hematopoiesis, and the development of myelofibrosis were also seen. All groups observed constitutive activation of Jak2 kinase signaling and Stat5 phosphorylation in addition to cytokine-independent colony formation. These models demonstrated that JAK2V617F expression in vivo was sufficient to induce an MPN phenotype and indicated that genetic modifiers of *JAK2V617F*-mediated fibrosis exist (more prominent fibrosis was seen in the Balb/c strain compared with C57Bl/6 strain).[19]

Transgenic

Three groups generated transgenic *JAK2V617F* models in 2008, with the main goal of correlating disease phenotype with differences in *JAK2V617F* gene dosage.[23–25] Tiedt and colleagues[23] conditionally expressed human JAK2V617F from the endogenous human *JAK2* promoter and crossed with Vav-Cre or Mx1-Cre transgenic mice to induce hematopoietic specific JAK2V617F expression. The ratio of human JAK2V617F to murine wild-type Jak2 expression was quantified in mRNA. Xing and colleagues[24] expressed human JAK2V617F from the Vav promoter, whereas Shide and colleagues[25] expressed murine Jak2V617F from the H-2Kb promoter.

In the model of Tiedt and colleagues,[23] JAK2V617F Vav-Cre mice had constitutive and sustained Cre expression, low transgene copy number, and a *JAK2* mutant–to–wild-type ratio of approximately 0.5. In JAK2V617F MxCre mice, Cre expression was induced following treatment with polyinosinic:polycytidylic acid (pI:pC) to activate the interferon response. Transgene copy number was higher than in JAK2V617F Vav-Cre animals and the *JAK2* mutant–to–wild-type mRNA ratio was approximately 1.0. The lower copy number in Vav-Cre compared with MxCre was attributed to sustained Cre expression in the Vav-Cre model, leading to more efficient deletion of additional transgene copies. The phenotype of *JAK2V617F* Vav-Cre mice was more consistent with essential thrombocythemia (ET) (high platelets, normal white blood cell count, and hemoglobin), whereas the phenotype *JAK2V617F* MxCre animals more closely recapitulated polycythemia vera (PV) (elevated hemoglobin with suppressed erythropoietin, high white blood cell count and high platelets). In the model of Xing and colleagues, the level of mutant JAK2 expression was extremely low and the phenotype most consistent with ET.[24] In the model of Shide and colleagues,[25] the MPN was incompletely penetrant in the founder line in which mutant Jak2 was expressed at a lower level than wild-type Jak2. In a second founder line in which mutant Jak2 expression was higher than wild-type Jak2, an MPN with myelofibrotic transformation developed.

The major conclusion to be drawn from the transgenic models is that the level of JAK2V617F expression influences the MPN phenotype, with the suggestion that lower JAK2V617F expression results in an ET phenotype and higher JAK2V617F expression gives rise to a PV phenotype.[23,24] However, some of the MPN phenotypic differences observed by Tiedt and colleagues[23] could be related to tissue-specific Cre effects (ie, Vav-Cre versus Mx1-Cre). JAK2V617F expression is driven by exogenous promoters in some of these transgenic models,[24,25] which could also influence the MPN phenotype.

Knock-in

Four *JAK2V617F* knock-in models were published in 2010.[26–29] These were generated with the major goals of (1) recapitulating human MPN through physiologic Jak2V617F expression, (2) assessing the impact of *Jak2V617F* gene dosage on disease phenotype, and (3) evaluating the effects of *Jak2V617F* on the HSPC compartment.

The models of Akada,[26] Marty,[27] and Mullally[28] and their colleagues all expressed murine Jak2V617F from the endogenous murine *Jak2* promoter but each in a slightly different manner. Akada and colleagues[26] and Mullally and colleagues[28] generated conditional *Jak2V617F* knock-in models, whereas Jak2V617F expression was constitutive in the model of Marty and colleagues.[27] Human JAK2V617F was conditionally expressed from the endogenous murine *Jak2* promoter in the model of Li and colleagues.[29] In all of the models, the ratio of mutant to wild-type Jak2 expression was 1:1 or less. The model of Akada and colleagues[26] was the only one in which homozygous *Jak2* mutant mice were generated, but because the Jak2 mutant allele expressed at approximately 50% of the wild-type allele, the level of Jak2V617F expression in homozygous mice was relatively low. A summary of the *Jak2V617F* knock-in models is outlined in **Table 1**, and a schematic representation of the targeting strategies for each of the models is given in a recent review by Li and colleagues.[30]

The phenotype of the 3 models that expressed murine Jak2V617F was broadly similar.[26–28] In each of these models, mice heterozygous for the Jak2V617F mutation had profound erythrocytosis, leukocytosis, splenomegaly caused by extramedullary hematopoiesis, and myelofibrosis that developed over time (although this was only observed in transplant recipients by Mullally and colleagues[31]). Compared with the other models, the hematologic phenotype was relatively mild in the model of Li and colleagues.[29] Only a modest increase in platelets and hemoglobin, more reminiscent of ET than of PV, was observed (erythropoietin levels were not suppressed), whereas approximately 10% mice developed marked erythrocytosis with prolonged follow-up. In this model, human JAK2V617F was expressed from the endogenous murine *Jak2* promoter, and whether human JAK2V617F signals differently in murine cells remains undetermined.

In all of the models, the MPN was transplantable into secondary recipients, indicating that the MPN is cell autonomous. The ability to transplant the disease enabled a functional analysis of the stem cell properties of Jak2V617F-expressing HSCs. Recent reports on this analysis suggest that *Jak2V617F* mutant HSCs have a clonal advantage over wild-type HSCs.[31–33] Mullally and colleagues found that *Jak2V617F* mutant HSCs have a subtle competitive repopulating advantage over normal HSCs,[28,31] whereas Marty and colleagues[32] and Lundberg and colleagues[33] recently described a stronger competitive advantage for *Jak2V617F* mutant HSCs in a knock-in model and a transgenic model, respectively. The HSC phenotype in the knock-in model of Li and colleagues[29] differs from that of the other researchers in that LSK cell numbers were reduced in JAK2V617F mice and demonstrated decreased cell cycle and increased senescence. In competitive repopulation experiments, *JAK2V617F* mutant HSCs were outcompeted by wild-type cells in primary BMT recipients as early as 5 weeks post transplantation, preventing transplantation of the MPN. It remains unclear whether this finding is related to expression of human JAK2V617F from the endogenous murine *Jak2* promoter or to another cause such as increased replicative stress or immunologic rejection. Finally, by transplanting sorted populations of progenitor cells, Mullally and colleagues[28] found that expanded Jak2V617F progenitor cell populations such as megakaryocytic erythroid progenitor cells are incapable of reconstituting MPN in a transplanted animal. These results are consistent with previously published reports indicating that oncogenic kinase alleles are incapable of transforming progenitor cells.[34,35]

The main conclusions from the Jak2V617F knock-in models are that (1) physiologic heterozygote expression of murine Jak2V617F in mice causes a polycythemia phenotype,[26–28] (2) the *Jak2V617F* mutation seems to provide a clonal advantage to HSCs,[31–33] and (3) Jak2V617F does not confer self-renewal properties to committed myeloid progenitor cells.[28] Although these models closely recapitulate human MPNs, some differences remain, including the fact that although Jak2V617F expression is driven by the endogenous *Jak2* promoter in these knock-in models, the mutant allele is expressed in all hematopoietic cells, instead of in an MPN clone as occurs in humans.[36] It is also important to note that reconstitution in competitive repopulation experiments is polyclonal and occurs in a bone marrow niche that has been perturbed by irradiation.

Xenograft

To study *BCR-ABL*–negative MPN cells in vivo, xenograft models have been generated. These models enable a functional assessment of the repopulating capacity of primary human MPN CD34$^+$ cells, which possess the full germline and somatic genotype of human MPNs.

Peripheral blood CD34$^+$ cells from patients with myelofibrosis engraft NOD/SCID mice and show clonal hematopoiesis with myeloid skewing.[1] Two independent groups have found relatively poor engraftment of *JAK2V617F* mutant CD34$^+$ cells from patients with PV and ET,[2,3] and the ratio of *JAK2V617F* to *JAK2* wild-type SRCs was found to be higher in myelofibrosis than in PV.[3] Functionally, *JAK2V617F* SRCs did not gain a proliferative advantage compared with wild-type SRCs over time.[3]

The major conclusions from these studies are that (1) *JAK2V617F* is found in a functionally competent LT-HSC population,[1–3] (2) the functional *JAK2V617F* LT-HSC compartment is expanded in myelofibrosis compared with PV,[3] and (3) poor *JAK2V617F* CD34$^+$ engraftment in xenografts may be related to down-regulation of chemokine receptor 4 (CXCR4).[37] Its important to note that incompatibilities between human cytokine receptors and murine cytokines in xenograft models may be particularly relevant in assessing the in vivo functional effects of the *JAK2V617F* allele, which activates cytokine receptor signaling. In general, reliable xenotransplantation across a wide spectrum of genetically diverse MPN requires further optimization.

MPLW515L

A somatic activating mutation in *MPL* (*MPLW515L*) was originally identified in *JAK2V617F*–negative myelofibrosis patients[38] and *MPLW515L* or *MPLW515K* mutations were subsequently found in approximately 5% and 1% of patients with myelofibrosis and ET, respectively.[39] In a retroviral BMT assay, *MPLW515L* induced an MPN in mice, characterized by leukocytosis, thrombocytosis, splenomegaly, and reticulin fibrosis.[38] This model has subsequently been used to provide preclinical evidence in support of the use of JAK2 kinase inhibitors in patients with MPN who carry the *MPLW515L* mutation.[40,41]

TET2

TET2 deletions and loss-of-function mutations occur in up to 12% of patients with MPN.[42,43] Initial studies by Delhommeau and colleagues[42] indicated that *TET2-JAK2V617F* co-mutated CD34$^+$ cells from patients with MPN show an increased capacity compared with *JAK2V617F*-mutated CD34$^+$ cells to repopulate NOD/SCID mice, suggesting that loss of *TET2* enhances HSC self-renewal. These findings have been validated with the publication by several groups of *Tet2* conditional knock-out mice, which demonstrate that *Tet2* null HSCs have a competitive repopulating advantage compared with wild-type HSCs.[44–47] Future studies will likely focus on murine modeling of compound mutants (eg, *Jak2V617F/Tet2*) to evaluate the impact of loss of *Tet2* on the MPN phenotype, on MPN-propagating stem cell function, and on the therapeutic susceptibilities of *Jak2V617F/Tet2* compound mutant hematopoietic cells.

LNK

Heterozygote loss-of-function mutations in the inhibitory adaptor protein *LNK* were originally reported in *JAK2* wild-type patients with MPN.[48] Overall, the frequency of *LNK* mutations in MPN is low, and although mutations in *LNK* have been reported in *JAK2V617F*–positive MPN, it is not known if both mutations occur in the same clone.[49] Knock-out mice for *Lnk* were generated before the identification of *LNK* mutations in MPNs; *Lnk* null mice exhibit an MPN phenotype (CML-like disease), whereas heterozygous *Lnk* mice have an intermediate disease phenotype.[50,51] Lnk negatively regulates Mpl through its SH2 domain. Consistent with this, *Lnk* null mice exhibit potentiation of Jak2 signaling in response to thrombopoietin, increased HSC quiescence, and decelerated HSC cell-cycle kinetics.[52] Lnk retains the ability to bind and inhibit Jak2V617F and, consistent with this, loss of Lnk exacerbates JAK2V617F-mediated MPN and accelerates the development of JAK2V617F-induced myelofibrosis, through the potentiation of JAK2V617F signaling.[51] These studies in *Lnk* null mice have provided important insights into the role of the thrombopoietin/Mpl/Jak2/Lnk pathway in regulating HSC self-renewal and quiescence and informed the understanding of MPN stem cell kinetics.

c-CBL

Mutations in *c-CBL* were identified in patients with myelofibrosis in a region of acquired uniparental disomy on chromosome 11q.[53] Most variants were missense substitutions in the RING or linker domains that abrogated CBL ubiquitin ligase activity.[53] These mutations were modeled in mice using retroviral overexpression in *c-Cbl* null cells and were demonstrated to further augment the enhanced cytokine sensitivity of *c-Cbl* null HSPCs, indicating a gain-of-function activity greater than that seen in *c-Cbl* null cells alone.[54] Subsequent *c-Cbl* mutant knock-in models have demonstrated that mutations in the *c-Cbl* RING finger domain (but not germline deletion of *c-Cbl*) cause loss of E3 ubiquitin ligase activity and an inability of c-Cbl to interact with target receptor tyrosine kinases, such as Flt3. This, in turn, causes activation of downstream signaling pathways and the development of an MPN in vivo, which is dependent on Flt3 signaling for the maintenance of disease.[55]

Other Genetic Lesions in MPNs

Other genetic lesions have been described in the epigenetic machinery in MPNs such as in *ASXL1*,[56] *EZH2*,[56,57] and *DNMT3A*.[58,59] *IDH1* and *IDH2* mutations have been identified at low frequency in MPNs.[60] Genetic murine models exist for some of these genetic abnormalities,[61,62] whereas others are in development.

Other MPN Animal Models

Additional murine models have an MPN phenotype, although they are driven by alleles that are not common, somatically mutated drivers of MPN in humans. These include the K-Ras^{G12D} knock-in model, in which oncogenic K-Ras was conditionally expressed from its endogenous murine promoter,[63,64] and the *FLT3* internal tandem duplication (ITD) knock-in model, in which an *FLT3*-ITD mutation was engineered into the *Flt3* locus and expressed from the endogenous murine *Flt3* promoter.[65,66] RAS and FLT3 are both recurrently mutated in human AML, but K-Ras^{G12D} and Flt3^{ITD} mice both develop MPNs, indicating that these genetic lesions alone are insufficient to induce AML. K-Ras^{G12D} mice develop an MPN characterized by leukocytosis, extramedullary hematopoiesis, and growth factor hypersensitivity, whereas Flt3^{ITD} mice develop MPNs reminiscent of human chronic myelomonocytic leukemia, with prominent monocytosis and splenomegaly.

The activator protein 1 transcription factor, JunB, is a transcriptional regulator of myelopoiesis and its expression is downregulated in AML.[67] Inactivation of *JunB* in postnatal mice results in LT-HSC expansion and an MPN resembling early CML.[68] Murine models of some of the genetic lesions found in human juvenile myelomonocytic leukemia have been developed, and these also result in an MPN phenotype in mice. Conditional deletion of *Nf1* and conditional activation of *Ptpn11*[D61Y] both induce an MPN characterized by leukocytosis and hypersensitivity to granulocyte-macrophage colony-stimulating factor.[69,70]

Each of these in vivo models has advanced the biologic understanding of these genetic abnormalities, particularly with respect to their effects on the HSPC compartment, and they continue to serve as useful preclinical models for testing novel pharmacologic agents.[71]

THE USE OF *JAK2V617F* MODELS IN THE PRECLINICAL DEVELOPMENT OF MPN THERAPIES

JAK2V617F and *MPLW515L* models have been used extensively in the preclinical development of MPN therapies. These studies have provided the following insights:

1. Provision of a "proof of concept" that JAK2 inhibitors could be safe and efficacious in the treatment of *JAK2V617F*-[72,73] and *MPLW515L*-mediated MPNs[40,41]
2. Demonstration that MPN-propagating stem cells are not effectively targeted with JAK2 inhibitor monotherapy[28]
3. Identification of heat shock protein 90 as a promising therapeutic target in *JAK2*-driven neoplasms[74,75]
4. Demonstration of the efficacy of the histone deacetylase inhibitor vorinostat for the treatment of *JAK2V617F*-mediated MPNs[76]
5. Indication that pharmacologic inhibition of STAT5 (if possible in patients with MPN) has the potential to be efficacious in treating *JAK2V617F*-mediated MPNs[77]

These insights have facilitated the clinical advancement of JAK2 kinase inhibitors, provided a rationale for clinical trials of heat shock protein 90 inhibitors in *JAK2*-driven cancers and offered supportive evidence for the use of histone deacetylase inhibitors in patients with MPN. No doubt, these models will continue to be used in the evaluation of future MPN therapies.

THE BONE MARROW MICROENVIRONMENT IN MPNS

The bone marrow microenvironment is perturbed in MPNs (at least in the late stages of the disease), sometimes to such an extent that myelofibrosis and bone marrow failure develop. Murine models in this area have helped advance understanding in 3 main areas:

1. Demonstration that genetic alterations in bone marrow stroma are sufficient to induce MPNs

In 2007, Walkley and colleagues showed in 2 separate genetic models that MPNs could be induced as a result of perturbation of the bone marrow microenvironment.[78,79] In the first model, germline deletion of the nuclear hormone receptor retinoic acid receptor γ resulted in an MPN that was tumor necrosis factor α (TNFα) mediated,[78] whereas in the second model, an MPN developed following conditional inactivation of the negative cell cycle regulator *Rb* in hematopoiesis using Mx1-Cre.[79] In both scenarios, the MPN could not be propagated into secondary recipients and could not be rescued by transplantation with wild-type HSCs, indicating that the disease phenotypes were cell extrinsic.

2. Investigation of the biologic mechanisms underlying myelofibrosis development

Before the advent of the *JAK2V617F* murine models, the main genetic models of myelofibrosis were GATA1^{low},[80] thrombopoietin (*THPO*) transgenic,[81] and Tri21 mice.[82] These models are all characterized by marked megakaryocytic hyperplasia, underpinning the central role of the megakaryocytic lineage in the development of a fibrosis phenotype. A retroviral *THPO* overexpression murine model of myelofibrosis[83] has facilitated the demonstration that transforming growth factor β1 is required,[84] whereas thrombospondin is redundant,[85] for THPO-induced myelofibrosis, and that osteoprotegerin is required for osteosclerotic transformation.[86] Although much data exist on the abnormal production of proinflammatory cytokines in patients with myelofibrosis, it is unclear which cytokines are the real drivers of fibrotic transformation in MPNs. Cytokine profiling has been performed in the retroviral *JAK2V617F* and *MPLW515L* models,[40,73] and further investigation of the specific contributions of individual cytokines to fibrotic transformation in *JAK2V617F*-mediated MPN will likely follow. There has been some heterogeneity in the fibrosis phenotype between the *Jak2V617F* knock-in models, which may be related to the level of Jak2V617F expression.

3. Investigation of cell nonautonomous contributions to clonal expansion in MPNs

A positive paracrine loop involving IL-6 was recently identified in a genetic model of CML, in which IL-6 produced by expanded CML myeloid cells was shown to act on leukemic multipotent progenitors and drive further myeloid expansion.[12] Using the same inducible transgenic *BCR-ABL* model, Zhang and colleagues[13] also recently demonstrated that altered cytokine expression (including that of IL-1, IL-6, and TNFα) in CML bone marrow was associated with selective impairment of normal LT-HSC growth and a growth advantage to CML LT-HSCs. In a retroviral *JAK2V617F* model, TNFα has been demonstrated to facilitate the preferential expansion of *JAK2V617F* mutant cells.[87] In aggregate, these studies indicate that differential microenvironmental regulation of HSPC populations in MPNs and normal bone marrow contributes to clonal expansion in MPNs.

SUMMARY

As the genetic landscape of MPNs has been defined, corresponding genetically engineered murine models have been developed. Going forward, mutations that co-occur in humans will be modeled in the mouse to investigate the functional effects and therapeutic susceptibilities of compound genetic lesions in MPNs. These models will also be useful in understanding the differential molecular dependencies and niche interactions of MPN-propagating stem cells and in studying fibrotic transformation in MPNs. Given the recent identification of a nuclear role for JAK2,[88] evaluation of the effects of noncanonical JAK2V617F signaling in vivo will be another important focus. These models will continue to be used in preclinical studies, particularly for the evaluation of combinatorial therapeutic strategies, aimed at targeting MPN-propagating stem cells and/or circumventing JAK2 kinase inhibitor resistance.

REFERENCES

1. Xu M, Bruno E, Chao J, et al. The constitutive mobilization of bone marrow-repopulating cells into the peripheral blood in idiopathic myelofibrosis. Blood 2005;105(4):1699–705.

2. Ishii T, Zhao Y, Sozer S, et al. Behavior of CD34+ cells isolated from patients with polycythemia vera in NOD/SCID mice. Exp Hematol 2007;35(11):1633–40.
3. James C, Mazurier F, Dupont S, et al. The hematopoietic stem cell compartment of JAK2V617F-positive myeloproliferative disorders is a reflection of disease heterogeneity. Blood 2008;112(6):2429–38.
4. Ishikawa F, Yasukawa M, Lyons B, et al. Development of functional human blood and immune systems in NOD/SCID/IL2 receptor {gamma} chain(null) mice. Blood 2005;106(5):1565–73.
5. Daley GQ, Van Etten RA, Baltimore D. Induction of chronic myelogenous leukemia in mice by the P210bcr/abl gene of the Philadelphia chromosome. Science 1990;247(4944):824–30.
6. Kelliher MA, McLaughlin J, Witte ON, et al. Induction of a chronic myelogenous leukemia-like syndrome in mice with v-abl and BCR/ABL. Proc Natl Acad Sci U S A 1990;87(17):6649–53.
7. Hu Y, Swerdlow S, Duffy TM, et al. Targeting multiple kinase pathways in leukemic progenitors and stem cells is essential for improved treatment of Ph+ leukemia in mice. Proc Natl Acad Sci U S A 2006;103(45):16870–5.
8. Heidel FH, Bullinger L, Feng Z, et al. Genetic and pharmacologic inhibition of beta-catenin targets imatinib-resistant leukemia stem cells in CML. Cell Stem Cell 2012;10(4):412–24.
9. Perez-Caro M, Cobaleda C, Gonzalez-Herrero I, et al. Cancer induction by restriction of oncogene expression to the stem cell compartment. EMBO J 2009;28(1):8–20.
10. Koschmieder S, Gottgens B, Zhang P, et al. Inducible chronic phase of myeloid leukemia with expansion of hematopoietic stem cells in a transgenic model of BCR-ABL leukemogenesis. Blood 2005;105(1):324–34.
11. Schemionek M, Elling C, Steidl U, et al. BCR-ABL enhances differentiation of long-term repopulating hematopoietic stem cells. Blood 2010;115(16):3185–95.
12. Reynaud D, Pietras E, Barry-Holson K, et al. IL-6 controls leukemic multipotent progenitor cell fate and contributes to chronic myelogenous leukemia development. Cancer Cell 2011;20(5):661–73.
13. Zhang B, Ho YW, Huang Q, et al. Altered microenvironmental regulation of leukemic and normal stem cells in chronic myelogenous leukemia. Cancer Cell 2012;21(4):577–92.
14. Zhang B, Strauss AC, Chu S, et al. Effective targeting of quiescent chronic myelogenous leukemia stem cells by histone deacetylase inhibitors in combination with imatinib mesylate. Cancer Cell 2010;17(5):427–42.
15. Sirard C, Lapidot T, Vormoor J, et al. Normal and leukemic SCID-repopulating cells (SRC) coexist in the bone marrow and peripheral blood from CML patients in chronic phase, whereas leukemic SRC are detected in blast crisis. Blood 1996;87(4):1539–48.
16. Eisterer W, Jiang X, Christ O, et al. Different subsets of primary chronic myeloid leukemia stem cells engraft immunodeficient mice and produce a model of the human disease. Leukemia 2005;19(3):435–41.
17. Dazzi F, Capelli D, Hasserjian R, et al. The kinetics and extent of engraftment of chronic myelogenous leukemia cells in non-obese diabetic/severe combined immunodeficiency mice reflect the phase of the donor's disease: an in vivo model of chronic myelogenous leukemia biology. Blood 1998;92(4):1390–6.
18. James C, Ugo V, Le Couedic JP, et al. A unique clonal JAK2 mutation leading to constitutive signalling causes polycythaemia vera. Nature 2005;434(7037):1144–8.

19. Wernig G, Mercher T, Okabe R, et al. Expression of Jak2V617F causes a polycythemia vera-like disease with associated myelofibrosis in a murine bone marrow transplant model. Blood 2006;107(11):4274–81.

20. Lacout C, Pisani DF, Tulliez M, et al. JAK2V617F expression in murine hematopoietic cells leads to MPD mimicking human PV with secondary myelofibrosis. Blood 2006;108(5):1652–60.

21. Zaleskas VM, Krause DS, Lazarides K, et al. Molecular pathogenesis and therapy of polycythemia induced in mice by JAK2 V617F. PLoS One 2006;1:e18.

22. Bumm TG, Elsea C, Corbin AS, et al. Characterization of murine JAK2V617F-positive myeloproliferative disease. Cancer Res 2006;66(23):11156–65.

23. Tiedt R, Hao-Shen H, Sobas MA, et al. Ratio of mutant JAK2-V617F to wild-type Jak2 determines the MPD phenotypes in transgenic mice. Blood 2008;111(8):3931–40.

24. Xing S, Wanting TH, Zhao W, et al. Transgenic expression of JAK2V617F causes myeloproliferative disorders in mice. Blood 2008;111(10):5109–17.

25. Shide K, Shimoda HK, Kumano T, et al. Development of ET, primary myelofibrosis and PV in mice expressing JAK2 V617F. Leukemia 2008;22(1):87–95.

26. Akada H, Yan D, Zou H, et al. Conditional expression of heterozygous or homozygous Jak2V617F from its endogenous promoter induces a polycythemia vera-like disease. Blood 2010;115(17):3589–97.

27. Marty C, Lacout C, Martin A, et al. Myeloproliferative neoplasm induced by constitutive expression of JAK2V617F in knock-in mice. Blood 2010;116(5):783–7.

28. Mullally A, Lane SW, Ball B, et al. Physiological Jak2V617F expression causes a lethal myeloproliferative neoplasm with differential effects on hematopoietic stem and progenitor cells. Cancer Cell 2010;17(6):584–96.

29. Li J, Spensberger D, Ahn JS, et al. JAK2 V617F impairs hematopoietic stem cell function in a conditional knock-in mouse model of JAK2 V617F-positive essential thrombocythemia. Blood 2010;116(9):1528–38.

30. Li J, Kent DG, Chen E, et al. Mouse models of myeloproliferative neoplasms: JAK of all grades. Dis Model Mech 2011;4(3):311–7.

31. Mullally A, Poveromo L, Schneider R, et al. Distinct roles for long-term hematopoietic stem cells and erythroid precursor cells in a murine model of Jak2V617F-mediated polycythemia vera. Blood 2012;120(1):166–72 [Epub 2012 May 24].

32. Marty C, Lacout C, Cuingnet M, et al. JAK2V617F promotes stem cell amplification driving MPN clonal dominance in mice and treatment by IFNa prevents this effect. Blood 2011;118:616.

33. Lundberg P, Kubovcakova L, Takizawa H, et al. JAK2-V617F expressing stem cells display a competitive advantage at low limiting dilution and are capable of initiating MPN phenotype. Blood 2011;118:615.

34. Jaiswal S, Traver D, Miyamoto T, et al. Expression of BCR/ABL and BCL-2 in myeloid progenitors leads to myeloid leukemias. Proc Natl Acad Sci U S A 2003;100(17):10002–7.

35. Huntly BJ, Shigematsu H, Deguchi K, et al. MOZ-TIF2, but not BCR-ABL, confers properties of leukemic stem cells to committed murine hematopoietic progenitors. Cancer Cell 2004;6(6):587–96.

36. Levine RL, Belisle C, Wadleigh M, et al. X-inactivation-based clonality analysis and quantitative JAK2V617F assessment reveal a strong association between clonality and JAK2V617F in PV but not ET/MMM, and identifies a subset of JAK2V617F-negative ET and MMM patients with clonal hematopoiesis. Blood 2006;107(10):4139–41.

37. Cho SY, Xu M, Roboz J, et al. The effect of CXCL12 processing on CD34+ cell migration in myeloproliferative neoplasms. Cancer Res 2010;70(8):3402–10.
38. Pikman Y, Lee BH, Mercher T, et al. MPLW515L is a novel somatic activating mutation in myelofibrosis with myeloid metaplasia. PLoS Med 2006;3(7):e270.
39. Pardanani AD, Levine RL, Lasho T, et al. MPL515 mutations in myeloproliferative and other myeloid disorders: a study of 1182 patients. Blood 2006;108(10): 3472–6.
40. Koppikar P, Abdel-Wahab O, Hedvat C, et al. Efficacy of the JAK2 inhibitor INCB16562 in a murine model of MPLW515L-induced thrombocytosis and myelo-fibrosis. Blood 2010;115(14):2919–27.
41. Wernig G, Kharas MG, Mullally A, et al. EXEL-8232, a small-molecule JAK2 inhib-itor, effectively treats thrombocytosis and extramedullary hematopoiesis in a murine model of myeloproliferative neoplasm induced by MPLW515L. Leukemia 2011;26(4):720–7.
42. Delhommeau F, Dupont S, Della Valle V, et al. Mutation in TET2 in myeloid cancers. N Engl J Med 2009;360(22):2289–301.
43. Abdel-Wahab O, Mullally A, Hedvat C, et al. Genetic characterization of TET1, TET2, and TET3 alterations in myeloid malignancies. Blood 2009;114(1):144–7.
44. Moran-Crusio K, Reavie L, Shih A, et al. Tet2 loss leads to increased hematopoietic stem cell self-renewal and myeloid transformation. Cancer Cell 2011;20(1):11–24.
45. Quivoron C, Couronne L, Della Valle V, et al. TET2 inactivation results in pleio-tropic hematopoietic abnormalities in mouse and is a recurrent event during human lymphomagenesis. Cancer Cell 2011;20(1):25–38.
46. Li Z, Cai X, Cai CL, et al. Deletion of Tet2 in mice leads to dysregulated hemato-poietic stem cells and subsequent development of myeloid malignancies. Blood 2011;118(17):4509–18.
47. Ko M, Bandukwala HS, An J, et al. Ten-Eleven-Translocation 2 (TET2) negatively regulates homeostasis and differentiation of hematopoietic stem cells in mice. Proc Natl Acad Sci U S A 2011;108(35):14566–71.
48. Oh ST, Simonds EF, Jones C, et al. Novel mutations in the inhibitory adaptor protein LNK drive JAK-STAT signaling in patients with myeloproliferative neoplasms. Blood 2010;116(6):988–92.
49. Pardanani A, Lasho T, Finke C, et al. LNK mutation studies in blast-phase myelo-proliferative neoplasms, and in chronic-phase disease with TET2, IDH, JAK2 or MPL mutations. Leukemia 2010;24(10):1713–8.
50. Velazquez L, Cheng AM, Fleming HE, et al. Cytokine signaling and hematopoietic homeostasis are disrupted in Lnk-deficient mice. J Exp Med 2002;195(12): 1599–611.
51. Bersenev A, Wu C, Balcerek J, et al. Lnk constrains myeloproliferative diseases in mice. J Clin Invest 2010;120(6):2058–69.
52. Bersenev A, Wu C, Balcerek J, et al. Lnk controls mouse hematopoietic stem cell self-renewal and quiescence through direct interactions with JAK2. J Clin Invest 2008;118(8):2832–44.
53. Grand FH, Hidalgo-Curtis CE, Ernst T, et al. Frequent CBL mutations associated with 11q acquired uniparental disomy in myeloproliferative neoplasms. Blood 2009;113(24):6182–92.
54. Sanada M, Suzuki T, Shih LY, et al. Gain-of-function of mutated C-CBL tumour suppressor in myeloid neoplasms. Nature 2009;460(7257):904–8.
55. Rathinam C, Thien CB, Flavell RA, et al. Myeloid leukemia development in c-Cbl RING finger mutant mice is dependent on FLT3 signaling. Cancer Cell 2010; 18(4):341–52.

56. Abdel-Wahab O, Pardanani A, Patel J, et al. Concomitant analysis of EZH2 and ASXL1 mutations in myelofibrosis, chronic myelomonocytic leukemia and blast-phase myeloproliferative neoplasms. Leukemia 2011;25(7):1200–2.

57. Guglielmelli P, Biamonte F, Score J, et al. EZH2 mutational status predicts poor survival in myelofibrosis. Blood 2011;118(19):5227–34.

58. Abdel-Wahab O, Pardanani A, Rampal R, et al. DNMT3A mutational analysis in primary myelofibrosis, chronic myelomonocytic leukemia and advanced phases of myeloproliferative neoplasms. Leukemia 2011;25(7):1219–20.

59. Stegelmann F, Bullinger L, Schlenk RF, et al. DNMT3A mutations in myeloproliferative neoplasms. Leukemia 2011;25(7):1217–9.

60. Tefferi A, Lasho TL, Abdel-Wahab O, et al. IDH1 and IDH2 mutation studies in 1473 patients with chronic-, fibrotic- or blast-phase essential thrombocythemia, polycythemia vera or myelofibrosis. Leukemia 2010;24(7):1302–9.

61. Neff T, Sinha AU, Kluk MJ, et al. Polycomb repressive complex 2 is required for MLL-AF9 leukemia. Proc Natl Acad Sci U S A 2012;109(13):5028–33.

62. Challen GA, Sun D, Jeong M, et al. Dnmt3a is essential for hematopoietic stem cell differentiation. Nat Genet 2011;44(1):23–31.

63. Braun BS, Tuveson DA, Kong N, et al. Somatic activation of oncogenic Kras in hematopoietic cells initiates a rapidly fatal myeloproliferative disorder. Proc Natl Acad Sci U S A 2004;101(2):597–602.

64. Chan IT, Kutok JL, Williams IR, et al. Conditional expression of oncogenic K-ras from its endogenous promoter induces a myeloproliferative disease. J Clin Invest 2004;113(4):528–38.

65. Lee BH, Tothova Z, Levine RL, et al. FLT3 mutations confer enhanced proliferation and survival properties to multipotent progenitors in a murine model of chronic myelomonocytic leukemia. Cancer Cell 2007;12(4):367–80.

66. Li L, Piloto O, Nguyen HB, et al. Knock-in of an internal tandem duplication mutation into murine FLT3 confers myeloproliferative disease in a mouse model. Blood 2008;111(7):3849–58.

67. Dorsam ST, Ferrell CM, Dorsam GP, et al. The transcriptome of the leukemogenic homeoprotein HOXA9 in human hematopoietic cells. Blood 2004;103(5):1676–84.

68. Passegue E, Wagner EF, Weissman IL. JunB deficiency leads to a myeloproliferative disorder arising from hematopoietic stem cells. Cell 2004;119(3):431–43.

69. Le DT, Kong N, Zhu Y, et al. Somatic inactivation of Nf1 in hematopoietic cells results in a progressive myeloproliferative disorder. Blood 2004;103(11):4243–50.

70. Chan G, Kalaitzidis D, Usenko T, et al. Leukemogenic Ptpn11 causes fatal myeloproliferative disorder via cell-autonomous effects on multiple stages of hematopoiesis. Blood 2009;113(18):4414–24.

71. Lyubynska N, Gorman MF, Lauchle JO, et al. A MEK inhibitor abrogates myeloproliferative disease in Kras mutant mice. Sci Transl Med 2011;3(76):76ra27.

72. Wernig G, Kharas MG, Okabe R, et al. Efficacy of TG101348, a selective JAK2 inhibitor, in treatment of a murine model of JAK2V617F-induced polycythemia vera. Cancer Cell 2008;13(4):311–20.

73. Tyner JW, Bumm TG, Deininger J, et al. CYT387, a novel JAK2 inhibitor, induces hematologic responses and normalizes inflammatory cytokines in murine myeloproliferative neoplasms. Blood 2010;115(25):5232–40.

74. Marubayashi S, Koppikar P, Taldone T, et al. HSP90 is a therapeutic target in JAK2-dependent myeloproliferative neoplasms in mice and humans. J Clin Invest 2010;120(10):3578–93.

75. Weigert O, Lane AA, Bird L, et al. Genetic resistance to JAK2 enzymatic inhibitors is overcome by HSP90 inhibition. J Exp Med 2012;209(2):259–73.

76. Akada H, Akada S, Gajra A, et al. Efficacy of vorinostat in a murine model of polycythemia vera. Blood 2012;119(16):3779–89.

77. Yan D, Hutchison RE, Mohi G. Critical requirement for Stat5 in a mouse model of polycythemia vera. Blood 2012;119(15):3539–49.

78. Walkley CR, Olsen GH, Dworkin S, et al. A microenvironment-induced myeloproliferative syndrome caused by retinoic acid receptor gamma deficiency. Cell 2007;129(6):1097–110.

79. Walkley CR, Shea JM, Sims NA, et al. Rb regulates interactions between hematopoietic stem cells and their bone marrow microenvironment. Cell 2007;129(6): 1081–95.

80. Vannucchi AM, Bianchi L, Cellai C, et al. Development of myelofibrosis in mice genetically impaired for GATA-1 expression (GATA-1(low) mice). Blood 2002; 100(4):1123–32.

81. Kakumitsu H, Kamezaki K, Shimoda K, et al. Transgenic mice overexpressing murine thrombopoietin develop myelofibrosis and osteosclerosis. Leuk Res 2005;29(7):761–9.

82. Kirsammer G, Jilani S, Liu H, et al. Highly penetrant myeloproliferative disease in the Ts65Dn mouse model of down syndrome. Blood 2008;111(2):767–75.

83. Villeval JL, Cohen-Solal K, Tulliez M, et al. High thrombopoietin production by hematopoietic cells induces a fatal myeloproliferative syndrome in mice. Blood 1997;90(11):4369–83.

84. Chagraoui H, Komura E, Tulliez M, et al. Prominent role of TGF-beta 1 in thrombopoietin-induced myelofibrosis in mice. Blood 2002;100(10):3495–503.

85. Evrard S, Bluteau O, Tulliez M, et al. Thrombospondin-1 is not the major activator of TGF-beta1 in thrombopoietin-induced myelofibrosis. Blood 2011;117(1):246–9.

86. Chagraoui H, Tulliez M, Smayra T, et al. Stimulation of osteoprotegerin production is responsible for osteosclerosis in mice overexpressing TPO. Blood 2003;101(8): 2983–9.

87. Fleischman AG, Aichberger KJ, Luty SB, et al. TNFalpha facilitates clonal expansion of JAK2V617F positive cells in myeloproliferative neoplasms. Blood 2011; 118(24):6392–8.

88. Dawson MA, Bannister AJ, Gottgens B, et al. JAK2 phosphorylates histone H3Y41 and excludes HP1alpha from chromatin. Nature 2009;461(7265):819–22.

Therapy with JAK2 Inhibitors for Myeloproliferative Neoplasms

Fabio P.S. Santos, MD[a], Srdan Verstovsek, MD, PhD[b],*

KEYWORDS

- Polycythemia vera • Essential thrombocythemia • Myelofibrosis • JAK2 inhibitor
- JAK2 V617F

KEY POINTS

- Activation of JAK-STAT pathway is at the center of pathogenesis of most cases of Philadelphia-negative myeloproliferative neoplasms.
- Activation of JAK-STAT in these disorders is dependent on JAK2, which can be activated either directly or indirectly through activating mutations of JAK2 and related molecules.
- Therapy with JAK2 inhibitors in myelofibrosis is associated with significant improvements in splenomegaly, constitutional symptoms, leukocytosis, and thrombocytosis.
- No significant improvement in bone marrow fibrosis and JAK2 allelic burden is usually seen with these drugs.
- Cytopenias are the most common side effects observed with JAK2 inhibitors.

INTRODUCTION

Philadelphia-negative myeloproliferative neoplasms (Ph-negative MPN) are a group of neoplasms that share some common features, including increased tendency to thrombosis and hemorrhage and an increased risk of transforming to acute myeloid leukemia (AML).[1] The classic Ph-negative MPN include polycythemia vera (PV), essential thrombocythemia (ET), and primary myelofibrosis (PMF). MF can also develop secondary to PV (post-PV MF) and ET (post-ET MF).[2]

In 2005, 4 independent groups reported on the presence of an activating mutation of the JAK2 gene (JAK2V617F) in approximately 90% of patients with PV and 60% of patients with ET and MF.[3–6] The JAK2V617F mutation leads to constitutive activation of the JAK2 tyrosine kinase (TK) and increased signaling through the JAK-STAT (Signal

Conflicts of interest: F.P.S.S. has received research funding from Novartis; S.V. has received research support from Incyte.
[a] Hematology and Oncology Center, Hospital Israelita Albert Einstein, Avenida Albert Einstein, 627/701, Building A, Sao Paulo, SP 05651-901, Brazil; [b] Department of Leukemia, The University of Texas MD Anderson Cancer Center, 1515 Holcombe Boulevard, Unit 0428, Houston, TX 77030, USA
* Corresponding author.
E-mail address: sverstov@mdanderson.org

Hematol Oncol Clin N Am 26 (2012) 1083–1099
http://dx.doi.org/10.1016/j.hoc.2012.07.008
0889-8588/12/$ – see front matter © 2012 Elsevier Inc. All rights reserved.

Transducer and Activator of Transcription) pathway, causing hyperresponsiveness to cytokine signaling, increased cellular proliferation, resistance to apoptosis, and DNA damage.[3–7] Following discovery of the JAK2V617F, other mutations were discovered in patients with JAK2V617F-negative MPN, including JAK2 exon 12 mutations (in 3% of PV patients), MPL W515K/L (in 5%–10% of patients with ET and MF), and CBL mutations (in 6% of MF patients).[8,9] These mutations share the common theme of leading to deregulation of the JAK-STAT pathway, further underscoring the importance of this pathway in the pathogenesis of Ph-negative MPN.[10]

JAK2V617F formed the rationale for the development of TK inhibitors (TKI) for treating patients with Ph-negative MPN, akin to imatinib and other successfully developed TKI for treatment of malignant neoplasms. The first clinical trials started in mid-2007, and in November 2011 the US Food and Drug Administration (FDA) approved the first JAK2 inhibitor (ruxolitinib; Jakafi) for treatment of MF, which is also the first drug to be approved for this disorder.[11] Although these drugs do not eradicate the neoplastic clone, as is seen with imatinib in chronic myelogenous leukemia, they lead to significant improvements in splenomegaly and systemic symptoms, and may possibly improve survival of patients with MF. Thus, there is great benefit to be gained from these compounds. This article reviews the rationale for using these drugs, and the most recent clinical results.

THE JAK KINASES

The JAK family of TK includes JAK1, JAK2, JAK3, and TYK2. These kinases were discovered in 1989 and were named after the two-faced Roman god Janus.[12] Structurally, JAK kinases share some common domains (**Fig. 1**).[13] The JH1 domain is the TK domain, responsible for the phosphorylating activity of JAK kinases.[14] The adjacent JH2 domain, also called the pseudokinase domain, regulates the activity of the JH1 domain.[15] Mutant JAK kinases lacking the JH2 domain display increased TK activity and phosphorylation of downstream messengers such as STAT molecules.[15] It was thought that the JH2 domain did not have true kinase activity. Recent evidence, however, has proved this to be not true. The JH2 domain is a dual-specificity kinase that phosphorylates key residues S523 and Y570, inhibiting the JH1 TK activity.[16] The V617F mutation locates in the JH2 domain and leads to loss of its kinase activity, thus explaining why JAK2V617F causes increased activity of the JAK2 kinase.[16]

JAK kinases associate with the intracellular portion of cytokine receptors that lack intrinsic TK activity, such as receptors for erythropoietin (EPOR), thrombopoietin (MPL), and interferon (IFNR).[17] Binding of the putative ligand leads to receptor dimerization and activation of associated JAK kinases, followed by activation of multiple intracellular signaling pathways.[17] The various JAK kinases bind to different cytokine receptors. Animal models and reports of patients with germline JAK mutations have proved to be very instructive in our understanding of the specificity of these kinases. JAK1 mutations are essential for signaling through both interferon type-1 (IFN-α/β) and

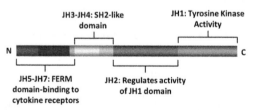

Fig. 1. Structure of JAK kinases and domains.

type-2 (IFN-γ) receptors, and also receptors containing glycoprotein 130 (gp130; eg, receptors for interleukin [IL]-6 and related cytokines) and the common γc chain (eg, receptors for IL-2, IL-7, IL-9, and IL-15).[18] JAK2 is essential for erythropoiesis, as mice embryo devoid of JAK2 die during embryonic life owing to failure of developing hematopoiesis.[19,20] Accordingly, JAK2 is associated with receptors for EPO, thrombopoietin, and receptors using the common β chain (eg, IL-3 receptor, granulocyte-macrophage colony-stimulating factor [GM-CSF] receptor), which are essential for granulopoiesis.[19,20] The JAK3 TK is associated with receptors of the IL-2 receptor family that share the common γc chain.[21,22] JAK3 deficiency impairs development of both T and B lymphocytes, as well as natural killer (NK) cells, and JAK3 mutations have been described in patients with severe combined immunodeficiency, a form of primary immunodeficiency.[21–23] TYK2 mediates signaling of receptors for type-1 IFN (IFN-α/β) and IL-12.[24,25]

JAK KINASES AS CENTRAL MOLECULES IN THE PATHOGENESIS OF PH-NEGATIVE MPN

The first hints for a role of JAK kinases in MPN came from studies conducted in the *Drosophila melanogaster* fruit fly. It was found that an activating mutation (E695K) in the JH2 domain of the protein encoded by the *Hopscotch* gene, the JAK equivalent in *Drosophila*, led to an increased proliferation of hemocytes (fly blood cells) and a clinical picture reminiscent of a leukemia.[26] Increased kinase activation was demonstrated, as well as increased phosphorylation of downstream target STAT92E.

Experimental studies demonstrated that the JAK2V617F oncogenic mutation leads to increased cellular proliferation and resistance to apoptosis.[4] Expression of JAK2V617F in Ba/F3 cells expressing EPOR leads to increased cell proliferation and hyperresponsiveness to EPO.[6] Several animal models of JAK2V617F-positive MPN have been published.[27–37] Mice harboring hematopoietic stem cells and progenitor cells expressing JAK2V617F develop a PV-like disease with bone marrow hypercellularity, increased hematocrit, and splenomegaly, and some mice eventually develop a clinical picture compatible with MF.[29,35]

The phenotype acquired with the JAK2V617F mutation is secondary to activation of intracellular oncogenic signaling pathways. Central among these is the JAK-STAT pathway. JAK2V617F phosphorylates latent cytoplasmic transcription factors STAT3 and STAT5.[4,6] This process leads to STAT dimerization and translocation to the nucleus where they induce expression of several genes relevant to the neoplastic phenotype, including *CCND1*, *BCLXL*, and *BIRC5A*.[38,39] The role of STATs as central mediators of JAK2-aberrant signaling in MPN has been demonstrated in recent publications. In a PV mouse model, inducible deletion of STAT5 through a Cre-recombinase–mediated mechanism essentially abolished all signs and symptoms of the disease, with normalization of the red cell mass, splenomegaly, and bone marrow cellularity.[40] Rescuing the STAT5 deletion with expression of only one allele restored disease features, underscoring the important role of STAT5 in the pathophysiology of MPN. Other reports have confirmed that STAT5 is an essential mediator of JAK2V617F-mutated disease.[41] Besides STATs, JAK2V617F can activate the oncogenic pathways PI3K-Akt-mTOR (phosphatidylinositol 3-kinase–Akt–mammalian target of rapamycin) and Ras-Raf-MEK-ERK (MAPK; mitogen-activated protein kinases).[42–44] Patients with JAK2V617F-negative MPN also have increased STAT5, Akt, and Erk phosphorylation, demonstrating that activation of these pathways is a common feature of all patients with Ph-negative MPN.[10]

JAK kinases may also contribute to oncogenesis by inducing epigenetic changes in the genome. It has been demonstrated that activated JAK can be found in the nucleus of hematopoietic cells, where it phosphorylates histone H3 at residue Y41.[45] This process inhibits binding of heterochromatin protein 1α (HP1α), which is responsible for gene silencing through epigenetic mechanisms. This epigenetic deregulation induced by JAK2 increases expression of oncogene *LMO2*, and inhibiting JAK2 increased HP1α phosphorylation and decreased *LMO2* expression.[45] Nuclear JAK2 has been demonstrated in the CD34+ cells of patients with Ph-negative MPN.[46] Thus, JAK2 may regulate gene expression not only through activation of oncogenic molecules, such as STAT5, but also through epigenetic deregulation.

More recently, the role of cytokines has gained greater importance in the pathophysiology of Ph-negative MPN, particularly MF. Several proinflammatory and profibrotic cytokines (eg, transforming growth factor β, IL-1b, IL-2, IL-6, IL-8, IL-12, IL-15, tumor necrosis factor α [TNF-α]) have been found to be elevated in patients with MF and PV.[47,48] Cells that are responsible for cytokine production include neoplastic megakaryocytes, monocytes, and bone marrow stromal cells.[49,50] These cytokines are associated with many of the clinical features of Ph-negative MPN, including bone marrow fibrosis, osteosclerosis, constitutional symptoms, hematopoietic stem cell mobilization, and transfusion-dependent anemia.[47] In one recent report, increased levels of cytokines IL-8, IL-2 receptor, IL-12, IL-15, and IP-10 (IFN-γ–inducible protein 10) were found to be associated with decreased overall survival in patients with MF.[47] Several of these cytokines are dependent on the JAK-STAT for intracellular signaling, and STAT3 activation increases autocrine production of proinflammatory cytokines such as IL-6.[51] In addition, increased cytokine signaling may lead to resistance to JAK2 inhibitors. Knock-down of the JAK2V617F gene with small interfering RNA inhibited proliferation of JAK2V617F-positive cells or CD34+ cells from patients with MPN.[52] However, addition of IL-3 and thrombopoietin impeded growth inhibition and increased STAT5 activation. In another study, coculture of JAK2V617F cells with bone marrow stromal cells blocked JAK2 inhibition by the compound atiprimod.[53] This protective effect of stromal cells was due to their production of proinflammatory cytokines IL-6 and IP-10.

In conclusion, the following picture emerges from our current understanding of the pathophysiology of Ph-negative MPN (**Fig. 2**). These disorders are caused by mutations that lead to chronic, persistent activation of the JAK-STAT pathway in hematopoietic stem cells. Mutations can either directly activate the JAK2 kinase (eg, JAKV617F, JAK2 exon 12 mutation) or indirectly (eg, MPL mutation, CBL mutation). Activation of the JAK-STAT pathway leads to increased cellular proliferation, resistance to apoptosis, genetic instability, and acquisition of further mutations. Epigenetic effects of JAK activation and the balance between STAT1 and STAT5 activation are likely related to the different disease phenotypes associated with these various mutations.[54] Chronic JAK-STAT activation also leads to increased production of proinflammatory cytokines, which further contribute to disease pathogenesis and activation of the pathway. Although the JAK2V617F mutation is not detected in all patients with Ph-negative MPN, activation of JAK kinases (mutated or wild-type) remains at the center of the pathogenesis of probably most patients with these disorders.[10] Thus, the development of drugs with ability to inhibit chronic JAK-STAT signaling is an important step toward achieving effective therapeutic agents for these patients.

RESULTS OF JAK2 INHIBITORS IN MYELOFIBROSIS

Several JAK2 inhibitors are currently under development for the treatment of Ph-negative MPN (**Table 1**). These inhibitors differ in their specificity against JAK2 kinases, and their main therapeutic benefits in patients with MF are reduction of splenomegaly and improvement in systemic symptoms.

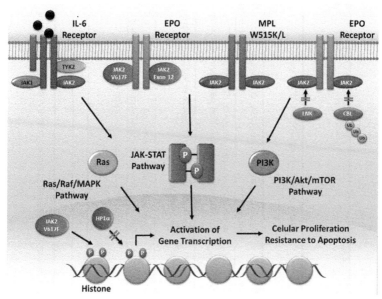

Fig. 2. Central role of JAK kinases in the pathogenesis of Philadelphia-negative myeloproliferative neoplasms (Ph-negative MPN). JAK-STAT signaling is activated in most, if not all, patients with the classic Ph-negative MPN. This process can be due to direct (JAK2 exon 12, JAK2V617F) or indirect (MPLW515L/K, LNK, and CBL mutations) activation of the JAK2 kinase. The presence of proinflammatory cytokines such as IL-6 also contributes to STAT activation. Besides STATs, JAK2 kinases can also activate other oncogenic pathways such as the PI3K and MAPK pathways. Nuclear JAK2 leads to epigenetic deregulation by phosphorylating histone proteins and blocking binding of epigenetic regulators such as HP1α. The final consequence of activation of these pathways is expression of genes associated with cellular proliferation and resistance to apoptosis. EPO, erythropoietin; HP1α, heterochromatin protein 1α; IL-6, interleukin-6; MAPK, mitogen-activated protein kinase; mTOR, mammalian target of rapamycin; PI3K, phosphatidylinositol 3-kinase.

Ruxolitinib

Ruxolitinib (formerly known as INCB018424; Incyte, Wilmington, DE) is an orally available, dual JAK1 and JAK2 inhibitor that has been recently approved as therapy for patients with intermediate or high-risk MF, either primary or post-PV/ET. In preclinical evaluation, ruxolitinib inhibited both JAK1 (half-maximal concentration [IC_{50}] = 3.3 nM) and JAK2 (IC_{50} = 2.8 nM), while sparing JAK3 (IC_{50} = 322 nM).[55] Ruxolitinib inhibited proliferation of JAK2V617F-positive cell lines and CD34$^+$ cells from patients with MPN, and this was associated with decreased phosphorylation of STAT3.[55] In mouse models, ruxolitinib led to spleen reduction, weight gain, and improved cytokine profile.

A phase I/II clinical trial recruited 153 patients with MF to be treated with ruxolitinib at different doses and schedules.[56] The dose-limiting toxicity (DLT) was thrombocytopenia, and maximum tolerated doses were 25 mg twice daily or 50 mg once daily. However, a dose-adjusted schedule whereby patients started with 15 mg twice daily (10 mg if platelet count between 100×10^9/L and 200×10^9/L) with further monthly dose increments if there was no response or side effect led to the best balance between efficacy and toxicity. A total of 61 among 140 patients had a clinical improvement in spleen size by the International Working Group for Myelofibrosis Research and Treatment (IWG-MRT) response criteria (ie, ≥50% spleen size reduction by physical

Table 1
JAK2 inhibitors for the treatment of Ph-negative MPN

Compound	Disease	Target	Responses	Toxicity
Ruxolitinib[60,61]	MF	JAK1, JAK2	Splenomegaly 28%–44% Improvement in MF-related symptoms, leukocytosis, thrombocytosis, overall survival	Anemia, thrombocytopenia, dizziness Headache
Ruxolitinib[77]	PV/ET	JAK1, JAK2	PV-ORR 97% (CR 50%) ET-ORR 90% (CR 26%)	Anemia, thrombocytopenia, dizziness Headache
SAR302503[65]	MF	JAK2	Splenomegaly 39% Improvement in MF-related symptoms, leukocytosis, thrombocytosis, JAK2V617F allelic burden	Anemia, thrombocytopenia, diarrhea Nausea, vomiting, elevated pancreatic enzymes
CYT387[68]	MF	JAK1, JAK2, TYK2	Splenomegaly 31% Improvement in MF-related symptoms Transfusion independence 46%	Thrombocytopenia, first-dose effect, peripheral neuropathy
Pacritinib[70]	MF	JAK2, FLT3	Splenomegaly 39% Improvement in MF-related symptoms	Diarrhea, nausea, vomiting Can be safely used in patients with cytopenias
LY2784544[72]	MF	JAK2V617F	Splenomegaly 41% Improvement in MF-related symptoms, bone marrow fibrosis	Tumor lysis syndrome, creatinine increase
NS-018[73]	MF	JAK2, SRC kinases	NA	NA
BMS-911453[74]	MF	JAK2	NA	NA

Abbreviations: CR, complete response; ET, essential thrombocythemia; MF, myelofibrosis; NA, not available; ORR, overall response rate; PV, polycythemia vera.

examination).[57] This figure corresponded to a 35% decrease in spleen volume by magnetic resonance imaging (MRI). Responses were observed in JAK2V617F-positive and -negative patients. After 1 year, 73% of patients who started with 15 mg twice daily and 78% of patients who started with 25 mg twice daily maintained their response. There was substantial improvement in systemic symptoms, including night sweats, pruritus, fatigue, bone pain, and abdominal pain, as well as improved ability to walk.[56] Improvement in symptoms was accompanied by a decrease in proinflammatory cytokine levels (eg, TNF-α, IL-6, IL-1ra). Reduction in intracellular phosphorylated STAT3 was observed after treatment with ruxolitinib, consistent with on-target activity.

More recently, 2 reports have focused on longer follow-up of patients who were enrolled in the phase I/II trial.[58,59] In one report, the outcomes of 107 patients with MF who were enrolled and treated at M.D. Anderson Cancer Center (MDACC) was compared with an historical cohort of 310 patients identified from 3 large MPN databases.[58] The historical cohort was matched to the MDACC cohort based on eligibility criteria for the phase I/II trial. In the MDACC cohort, after a median follow-up of 32 months, 54% of patients remained on study. Median duration of spleen response had not been reached at the time of report. Most common reasons for discontinuation were death (12.1%) and progressive disease (11.2%). Compared with the historical cohort, therapy with ruxolitinib significantly improved survival outcomes, with a hazard ratio (HR) of 0.61 (95% confidence interval [CI] 0.41–0.89; $P = .022$) for overall survival (OS).[58] This effect was more pronounced in the subgroup of patients at high risk according to the International Prognostic Scoring System (IPSS) (HR = 0.50; 95% CI 0.31–0.81; $P = .006$).[58] By contrast, the report from the Mayo Clinic on 51 patients treated with ruxolitinib at that center did not reveal an improvement in OS compared with a cohort of 410 patients with MF from all IPSS risk categories treated with standard therapy (unadjusted $P = .43$; $P = .58$ after adjusting for the Dynamic IPSS-Plus score).[59] The rate of treatment discontinuation was very high in the Mayo Clinic cohort (51% at 1 year, 89% at 3 years), and this may have affected the results obtained.[59] Most common reasons for discontinuation in the Mayo cohort were patient withdrawal of consent (29.4%), physician decision (23.5%), and disease progression (19.6%).

Ruxolitinib was further evaluated in 2 phase III trials for patients with MF. In the trial conducted in North America and Australia (COMFORT-I), 309 patients with MF and Int-2/High IPSS risk were randomized among ruxolitinib and placebo in a 1:1 fashion.[60] Starting dose was 15 mg twice daily for those patients with a platelet count between 100 and 200 $\times$ 10^9/L, and 20 mg twice daily for those patients with a platelet count higher than 200 $\times$ 10^9/L. The primary end point was the percentage of patients with a reduction in spleen volume by MRI of at least 35% at 24 weeks. After a median follow-up of 32 weeks, the primary end point had been reached in 41.9% of patients in the ruxolitinib group versus 0.7% of patients in the placebo group ($P<.0001$).[60] Patients receiving ruxolitinib had a mean decrease in spleen volume of 31.6% versus an increase of 8.1% in patients receiving placebo. Similar to phase I/II trial data, there were significant improvements in symptoms related to MF.[60] The Myelofibrosis Symptom Assessment Form Total Symptom Score (TSS; sum of scores for itching, night sweats, bone/muscle pain, abdominal discomfort, pain under the ribs on the left, and early satiety) decreased by 50% or greater in 46% of patients in the ruxolitinib arm versus 5.3% of patients in the placebo arm ($P<.001$). The efficacy of ruxolitinib in decreasing splenomegaly and improving systemic symptoms was independent of the presence of the JAK2V617F mutation. There was reduction in proinflammatory cytokines, and an increase in leptin and EPO levels. After a median follow-up of 51 weeks, a planned data cutoff analysis for safety revealed that ruxolitinib improved survival compared with placebo (HR 0.5; P = .04).[60]

In the companion trial COMFORT-II, 219 patients with Int-2/High-risk MF were randomized 2:1 to receive ruxolitinib or best available therapy.[61] The primary end point was percentage of patients with a reduction of at least 35% in spleen volume by MRI at 48 weeks. In the ruxolitinib arm, 28% of patients reached the primary end point, versus 0% in control arm (P<.001).[61] Responses were durable, and after 12 months of follow-up 80% of responding patients receiving ruxolitinib still maintained a response. There was also significant improvement in quality of life and symptoms associated with MF, including fatigue, insomnia, and appetite loss in patients receiving ruxolitinib, whereas a worsening of these symptoms were observed in patients in the best available therapy group.[61] There was no improvement in OS in patients receiving ruxolitinib, but the study was underpowered to detect such a difference.

Ruxolitinib is a relatively well tolerated medication. Most nonhematologic side effects are grade 1 to 2 in severity, and treatment discontinuations attributable to side effects were uncommon in both phase III trials (11% and 8%).[60,61] Side effects that occurred more frequently with ruxolitinib than with placebo in the COMFORT-I study included ecchymosis (18.7% vs 9.3%), headache (14.8% vs 5.3%), and dizziness (14.8% vs 6.6%). These side effects were all grade 1 to 2 in severity, with the exception of one case of dizziness grade 3 to 4.[60] Because of its mechanism of action, cytopenias are a common side effect of ruxolitinib. Compared with placebo, anemia grade 3 to 4 occurred in 25% more patients in the ruxolitinib arm of the COMFORT-I phase III trial, while thrombocytopenia grade 3 to 4 was documented in an excess of 12% of cases.[60] Severe (grade 3–4) neutropenia was uncommon (7% in one trial).[60] Data from both phase III trials demonstrated a clear time-dependent pattern of anemia severity during therapy with ruxolitinib: hemoglobin drops approximately 1.5 g/dL during the first 8 to 12 weeks of therapy, reaching a mean nadir value of 9.4 g/dL. By 24 weeks of therapy, hemoglobin increased to a new mean steady state of 10.1 g/dL. This pattern was independent of transfusions and dose modifications. Most cases of thrombocytopenia grade 3 to 4 happened during the first 8 weeks of therapy with ruxolitinib, and were managed with dose reductions and treatment interruptions. The monthly prevalence of thrombocytopenia decreased to placebo levels with 24 weeks of therapy.[60] Bleeding episodes of grade 3 to 4 happened in 3.9% of patients being treated with ruxolitinib and 3.3% of patients in the placebo arm. Despite its high incidence, few patients (only 1 in each trial) discontinued ruxolitinib because of cytopenias.[60,61]

Patients who discontinue ruxolitinib have a rapid relapse of symptoms, usually within 7 days of therapy interruption.[60] One report has stated that patients who discontinue therapy with ruxolitinib may develop a cytokine rebound syndrome, with acute spleen enlargement and a shock-like syndrome.[62] In the COMFORT-I trial, adverse events after treatment interruption were not more commonly seen with ruxolitinib. Grade-3 events occurred in 16% of patients in the ruxolitinib arm compared with 13% of patients in the placebo arm.[60] No clear pattern suggestive of a withdrawal effect was seen. Severe adverse events occurred in only 3 patients in each treatment arm (6.1% [ruxolitinib] vs 5.6% [placebo]).[60] Eleven percent of patients in each arm of the COMFORT-I study discontinued therapy because of side effects.

The FDA approved ruxolitinib for the treatment of patients with intermediate-risk and high-risk MF. Despite this, ruxolitinib is still being evaluated in clinical trials. Alternative dose schedules for patients with thrombocytopenia (50–100 × 10^9/L) are being studied (NCT01348490, NCT01317875), as well as a sustained-release formulation (NCT01340651). Combination trials with lenalidomide (NCT01375140) and panobinostat (NCT01433445) have recently started.

SAR302503

SAR302503 (formerly known as TG101348; Sanofi S.A., Paris, France) is an orally available TKI that has selective activity versus JAK2 (IC_{50} = 3 nM).[63,64] SAR302503 has limited activity against JAK1 (IC_{50} = 105 nM) and no activity against JAK3 (IC_{50} = 996 nM). Preclinical evaluation of SAR302503 demonstrated it to be a potent inhibitor of JAK2V617F oncogenic signaling, and it had in vivo activity in a mouse model of JAK2V617F-positive MPN.[63,64]

SAR302503 has been evaluated in a phase I/II clinical trial that recruited 59 patients with MF, the majority of whom (86%) was JAK2V617F-positive.[65] The maximum tolerated dose (MTD) was determined to be 680 mg once daily, and DLT included asymptomatic hyperamylasemia and hyperlipasemia grade 3 to 4. After 6 cycles of therapy, a spleen response by IWG-MRT criteria was seen in 39% of patients, and the spleen response was 45% in the MTD cohort.[65] Median time to response was 113 days and the mean duration of spleen response was 315 days. SAR302503 led to normalization of leukocytosis and thrombocytosis in 56% and 90% of cases, respectively. The drug led to improvements in systemic symptoms, including cough, early satiety, fatigue, night sweats, and pruritus.[65] No decrease in proinflammatory cytokines was observed in this trial, suggesting that this drug has more of an antiproliferative than an anticytokine effect.[65] A decrease in JAK2V617F allele burden has been reported with this drug. At baseline, the median allele burden was 20% (range 3%–100%), which decreased to 9% (range 0%–100%; P = .03) after 24 cycles of treatment.[65] A similar effect was seen in patients who presented with baseline JAK2V617F burden greater than 20% (baseline median 60% [range 23%–100%]; after 24 cycles of therapy, median 21% [range 6%–100%]; P = .03).[65]

Toxicities of SAR302503 include cytopenias, gastrointestinal toxicity, and elevation of pancreatic enzymes. In the phase I/II study, anemia was reported in 43.2% of patients, and it was grade 3 to 4 in 35% of cases.[65] Thrombocytopenia occurred in 40.7% (grade 3–4 23.7%) and neutropenia in 4.4% (grade 3–4 1%). Among nonhematological adverse events, diarrhea (all grades 64%, grade 3–4 10%), nausea (all grades 69.5%, grade 3–4 3.4%), and vomiting (all grades 57.6%, grade 3–4 3.4%) were the most commonly reported. In the MTD cohort of patients (n = 40), 70% of patients required dose reductions during the first 6 cycles of therapy, more commonly because of gastrointestinal toxicity or cytopenias (32.5% of cases).[65]

SAR302503 is highly effective for treating patients with MF, but has a relatively high incidence of side effects at the MTD. A lower starting dose may provide similar efficacy with more manageable toxicity. At present, a randomized trial (NCT01437787) of SAR302503 versus placebo for patients with Int-2/high-risk MF is recruiting, and patients randomized to the drug will receive SAR302503 at doses of 400 or 500 mg once daily.

CYT387

The compound CYT387 (YM Biosciences, Mississauga, Canada) is an orally available JAK1 (IC_{50} = 11 nM), JAK2 (IC_{50} = 17 nM), and TYK2 (IC_{50} = 17 nM) inhibitor.[66] Preclinical activity of CYT387 was demonstrated against both JAK2V617F- and MPL-mutated cell lines.[66,67]

A phase I/II clinical trial of CYT387 reported on 166 patients with MF (primary = 65%; post-PV = 22%; post-ET = 14%) treated with CYT387 at different doses and schedules.[68] The MTD was 300 mg once daily, and DLTs were headache and hyperlipasemia. After a median follow-up of 10.4 months, the response rate on splenomegaly by IWG-MRT criteria was 31%.[68] Responses were rapid, occurring at a median of 15 days after the start of treatment. There was also significant improvement in MF-related symptoms, including bone pain (49% improvement), cough (49%), fever (100%), night sweats (80%), and pruritus (74%). An improvement in erythropoiesis and transfusion dependency has been seen with this drug. Among 68 patients (41%) who were transfusion-dependent at baseline, according to IWG-MRT criteria, 46% achieved transfusion independence and a hemoglobin level of 8 g/dL or higher.[68] Median time to transfusion independence was 84 days. Median duration has not been reached.

Similar to other compounds of this class, CYT387 can induce thrombocytopenia (all grades 33%, grade 3–4 17%).[68] Neutropenia and anemia have also been reported, albeit at much lower rates (grade 3–4 3% and 1%, respectively). The first dose effect is a transient dizziness and lightheadedness that may be accompanied by hypotension, and occurs after the patient takes the first dose of the drug.[68] It has been reported in 20% of patients, and is usually grade 1 in severity. Peripheral neuropathy (grade 1–2 only, 20%), nausea (grade 1–2 17%), and diarrhea (grade 1–2 18%) have also occurred with this medication.

The compound CYT387 is highly effective for inducing spleen responses and improvement in constitutional symptoms, while possessing a relatively favorable side-effect profile, similar to other JAK2 inhibitors. The reported rates of transfusion independence are encouraging and need to be further explored in additional trials. Despite this, it should be mentioned that the IWG-MRT criteria for transfusion independence are suboptimal, because in the COMFORT-I trial a transfusion independence rate of 47% was reported in patients in the placebo, underscoring the need for better and improved criteria.[60]

Other JAK2 Inhibitors in Clinical Development

The JAK2 inhibitor pacritinib (formerly known as SB1518; Cell Therapeutics, Inc, Seattle, WA) has selective activity against JAK2 (IC_{50} = 19 nM) and is in clinical trials at the moment.[69] Phase I studies determined the MTD to be 500 mg/d, but pharmacokinetic analysis recommended a dose of 400 mg/d because no increase in plasma level is seen above this dosage. A phase II study has recruited 31 patients, and recently presented data demonstrated that pacritinib improves splenomegaly (39% by physical examination; 55% had a $\geq$25% reduction in spleen volume by MRI) and constitutional symptoms (31%–78% improvement in Myelofibrosis Symptom Assessment Form scores by the 7th–10th cycle).[70] Adverse events consisted mostly of diarrhea (all grades 87%; grade 3–4 10%), nausea (all grades 45%; grade 3–4 6%), and vomiting (all grades 29%; grade 3–4 3%). Pacritinib appears to induce few treatment-related cytopenias. Rates of thrombocytopenia and anemia grade 3 to 4 are low (14% and 5%, respectively), and the drug could be safely used in patients with a platelet count less than 100×10^9/L.[70] Spleen response was not affected by pretreatment platelet counts (35% [platelet $<150 \times 10^9$/L] vs 39% [all patients]).

LY2784544 (Eli Lilly, Indianapolis, IN) is an orally available, selective inhibitor of JAK2V617F (IC_{50} = 55 nM), harboring no activity against wild-type JAK2 (IC_{50} = 2.26 μM).[71] Preclinical studies demonstrated that LY2784544 inhibited JAK2V617F and STAT5 phosphorylation, induced cell-cycle arrest and apoptosis, and reduced growth of Ba/F3-JAKV617F-GFP tumor cells xenografts in mice.[71] At the same time, LY2784544 did not inhibit proliferation of cells expressing wild-type JAK2 (IC_{50} = 1.356 μM).[71] Preliminary results of a phase I clinical trial of LY2784544 have been presented in abstract form.[72] Nineteen patients (MF = 18, PV = 1) were recruited, and the MTD was reported to be 120 mg. DLTs included hyperuricemia and creatinine increase. There were 4 cases of tumor lysis syndrome, 3 of which had clinical consequences.[72]

Regarding response rates, of 17 evaluable patients, 41% had a reduction in spleno-megaly of 50% or greater.[72] A reduction in MPN-related symptoms of 50% or more was observed in 59% of patients. In addition, very preliminary observations suggest that an improvement in bone marrow fibrosis might be obtained, as 3 of 5 patients with follow-up bone marrow biopsies had a reduction in the severity of marrow fibrosis.[72] The study is ongoing and alternative dose schedules to decrease toxicity will be explored.

NS-018 (Nippon Shinyaku Co. Ltd, Kyoto, Japan) is a JAK2-specific inhibitor that also has activity against kinases of the Src family.[73] In vitro, NS-018 inhibits JAK2 ($IC_{50} = 0.72$ nM), has limited activity against JAK1, JA3, and TYK2, and can inhibit several Src-family kinases including SRC, FYN, and YES.[73] NS-018 inhibits JAK2 phosphorylation in Ba/F3 cells expressing EPOR and JAK2V617F, and demonstrated activity in a mouse model of JAK2V617F-induced MPN, with resolution of spleno-megaly, extramedullary hematopoiesis, and leukocytosis.[73] NS-018 is being tested in a phase I/II clinical trial in patients with MF (NCT01423851).

BMS-911543 (Bristol-Myers Squibb, New York, NY) is a JAK2 kinase selective inhib-itor ($IC_{50} = 1$ nM) that has virtually no activity against other JAK family members and other target kinases.[74] BMS-911543 inhibited proliferation of cells expressing JAK2V617F, and had no effect in cell lines dependent on JAK3 for proliferation. The drug inhibited proliferation of primary CD34$^+$ cells from patients with MPN ($IC_{50} = 0.15–0.9$ μM) while having a limited effect against control CD34$^+$ cells ($IC_{50} = 1.5$ μM).[74] A phase I/II clinical trial in patients with MF (NCT01236352) will provide further information on the clinical activity of BMS-911543.

CLINICAL RESULTS IN POLYCYTHEMIA VERA AND ESSENTIAL THROMBOCYTHEMIA

Most clinical studies with JAK2 inhibitors have focused on patients with MF, who usually have few available therapeutic options. Patients with PV and ET usually have a more benign clinical course than those with MF, and are typically managed with phlebotomies (for PV), aspirin, and cytoreductive agents such as hydroxyurea and pegylated IFN-α2a. The role of JAK2 inhibitors for these patients is unclear. However, a fraction of patients with PV/ET who need cytoreductive therapy will be either intolerant or resistant to currently available agents.[75,76] A phase I/II trial evalu-ated ruxolitinib in this population of patients.[77] Inclusion criteria were a diagnosis of ET or PV with need for cytoreduction and intolerance or resistance to hydroxyurea, the most commonly used agent for this purpose. Additional inclusion criteria were hematocrit greater than 45% and/or phlebotomy dependence (for PV), and platelet count greater than 650×10^9/L (for ET).

A total of 73 patients were recruited (PV = 34, ET = 39). The MTD was 10 mg twice daily (PV) and 25 mg twice daily (ET).[77] The JAK2V617F mutation was present in 100% of PV patients and 67% of ET patients. In PV, therapy with ruxolitinib led to a decrease in hematocrit with phlebotomy independence in 97% of patients, and all continued to maintain response at last follow-up.[77] A decrease in spleen size of 50% or more was seen in 80% of patients, as well as normalization of leukocytosis (73%) and thrombocytosis (69%) and improvements in pruritus, night sweats, and bone pain. The overall response rate (ORR) by European LeukemiaNet criteria[78] was 97%, including a complete remission (CR) rate of 50% and a partial response rate of 47%.[77] As expected from the ruxolitinib toxicity profile, most common side effects were anemia (grade 1–2 only, 74%), thrombocytopenia (all grades 29%, grade 3–4 6%), and leuko-penia (grade 1–2 only, 15%). A downward trend in the JAK2V617F allele burden was seen in 4 patients with PV. Responses did not correlate with JAK2V617F allele burden.

In patients with ET, ruxolitinib normalized platelet count after a median of 15 days in 49% of patients, and in 79% the platelet count went down to less than $600 \times 10^9/L$.[77] Four patients had palpable splenomegaly and had achieved a nonpalpable spleen (n = 3) or a 50% or more reduction in size (n = 1). The ORR was 90%, with a CR rate of 26% and a partial response rate of 64%.[77] The most frequent side effects in the ET cohort were anemia (grade 1–2 only, 74%) and weight increase (grade 1–2 only, 23%).

Despite these excellent results, there is still uncertainty regarding the role of JAK2 inhibitors in the routine management of patients with PV and ET. At present there is a randomized, open-label phase III trial evaluating ruxolitinib (10 mg twice daily) against best available therapy in patients with hydroxyurea-resistant or hydroxyurea-intolerant patients with PV (RESPONSE trial; NCT01243944). The primary end point is the proportion of patients who achieve a response (absence of phlebotomy and reduction in spleen volume of 35% or more as determined by MRI or computed tomography) at 32 weeks of therapy. The results of this trial will help to determine if ruxolitinib is superior to alternative agents in this population of patients with PV.

RESISTANCE TO JAK2 INHIBITORS

At present, the exact mechanisms of resistance to JAK2 inhibitors in patients with MF and other Ph-negative MPN remain largely unknown. In chronic myelogenous leukemia, resistance to imatinib is often (40%–50%) associated with point mutations in the kinase domain of BCR-ABL1. These mutations interfere with the binding of imatinib to BCR-ABL1, or change the oncoprotein conformation to an active state that imatinib cannot bind. In vitro exposure of JAK2V617F-positive cells to JAK2 inhibitors can induce mutations associated with resistance to JAK2 inhibitors.[79] The most relevant mutations include Y931C, G935R, R938L, I960V, and E985K. These mutations interfere with binding of JAK2 inhibitors to the kinase domain of JAK2, and confer resistance to all available JAK2 inhibitors.[79] The gatekeeper mutation M929I in JAK2 is homologous to the T315I mutation described in BCR-ABL1, but it only alters sensitivity to ruxolitinib, with no cross-resistance to other JAK2 inhibitors.[79] No studies have been published thus far demonstrating the presence of JAK2 mutations associated with resistance to JAK2 inhibition in patients treated with these compounds.

Besides mutation of JAK2, other mechanisms may operate that are associated with resistance to these drugs. It is known that JAK2 inhibition does not seem to eradicate the malignant clone, as evidenced by the lack of significant reduction in JAK2V617F allele burden in most clinical trials in MF, absence of improvement in fibrosis, and the rapid relapse in symptoms and splenic enlargement once therapy is discontinued. This persistence of malignant cells suggests maintenance of JAK2 signaling in the setting of chronic JAK2 inhibition. To further elucidate this aspect, in one study the investigators generated mutant JAK2/MPL cells that had persistent JAK2 signaling in the presence of JAK inhibitors (eg, ruxolitinib, SAR302503).[80] Evaluation of intracellular signaling pathways revealed that JAK2 was activated in trans by other JAK kinases, such as JAK1 and TYK2, and there was increased heterodimerization of JAK2 with other JAK kinases.[80] Increased expression of JAK2 was found in JAK2/MPL-persistent cells, as well as in samples from patients treated with JAK2 inhibitors who did not have a response to the drug, indicating that the cells remained dependent on JAK2 for survival.[80] This increased expression was secondary to epigenetic abnormalities and changes in histone methylation in the JAK2 gene locus. Targeting JAK2 degradation by other pathways such as Heat Shock Protein 90 inhibition may lead to signaling inhibition and may be potentially used as therapeutic agents in conjunction with JAK2 inhibitors.[81]

SUMMARY

The results of clinical trials have demonstrated that JAK2 inhibitors are a significant addition to the roster of therapeutic agents for MF. These drugs can significantly decrease spleen size, improve systemic symptoms, decrease leukocytosis and thrombocytosis, and improve patients' quality of life. Results of a randomized trial and a retrospective analysis compared with a historical cohort suggest that these drugs may also improve the survival of patients with MF, which has not been achieved with any conventional drug therapy for this disease to date.[58,60] These benefits, however, come at the cost of side effects, mainly cytopenias, which can lead to transfusion requirements in a percentage of patients. Fortunately, in most situations drug-induced cytopenias can be transient and are managed with drug interruptions and/or dose reduction. Better understanding of intrinsic and acquired mechanisms of resistance to these drugs is needed, as no major reduction in JAK2V671F allele burden has been observed during therapy with these drugs, and symptoms recur rapidly once the medication is stopped, indicating that JAK2 inhibitors do not eradicate the malignant clone. Future studies conducted with these compounds as single agents and in combination therapy will help to further improve on the results obtained with JAK2 inhibitors at present.

REFERENCES

1. Thiele J, Kvasnicka HM, Tefferi A, et al. Primary myelofibrosis. In: Swerdlow SH, Campo E, Harris NL, et al, editors. World health organization classification of tumours of haematopoietic and lymphoid tissues. Lyon (France): IARC Press; 2008. p. 44–7.
2. Vardiman JW, Thiele J, Arber DA, et al. The 2008 revision of the World Health Organization (WHO) classification of myeloid neoplasms and acute leukemia: rationale and important changes. Blood 2009;114:937–51.
3. Baxter EJ, Scott LM, Campbell PJ, et al. Acquired mutation of the tyrosine kinase JAK2 in human myeloproliferative disorders. Lancet 2005;365:1054–61.
4. James C, Ugo V, Le Couedic JP, et al. A unique clonal JAK2 mutation leading to constitutive signalling causes polycythaemia vera. Nature 2005;434:1144–8.
5. Kralovics R, Passamonti F, Buser AS, et al. A gain-of-function mutation of JAK2 in myeloproliferative disorders. N Engl J Med 2005;352:1779–90.
6. Levine RL, Wadleigh M, Cools J, et al. Activating mutation in the tyrosine kinase JAK2 in polycythemia vera, essential thrombocythemia, and myeloid metaplasia with myelofibrosis. Cancer Cell 2005;7:387–97.
7. Plo I, Nakatake M, Malivert L, et al. JAK2 stimulates homologous recombination and genetic instability: potential implication in the heterogeneity of myeloproliferative disorders. Blood 2008;112:1402–12.
8. Scott LM, Tong W, Levine RL, et al. JAK2 exon 12 mutations in polycythemia vera and idiopathic erythrocytosis. N Engl J Med 2007;356:459–68.
9. Pardanani AD, Levine RL, Lasho T, et al. MPL515 mutations in myeloproliferative and other myeloid disorders: a study of 1182 patients. Blood 2006;108:3472–6.
10. Anand S, Stedham F, Gudgin E, et al. Increased basal intracellular signaling patterns do not correlate with JAK2 genotype in human myeloproliferative neoplasms. Blood 2011;118:1610–21.
11. FDA approval of ruxolitinib. Available at: http://www.fda.gov/AboutFDA/CentersOffices/OfficeofMedicalProductsandTobacco/CDER/ucm280155.htm. Accessed on April 10, 2012.

12. Wilks AF. Two putative protein-tyrosine kinases identified by application of the polymerase chain reaction. Proc Natl Acad Sci U S A 1989;86:1603–7.

13. Giordanetto F, Kroemer RT. Prediction of the structure of human Janus kinase 2 (JAK2) comprising JAK homology domains 1 through 7. Protein Eng 2002;15:727–37.

14. Wilks AF, Harpur AG, Kurban RR, et al. Two novel protein-tyrosine kinases, each with a second phosphotransferase-related catalytic domain, define a new class of protein kinase. Mol Cell Biol 1991;11:2057–65.

15. Saharinen P, Silvennoinen O. The pseudokinase domain is required for suppression of basal activity of Jak2 and Jak3 tyrosine kinases and for cytokine-inducible activation of signal transduction. J Biol Chem 2002;277:47954–63.

16. Ungureanu D, Wu J, Pekkala T, et al. The pseudokinase domain of JAK2 is a dual-specificity protein kinase that negatively regulates cytokine signaling. Nat Struct Mol Biol 2011;18:971–6.

17. Leonard WJ, O'Shea JJ. Jaks and STATs: biological implications. Annu Rev Immunol 1998;16:293–322.

18. Rodig SJ, Meraz MA, White JM, et al. Disruption of the Jak1 gene demonstrates obligatory and nonredundant roles of the Jaks in cytokine-induced biologic responses. Cell 1998;93:373–83.

19. Neubauer H, Cumano A, Muller M, et al. Jak2 deficiency defines an essential developmental checkpoint in definitive hematopoiesis. Cell 1998;93:397–409.

20. Parganas E, Wang D, Stravopodis D, et al. Jak2 is essential for signaling through a variety of cytokine receptors. Cell 1998;93:385–95.

21. Nosaka T, van Deursen JM, Tripp RA, et al. Defective lymphoid development in mice lacking Jak3. Science 1995;270:800–2.

22. Thomis DC, Gurniak CB, Tivol E, et al. Defects in B lymphocyte maturation and T lymphocyte activation in mice lacking Jak3. Science 1995;270:794–7.

23. Russell SM, Tayebi N, Nakajima H, et al. Mutation of Jak3 in a patient with SCID: essential role of Jak3 in lymphoid development. Science 1995;270:797–800.

24. Karaghiosoff M, Neubauer H, Lassnig C, et al. Partial impairment of cytokine responses in Tyk2-deficient mice. Immunity 2000;13:549–60.

25. Shimoda K, Kato K, Aoki K, et al. Tyk2 plays a restricted role in IFN alpha signaling, although it is required for IL-12-mediated T cell function. Immunity 2000;13:561–71.

26. Luo H, Rose P, Barber D, et al. Mutation in the Jak kinase JH2 domain hyperactivates Drosophila and mammalian Jak-Stat pathways. Mol Cell Biol 1997;17:1562–71.

27. Akada H, Yan D, Zou H, et al. Conditional expression of heterozygous or homozygous Jak2V617F from its endogenous promoter induces a polycythemia vera-like disease. Blood 2010;115:3589–97.

28. Bumm TG, Elsea C, Corbin AS, et al. Characterization of murine JAK2V617F-positive myeloproliferative disease. Cancer Res 2006;66:11156–65.

29. Lacout C, Pisani DF, Tulliez M, et al. JAK2V617F expression in murine hematopoietic cells leads to MPD mimicking human PV with secondary myelofibrosis. Blood 2006;108:1652–60.

30. Li J, Spensberger D, Ahn JS, et al. JAK2 V617F impairs hematopoietic stem cell function in a conditional knock-in mouse model of JAK2 V617F-positive essential thrombocythemia. Blood 2010;116(9):1528–38.

31. Marty C, Lacout C, Martin A, et al. Myeloproliferative neoplasm induced by constitutive expression of JAK2V617F in knock-in mice. Blood 2010;116(5):783–7.

32. Mullally A, Lane SW, Ball B, et al. Physiological Jak2V617F expression causes a lethal myeloproliferative neoplasm with differential effects on hematopoietic stem and progenitor cells. Cancer Cell 2010;17:584–96.

33. Shide K, Shimoda HK, Kumano T, et al. Development of ET, primary myelofibrosis and PV in mice expressing JAK2 V617F. Leukemia 2008;22:87–95.
34. Tiedt R, Hao-Shen H, Sobas MA, et al. Ratio of mutant JAK2-V617F to wild-type Jak2 determines the MPD phenotypes in transgenic mice. Blood 2008;111:3931–40.
35. Wernig G, Mercher T, Okabe R, et al. Expression of Jak2V617F causes a polycythemia vera-like disease with associated myelofibrosis in a murine bone marrow transplant model. Blood 2006;107:4274–81.
36. Xing S, Wanting TH, Zhao W, et al. Transgenic expression of JAK2V617F causes myeloproliferative disorders in mice. Blood 2008;111:5109–17.
37. Zaleskas VM, Krause DS, Lazarides K, et al. Molecular pathogenesis and therapy of polycythemia induced in mice by JAK2 V617F. PLoS One 2006;1:e18.
38. Yu H, Jove R. The STATs of cancer—new molecular targets come of age. Nat Rev Cancer 2004;4:97–105.
39. Gu L, Chiang KY, Zhu N, et al. Contribution of STAT3 to the activation of survivin by GM-CSF in CD34+ cell lines. Exp Hematol 2007;35:957–66.
40. Yan D, Hutchison RE, Mohi G. Critical requirement for Stat5 in a mouse model of polycythemia vera. Blood 2012;119(15):3539–49.
41. Walz C, Ahmed W, Lazarides K, et al. Essential role for Stat5a/b in myeloproliferative neoplasms induced by BCR-ABL1 and Jak2V617F in mice. Blood 2012; 119(15):3550–60.
42. Al-Shami A, Naccache PH. Granulocyte-macrophage colony-stimulating factor-activated signaling pathways in human neutrophils. Involvement of Jak2 in the stimulation of phosphatidylinositol 3-kinase. J Biol Chem 1999;274:5333–8.
43. Bouscary D, Pene F, Claessens YE, et al. Critical role for PI 3-kinase in the control of erythropoietin-induced erythroid progenitor proliferation. Blood 2003;101:3436–43.
44. Mizuguchi R, Noto S, Yamada M, et al. Ras and signal transducer and activator of transcription (STAT) are essential and sufficient downstream components of Janus kinases in cell proliferation. Jpn J Cancer Res 2000;91:527–33.
45. Dawson MA, Bannister AJ, Gottgens B, et al. JAK2 phosphorylates histone H3Y41 and excludes HP1alpha from chromatin. Nature 2009;461:819–22.
46. Rinaldi CR, Rinaldi P, Alagia A, et al. Preferential nuclear accumulation of JAK2V617F in CD34+ but not in granulocytic, megakaryocytic or erythroid cells of patients with Philadelphia-negative myeloproliferative neoplasia. Blood 2010; 116(26):6023–6.
47. Tefferi A, Vaidya R, Caramazza D, et al. Circulating interleukin (IL)-8, IL-2R, IL-12, and IL-15 levels are independently prognostic in primary myelofibrosis: a comprehensive cytokine profiling study. J Clin Oncol 2011;29:1356–63.
48. Vaidya R, Sulai N, Rozell SA, et al. Comprehensive plasma cytokine profiling in polycythemia vera: comparison with myelofibrosis and clinical correlates [abstract]. Blood 2011;118:3850.
49. Emadi S, Clay D, Desterke C, et al. IL-8 and its CXCR1 and CXCR2 receptors participate in the control of megakaryocytic proliferation, differentiation, and ploidy in myeloid metaplasia with myelofibrosis. Blood 2005;105:464–73.
50. Rameshwar P, Narayanan R, Qian J, et al. NF-kappa B as a central mediator in the induction of TGF-beta in monocytes from patients with idiopathic myelofibrosis: an inflammatory response beyond the realm of homeostasis. J Immunol 2000;165:2271–7.
51. Huang WL, Yeh HH, Lin CC, et al. Signal transducer and activator of transcription 3 activation up-regulates interleukin-6 autocrine production: a biochemical and genetic study of established cancer cell lines and clinical isolated human cancer cells. Mol Cancer 2010;9:309.

52. Jedidi A, Marty C, Oligo C, et al. Selective reduction of JAK2V617F-dependent cell growth by siRNA/shRNA and its reversal by cytokines. Blood 2009;114:1842–51.

53. Manshouri T, Estrov Z, Quintas-Cardama A, et al. Bone marrow stroma-secreted cytokines protect JAK2(V617F)-mutated cells from the effects of a JAK2 inhibitor. Cancer Res 2011;71:3831–40.

54. Chen E, Beer PA, Godfrey AL, et al. Distinct clinical phenotypes associated with JAK2V617F reflect differential STAT1 signaling. Cancer Cell 2010;18:524–35.

55. Quintas-Cardama A, Vaddi K, Liu P, et al. Preclinical characterization of the selective JAK1/2 inhibitor INCB018424: therapeutic implications for the treatment of myeloproliferative neoplasms. Blood 2010;115:3109–17.

56. Verstovsek S, Kantarjian H, Mesa RA, et al. Safety and efficacy of INCB018424, a JAK1 and JAK2 inhibitor, in myelofibrosis. N Engl J Med 2010;363:1117–27.

57. Tefferi A, Barosi G, Mesa RA, et al. International Working Group (IWG) consensus criteria for treatment response in myelofibrosis with myeloid metaplasia, for the IWG for Myelofibrosis Research and Treatment (IWG-MRT). Blood 2006;108:1497–503.

58. Verstovsek S, Kantarjian HM, Estrov Z, et al. Comparison of outcomes of advanced myelofibrosis patients treated with ruxolitinib (INCB018424) to those of a historical control group: survival advantage of ruxolitinib therapy [abstracts]. Blood 2011;118:793.

59. Tefferi A, Litzow MR, Pardanani A. Long-term outcome of treatment with ruxolitinib in myelofibrosis. N Engl J Med 2011;365:1455–7.

60. Verstovsek S, Mesa RA, Gotlib J, et al. A double-blind, placebo-controlled trial of ruxolitinib for myelofibrosis. N Engl J Med 2012;366:799–807.

61. Harrison C, Kiladjian JJ, Al-Ali HK, et al. JAK inhibition with ruxolitinib versus best available therapy for myelofibrosis. N Engl J Med 2012;366:787–98.

62. Tefferi A, Pardanani A. Serious adverse events during ruxolitinib treatment discontinuation in patients with myelofibrosis. Mayo Clin Proc 2011;86:1188–91.

63. Wernig G, Kharas MG, Okabe R, et al. Efficacy of TG101348, a selective JAK2 inhibitor, in treatment of a murine model of JAK2V617F-induced polycythemia vera. Cancer Cell 2008;13:311–20.

64. Lasho TL, Tefferi A, Hood JD, et al. TG101348, a JAK2-selective antagonist, inhibits primary hematopoietic cells derived from myeloproliferative disorder patients with JAK2V617F, MPLW515K or JAK2 exon 12 mutations as well as mutation negative patients. Leukemia 2008;22:1790–2.

65. Pardanani A, Gotlib JR, Jamieson C, et al. Safety and efficacy of TG101348, a selective JAK2 inhibitor, in myelofibrosis. J Clin Oncol 2011;29:789–96.

66. Tyner JW, Bumm TG, Deininger J, et al. CYT387, a novel JAK2 inhibitor, induces hematologic responses and normalizes inflammatory cytokines in murine myelo-proliferative neoplasms. Blood 2010;115:5232–40.

67. Pardanani A, Lasho T, Smith G, et al. CYT387, a selective JAK1/JAK2 inhibitor: in vitro assessment of kinase selectivity and preclinical studies using cell lines and primary cells from polycythemia vera patients. Leukemia 2009;23:1441–5.

68. Pardanani A, Gotlib J, Gupta V, et al. An expanded multicenter phase I/II study of CYT387, a JAK-1/2 inhibitor for the treatment of myelofibrosis [abstract]. Blood 2011;118:3849.

69. Verstovsek S, Deeg HJ, Odenike O, et al. Phase 1/2 study of SB1518, a novel JAK2/FLT3 inhibitor, in the treatment of primary myelofibrosis [abstract]. Blood 2010;116:3082.

70. Deeg HJ, Odenike O, Scott BL, et al. Phase II study of SB1518, an orally available novel JAK2 inhibitor, in patients with myelofibrosis [abstract]. J Clin Oncol 2011; 29:6515.

71. Ma L, Zhao B, Walgren R, et al. Efficacy of LY2784544, a small molecule inhibitor selective for mutant jak2 kinase, in JAK2 V617F-induced hematologic malignancy models [abstract]. Blood 2010;116:4087.

72. Verstovsek S, Mesa RA, Rhoades SK, et al. Phase I study of the JAK2 V617F inhibitor, LY2784544, in patients with myelofibrosis (MF), polycythemia vera (PV), and essential thrombocythemia (ET) [abstract]. Blood 2011;118:2814.

73. Nakaya Y, Shide K, Niwa T, et al. Efficacy of NS-018, a potent and selective JAK2/Src inhibitor, in primary cells and mouse models of myeloproliferative neoplasms. Blood Cancer J 2011;1:e29.

74. Purandare AV, McDevitt TM, Wan H, et al. Characterization of BMS-911543, a functionally selective small-molecule inhibitor of JAK2. Leukemia 2012;26:280–8.

75. Alvarez-Larran A, Pereira A, Cervantes F, et al. Assessment and prognostic value of the European LeukemiaNet criteria for clinicohematologic response, resistance, and intolerance to hydroxyurea in polycythemia vera. Blood 2012;119: 1363–9.

76. Antonioli E, Guglielmelli P, Pieri L, et al. Hydroxyurea-related toxicity in 3,411 patients with Ph'-negative MPN. Am J Hematol 2012;87:552–4.

77. Verstovsek S, Passamonti F, Rambaldi A, et al. Durable responses with the JAK1/JAK2 inhibitor, INCB018424, in patients with polycythemia vera (PV) and essential thrombocythemia (ET) refractory or intolerant to hydroxyurea (HU) [abstract]. Blood 2010;116:313.

78. Barosi G, Birgegard G, Finazzi G, et al. Response criteria for essential thrombocythemia and polycythemia vera: result of a European LeukemiaNet consensus conference. Blood 2009;113:4829–33.

79. Deshpande A, Reddy MM, Schade GO, et al. Kinase domain mutations confer resistance to novel inhibitors targeting JAK2V617F in myeloproliferative neoplasms. Leukemia 2012;26:708–15.

80. Bhagwat N, Koppikar P, Kilpivaara O, et al. Heterodimeric JAK-STAT activation as a mechanism of persistence to JAK2 inhibitor therapy [abstract]. Blood 2011;118:122.

81. Weigert O, Lane AA, Bird L, et al. Genetic resistance to JAK2 enzymatic inhibitors is overcome by HSP90 inhibition. J Exp Med 2012;209:259–73.

Clinical Predictors of Outcome in MPN

Francesco Passamonti, MD*, Margherita Maffioli, MD,
Michele Merli, MD, Andrea Ferrario, MD,
Domenica Caramazza, MD

KEYWORDS

- Myelofibrosis • Polycythemia • Thrombocythemia • JAK2 • Prognosis

KEY POINTS

- Myeloproliferative neoplasms include 3 diseases: polycythemia vera (PV), essential thrombocythemia (ET), and primary myelofibrosis (PMF).
- PV and ET are dominated by a high risk of thrombosis and a late risk of clonal evolution into secondary MF and acute myeloid leukemia.
- Current risk prediction of PV and ET requires 2 parameters: age older than 60 years and prior history of thrombosis and, on the basis of these risk factors, patients are stratified as low risk or high risk.
- Patients with PMF may encounter many complications associated with disease progression or with PMF evolution.
- Concerning MF prognostication, the IPSS (International Prognostic Scoring System) model at diagnosis and the DIPSS (Dynamic IPSS) anytime during the course of the disease define survival of patients with MF; IPSS and DIPSS are based on age older than 65 years, presence of constitutional symptoms, hemoglobin level less than 10 g/dL, leukocyte count greater than 25 × 10^9/L, and circulating blast cells 1% or greater.

Myeloproliferative neoplasms (MPNs) include 3 main diseases: polycythemia vera (PV), essential thrombocythemia (ET), and primary myelofibrosis (PMF).[1] Patients with ET may slowly progress to PV, especially those carrying the *JAK2*(V617F) mutation.[2,3] Furthermore, PV and ET have a variable risk of transformation to secondary myelofibrosis (post-PV and post-ET MF)[4,5] and subsequently to acute myeloid leukemia (AML).[6] Eventually, AML may occur directly from ET and PV without the intermediate step of MF, in which case AML may lack *JAK2* mutation even if arising from

---

All authors have no relationship to disclose.
Division of Hematology, Department of Internal Medicine, Ospedale di Circolo e Fondazione Macchi, Viale Borri 57, 21100 Varese, Italy
* Corresponding author.
E-mail address: francesco.passamonti@ospedale.varese.it

Hematol Oncol Clin N Am 26 (2012) 1101–1116
http://dx.doi.org/10.1016/j.hoc.2012.07.009
0889-8588/12/$ – see front matter © 2012 Elsevier Inc. All rights reserved.

JAK2-positive MPN.[7] Evolution to post-PV and post-ET MF occurs at a rate of 10% to 20% after 15 to 20 years of follow-up.[5] Progression to AML is less frequent in PV and ET (2%–7%) than in PMF (8%–30%).[2,8–10] Although prognostication in PV and ET is mainly aimed at defining the risk of thrombosis, prognostic models in PMF are tailored to define survival.

PROGNOSIS IN ET

Survival of patients with ET is not significantly shortened when compared with that of the healthy population.[4,11] Disease-related complications affecting survival are mainly vascular events (thrombosis and hemorrhage) and transformation to MF or AML. In ET, the incidence of thrombosis, MF, and AML was estimated at 12.0, 1.6, and 1.2 × 1000 person-years.[4] Evolution to AML is difficult to predict, as it is a rare event, but advanced age (sign of genomic instability) and high leukocyte count (sign of myeloproliferation) at diagnosis are considered risk factors.[12] Concerning the role of chemotherapy on leukemia occurrence in MPNs, a recent population-based study on 11,039 MPNs proved that 25% of patients post-MPN AML were never exposed to cytotoxic drugs, and that hydroxyurea at any dose is not associated with an increased risk of AML, whereas an increasing cumulative dose of alkylators is.[13]

Prognostic Models in ET

As thrombosis is the most frequent complication in ET, there is a comprehensible rationale for stratifying patients according to the risk of thrombosis. There is a general agreement among investigators to consider age older than 60 years at diagnosis and presence of vascular events in the patient's history as the 2 prognostic factors in ET as well as in PV (**Table 1**).[14–17] Therefore, patients with 1 or 2 of these risk factors at diagnosis are considered as high risk, whereas those with none of them are considered as low risk. This risk classification guides therapeutic strategy. Cardiovascular (CV) risk factors (arterial hypertension, smoking, hypercholesterolemia, diabetes) do not enter in the risk stratification of ET,[18] but an appropriate strategy of prevention and management is recommended.

Other Risk Factors in ET

Mutational profile
The mutational profile of patients with ET includes the *JAK2*(V617F) mutation present in roughly 60% of patients, different mutations of *MPL* in 5%, and very few cases with *TET2* mutations only. Many studies, recently reviewed,[19] evaluated the relationship between the presence of the *JAK2*(V617F) mutation and thrombosis occurrence during follow-up. Meta-analyses indicated that the risk of venous thrombosis and arterial thrombosis is 2.09-fold and 1.96-fold higher in *JAK2*(V617F)-positive ET when compared with *JAK2*(V617F)-negative ET.[20,21] When studying allele burden, patients with homozygous mutations seem to have a higher risk of thrombosis (hazard ratio: 3.97) if compared with *JAK2*-wt[22]: it is notable that very few patients with ET (<2%)

Table 1 Risk categories in essential thrombocythemia and polycythemia vera	
Low Risk	Age <60 years and
	No history of thrombosis
High risk	Age ≥60 years, or
	History of thrombosis

have a homozygous mutation of *JAK2*. Mutations of *MPL* were reported in approximately 3% to 5% of patients with ET.[23–25] *MPL* mutations do not define a distinct phenotype in ET, although patients with MPL (W515L/K) presented lower hemoglobin levels and higher platelet counts than did MPLwt.[24] *MPL* mutation was demonstrated as a significant risk factor for microvessel disturbances, suggesting platelet hyperreactivity associated with constitutively active MPL. Studying bone marrow histopathology, patients with *MPL*(W515L/K) presented reduced total and erythroid bone marrow cellularity.[24,25] Finally, *MPL* mutations lacked prognostic significance with respect to thrombosis, major hemorrhage, myelofibrotic transformation, or survival.[25] *TET2* mutations (frameshift, nonsense, or missense), mostly involving exons 4 and 12, have been found in 5% of patients with ET (mutant *TET2* detected in 17%/7% of *JAK2* [V617F]positive/negative MPN cases, respectively).[26] The presence of mutant *TET2* does not affect survival, leukemic transformation, or thrombosis in MPNs.

Cytogenetic abnormalities
Karyotypic abnormalities in ET are uncommon and occur in fewer than 5% of cases, with trisomy 9 and 8, del(13q) and del(20q), and unbalanced translocations as most common.[27] A recent study of 402 patients with ET showed an association between abnormal cytogenetics at diagnosis and palpable splenomegaly, current tobacco use, venous thrombosis, and lower hemoglobin levels.[27] Nevertheless, it was noted that these patients did not have a shorter survival, or an increased transformation to AML or MF. Very uncommon cytogenetic abnormalities, such as der(1;7)(q10;p10), define a subgroup of patients with ET with an unfavorable prognosis.[28] Leukemic transformations are commonly associated with very poor prognostic abnormalities, including −5/5q− and −7/7q−.[12]

Leukocytosis
A large retrospective cohort of 1063 patients with ET (193 patients [18%] with prior thrombosis), had 118 major thromboses (2.3% patients per year) during up to 38 years of follow-up.[29] With regard to disease-related risk factors, the predictive role of baseline leukocyte levels was examined. Compared with patients having a leukocyte count lower than 8×10^9/L, those with leukocyte count greater than 11×10^9/L had a significantly higher risk of major thrombosis. This association seems particularly evident in younger and asymptomatic patients (low-risk category): ad hoc statistics indicated a higher risk of thrombosis in low-risk patients with leukocytosis, which figure was similar to that calculated in a conventionally defined high-risk group with a best leukocyte cutoff value of 9.4×10^9/L.[30] A study that dynamically evaluated the impact of leukocyte count variation over time in low-risk ET demonstrated that the increase of leukocytes implies a higher risk of subsequent thrombosis.[31] Although some investigators found the same correlation,[32,33] others did not disclose any relationship between leukocytosis and thrombosis.[2,34]

Thrombocytosis
Extreme thrombocytosis per se might provoke an excess of bleeding because of acquired von Willebrand disease, and platelet counts of more than 1500×10^9/L should be considered as a criterion to start cytoreduction in ET.[14]

Bone marrow histopathology
After the first Polycythemia Vera Study Group (PVSG) criteria,[35] the World Health Organization (WHO) dictated the new criteria for diagnosis of ET, which are essentially based on platelet count, histopathological features (normal age-matched bone marrow cellularity with dispersed large to giant megakaryocytes), and demonstration

of clonality.[1] The WHO histopathological criteria help to distinguish ET from another entity presenting with thrombocytosis: prefibrotic primary myelofibrosis (pPMF), characterized by increased age-matched bone marrow cellularity, dense to loose clustered atypical megakaryocytes, increased granulopoiesis, and reduced erythropoiesis. At first, the WHO histopathological criteria appeared not easy to apply, resulting in an insufficient distinction between ET and pPMF.[36] More recently, an overall blinded consensus ranging from 88% (295 cases, 2 European centers) to 93% (1104 cases, 7 international centers) has been achieved among pathologists to recognize the 2 entities.[11,37] The impact of a clear-cut identification of these 2 entities by histopathology is emphasized by clinical results of the international-based data collection of 1104 patients with a clinical phenotype of ET.[11] Patients with WHO-defined ET showed a lower risk of overt myelofibrosis, AML evolution, and better survival when compared with patients with pPMF: the 10-year figures were 0.7%, 0.8%, and 89.0% for ET and 5.8%, 12.3%, and 76.0% for pPMF, respectively.[11]

Model to Predict Survival in ET: International Prognostic System in ET

Very recently, a new prognostic score, International Prognostic System in ET (IPSET), has been developed.[38] The prognostic impact on survival of age, prior thrombosis, leukocyte count, platelet count, hemoglobin level, JAK2 mutational status, and splenomegaly was tested in 867 patients with WHO-defined ET. Age older than 60 years, leukocyte count greater than 11×10^9/L, and prior history of thrombosis were statistically significant on survival by multivariable analysis and were included in the new prognostic model. Each factor was assigned an integer weight close to the corresponding hazard ratio in the multivariable Cox regression: weight 2 for age older than 60 years; weight 1 for leukocyte count greater than 11×10^9/L and for prior thrombosis. So, the IPSET model allocated patients into 3 risk categories with significantly different survival: low (sum of points = 0; median survival not reached), intermediate (sum = 1–2; median survival 24.5 years), and high (sum = 3–4, median survival 13.8 years).

PROGNOSIS IN PV

PV is a clonal myeloproliferative disorder characterized by the excessive production of red blood cells (RBCs) that in some cases is accompanied by leukocytosis and/or thrombocytosis.[15] This deregulated proliferative pattern is sustained by the constitutive activation of the JAK-STAT signal transduction pathway through different mutations in the JAK2 gene: JAK2(V617F) in approximately 95% of patients with PV and mutations within JAK2 exon 12 in approximately 4%.[39–41] In a few cases, mutations of LNK or SOCS have been reported.[42,43] The molecular characterization of PV has further been enriched by the identification of mutations in other potential epigenetic regulators, such as EZH2[44] and TET2,[26,45,46] in approximately 3% of and in approximately 16% of JAK2(V617F)-positive patients with PV, respectively. Except for JAK2 exon 12 mutations, none of the above-cited molecular alterations is PV-specific.

Prognostic Models in PV

Patients with PV have a shortened life expectancy when compared with that of the general population.[4,47] The most frequent complication is thrombosis (with arterial thrombotic events being predominant),[48] with an incidence estimated at 18×1000 person-years and accounting for 45% of all deaths; whereas evolution to post-PV MF and to AML both occur with an incidence of 5×1000 person-years and account for 13% of all deaths.[4] Considering the type and frequency of disease-related complications, and the absence to date of effective long-term treatments able to significantly reduce or eliminate *JAK2*(V617F), patients tend to be stratified per thrombotic risk and treated accordingly.[15] Among others, the European Collaboration on Low-dose Aspirin in Polycythemia Vera (ECLAP) showed that age and history of thrombosis were the main predictors of CV events.[18] In detail, this study reported that patients younger than 65 years without prior thrombosis have an incidence of thrombosis of 2.5×100 persons per year, those older than 65 years or with prior thrombosis have an incidence of 5.0×100 persons per year, and patients older than 65 years with prior thrombosis have an incidence of 10.9×100 persons per year. The current risk stratification system includes age older than 60 years at diagnosis and previous history of vascular events: patients with at least one of these risk factors at diagnosis are considered high risk, as opposed to those with no risk factors, who are classified as low risk.[15] This risk stratification applies to all patients with PV, regardless of the type of *JAK2* mutation they harbor.[49]

Classic CV risk factors, such as arterial hypertension, smoking, hypercholesterolemia, diabetes, and obesity, although not included in the risk-stratification model, can enhance CV risk and should be minimized (smoking has been demonstrated to increase thrombotic risk in PV).[15]

Other Prognostic Risk Factors in PV

Hematocrit value and platelet count

The optimal hematocrit target to pursue in PV will be clarified by the ongoing CYTO-reductive Therapy to Prevent Cardiovascular Events in Patients with Polycythemia Vera trial[50]: for the time being the European LeukemiaNet guidelines suggest to lower the hematocrit below 45%,[14] even though the 2 largest studies in PV, namely the ECLAP[18] and the Polycythemia Vera Study Group-01[35] studies, did not identify a benefit in maintaining hematocrit values below 50% to 52%.

Thrombocytosis has not been demonstrated to increase thrombotic risk and, when platelets exceed $1500 \times 10^9/L$, may even confer an increased bleeding risk, owing to acquired von Willebrand disease, and therefore warrants caution.[15]

Leukocytosis

Many investigators have studied the relationship between leukocytosis and thrombosis. A positive correlation between these 2 factors has been found in some,[51] but not in all,[8,34] studies. The ECLAP study found a significant increase of myocardial infarction in patients with leukocyte counts exceeding $15 \times 10^9/L$ versus those having leukocyte counts below $10 \times 10^9/L$.[51] In addition, a leukocyte count exceeding $15 \times 10^9/L$ has been found associated with a higher risk of evolution into post-PV MF.[5]

Mutational status

Regarding *JAK2*(V617F) allele burden, one study reported that patients harboring greater than 75% *JAK2*(V617F) allele had significantly increased relative risk of total thrombosis (at diagnosis and in the follow-up) and of thrombosis occurring during follow-up, whereas the difference did not reach the significance levels for thrombosis occurring at diagnosis.[52] Other retrospective and prospective analysis revealed no correlation between thrombosis and increasing allele burden.[8,22]

Concerning *TET2* mutations, reported in 16% of all cases of PV, the presence of mutant *TET2* does not affect survival, leukemic transformation, or thrombosis.[26]

A recent and very interesting study has shown that individual genetic variability may play a role in AML transformation.[53] A polymorphism in the XPD gene (involved in the nucleotide excision repair pathway), namely Lys751Gln, has been found to be an independent risk factor for leukemic transformation in ET and PV. In detail, homozygous carriers of the minor allele (Gln/Gln) of this polymorphism have a nearly fivefold higher risk of progression to AML compared with patients harboring the other XPD genotypes.

Bone marrow fibrosis

Prevalence and prognostic relevance of bone marrow reticulin fibrosis was assessed in 526 patients with WHO-defined PV.[54] At diagnosis, 14% of the patients displayed grade 1 reticulin fibrosis. Patients with fibrosis were less prone to experience thrombosis during their clinical course (1.1 vs 2.7 per 100 patient-years) and more prone to develop post-PV MF (2.2 vs 0.8 per 100 patient-years). There was no significant difference between the 2 groups in terms of overall or leukemia-free survival.

Model to Predict Survival in PV

A model to predict survival has been reported in PV, indicating that advanced age, leukocytosis, and prior venous thrombosis affect survival. As an example, based on this model, a 60-year-old patient with PV with leukocytosis or with prior venous thrombosis has an expected median survival of approximately 11 years.

PROGNOSIS IN PMF

Among MPNs, PMF has the most heterogeneous clinical presentation, which may encompass anemia, splenomegaly, leukocytosis or leukopenia, thrombocytosis or thrombocytopenia, and constitutional symptoms. Median survival in PMF is estimated at 6 years, but it can range from a few months to many years.[55–58] Causes of death may be recapitulated into bone marrow failure (severe anemia, bleeding caused by thrombocytopenia, and infections because of leukopenia) in 25% to 30% of patients, leukemic transformation, named blast phase (BP), in 10% to 20% of patients, CV complications in 15% to 20%, and portal hypertension in 10%. Increasing rates of secondary malignancy have been reported in patients with a longer follow-up.[55,57]

Many factors affect survival in PMF, such as advanced age,[55,57,59–63] anemia,[55–61,64,65] RBC transfusion need,[57,66–68] leukopenia,[64] leukocytosis,[56,64,69] thrombocytopenia,[58,69,70] peripheral blast count,[55,59–61,63] systemic symptoms,[55,56,61,65] hepatic myeloid metaplasia,[71] decreased marrow cellularity with higher degree of fibrosis,[72] higher degree of microvessel density,[73] high number of circulating CD34-positive cells,[74–76] cytogenetic abnormalities,[55,57,58,60,62,77–80] the *JAK2* (V617F) mutation,[55,81–83] *EZH2* mutation,[84] and high level of some cytokines.[85]

Prognostic Models at Diagnosis of PMF

In the past years, many prognostic models have been developed in PMF, but the most used was the Lille score,[64] recently replaced with the International Prognostic scoring System (IPSS).[55] The progressive nature of PMF generated interest in defining new so-called dynamic models, such as the dynamic-IPSS (DIPSS) and the most recent DIPSS-Plus.

The Lille score

The Lille score model was designed on 195 patients with PMF, who had a median survival of 42 months.[64] The scoring system was based on hemoglobin less than 10 g/dL and leukocyte count lower than 4×10^9/L or greater than 30×10^9/L. Patients were grouped into 3 categories, low (0 factor), intermediate (1 factor), and high (2 factors) risk, associated with a median survival of 93, 26, and 13 months, respectively. The study also revealed that an abnormal karyotype (present in ~35% of patients) was associated with a shortened survival , especially in the low-risk group. Leukocyte count greater than 30 × 10⁹/L and abnormal karyotype predict evolution to BP.

The IPSS score

The IPSS was defined through the collaboration of 7 centers under the auspices of the International Working Group on MPN Research and Treatment (IWG-MRT) in 2009.[55] After a systematic individual case review, the database included 1054 patients with PMF defined according to the WHO classification system, excluding post-PV and post-ET MF and pPMF. This is the largest prognostic study ever performed in PMF. Median survival was 69 months. Multivariate analysis of parameters obtained at disease diagnosis identified age older than 65 years, presence of constitutional symptoms, hemoglobin level less than 10 g/dL, leukocyte count greater than 25×10^9/L, and circulating blast cells 1% or greater as predictors of shortened survival. Based on the presence of 0 (low risk), 1 (intermediate risk-1), 2 (intermediate risk-2), or greater than or equal to 3 (high risk) of these variables, 4 risk groups with no overlapping in their survival curves were generated (**Table 2**). The 4 risk categories were well balanced: 22% in low risk, 29% in intermediate risk-1, 28% in intermediate risk-2, and 21% in high risk. Median survivals were 135 months for low-risk patients, 95 months for intermediate-1 patients, 48 months for intermediate-2 patients, and 27 months for high-risk patients.

Among these patients, 409 patients had available cytogenetic analysis at diagnosis: an abnormal karyotype implies a shorter survival, primarily restricted to patients in the intermediate-1 and intermediate-2 risks. Concerning the *JAK2*(V617F) mutation, no association was observed between the JAK2 status and the prognostic score or the survival.

Other Prognostic Factors in PMF

Mutational profile

In PMF, the prognostic role of the *JAK2*(V617F) mutation has been widely assessed, whereas the prognostic role of other mutations, such as *TET2* or *MPL,* are less investigated and do not seem to affect survival.[26] A study on 152 PMFs showed that the *JAK2*(V617F) mutation was associated with inferior survival: to note that among 6 patients developing BP, 5 were V617F-positive.[86] This relationship was confirmed in a series of 174 genotyped PMFs[83]; however, when adjusting for conventional risk factors, only progression to splenomegaly and to BP were independently predicted

Table 2
Score values for International Prognostic Scoring System (IPSS) and Dynamic International Prognostic Scoring System (DIPSS)

Parameter	Scores	
	IPSS	DIPSS
Age >65 y	1	1
Hemoglobin <10 g/dL	1	2
Leukocyte count >25 × 10⁹/L	1	1
Blast cells ≥1%	1	1
Constitutional symptoms	1	1

IPSS: score 0 for low risk, score 1 for intermediate risk-1, score 2 for intermediate risk-2, score ≥3 for high risk; DIPSS: score 0 for low risk, score 1–2 for intermediate risk-1, score 3–4 for intermediate risk-2, score 5–6 for high risk.

by the *JAK2*(V617F) mutation. Three more recent studies, including 199, 186, and 174 patients each, showed no significant correlation between the presence of the V617F mutation and survival or leukemic transformation.[79,81,82] Concerning allele burden, data from the literature indicate that having a lower allele load implies a worse survival. In one study,[81] survival was significantly reduced in the lower quartile compared with upper quartiles and patients with *JAK2*wt, mostly because of infections. In the second article,[82] Kaplan-Meier plots revealed significantly shortened overall and leukemia-free survival for the lower quartile allele burden group, mostly deputed to AML transformation. Very intriguing results on the *JAK2*(V617F) mutation was obtained in patients with PMF who received allogeneic hematopoietic stem cell transplantation (HSCT).[87] In 139 of 162 patients with known *JAK2*(V617F) mutation status who received HSCT after reduced-intensity conditioning, overall survival was significantly reduced in patients harboring *JAK2*wt compared with patients with *JAK2* mutation. In addition, patients who cleared *JAK2* mutation level in peripheral blood 6 months after HSCT had a significantly lower risk of relapse.

After reports noted in 2009 describing an association between a *JAK2* haplotype (46/1) and *JAK2*(V617F)-positive MPN, 130 patients with PMF, assessed for the 46/1 haplotype, have been studied for survival.[88] Nullizygosity for the JAK2 46/1 haplotype was associated with shortened survival, which was not accounted for IPSS.

Mutations in the *EZH2* gene, modifying chromatin structure and rendering genes involved in apoptosis inaccessible for transcription, have been found in roughly 6% of PMF. Recently, in 370 PMFs, 148 post-PV/ET MFs genotyped for mutations of *EZH2*, a total of 25 different mutations were detected. Patients with PMF with *EZH2* mutations had significantly higher leukocyte counts, blast cell counts, and larger spleens at diagnosis, and most of them (52.6%) were in the high-risk IPSS category. Leukemia-free survival and overall survival were significantly reduced in patients with PMF with *EZH2* mutations.

Cytogenetic abnormalities

Cytogenetic analysis has a role to identify an abnormal profile that provides evidence of clonality. Although most the bone marrow aspirate of patients with PMF is "dry tap," karyotype analysis can be performed on peripheral blood.[89] Among MPN, PMF shows the highest aberration rate with approximately 30% of patients carrying an abnormal karyotype at diagnosis.[90] The most frequent isolated abnormalities in PMF involve chromosomes 1, 8, 9, 13, and 20.[77,79] Concerning prognostic relevance of cytogenetic changes in PMF, recent studies have been consistent in their reports on prognostic impact on survival.[58,77–79,91] Three studies, each comprising 202, 200, and 131 patients, showed a favorable prognostic value for sole 20q- or sole 13q-.[58,78,91] A further study of 433 patients with PMF refined a 2-tiered cytogenetic-risk stratification: unfavorable and favorable karyotype.[79] In detail, this study[79] identified a high-risk profile for cytogenetics when patients carry sole abnormalities of i(17q), −5/5q−, 12p−, 11q23 rearrangement, inv(3), sole +8 or sole −7/7q−, complex karyotype, and a low-risk profile when patients carry normal diploid, or sole abnormalities not included in high-risk profile. The respective 5-year survival rates were 8% and 51%, respectively. Multivariable analysis confirmed the IPSS-independent prognostic value of cytogenetic risk categorization. The presence of monosomal karyotype, which is defined as 2 or more autosomal monosomies or a single autosomal monosomy associated with at least one structural abnormality, identified a subset of patients with unfavorable karyotype (n = 17, 42% of the 41 patients with complex karyotype) associated with extremely poor overall and leukemia-free survival, as demonstrated by a study of 793 patients with PMF.[80]

RBC transfusion dependency

Criteria for RBC transfusion dependency in PMF has been published.[92] Experts considered a volume of 2 U of RBCs per month over 3 months to be the most appropriate observational interval and RBC-transfusion frequency to define a person as RBC-transfusion-dependent. In general, the cutoff level of hemoglobin to define the need for RBC transfusion is 8.5 g/dL. The prognostic impact of RBC transfusion need was examined in 254 consecutive patients, of whom 24% required RBC transfusions at diagnosis and 9% became RBC transfusion dependent during the first year after diagnosis.[67] RBC transfusion need clearly separated 2 groups with different survivals: 35 months (transfused from diagnosis), 25 months (transfused after 1 year), and 117 months (not transfused). RBC transfusion need had an IPSS-independent prognostic power downgrading or upgrading prognosis within specific IPSS categories. This result was confirmed by a study on 288 consecutive patients with PMF.[68]

Proinflammatory cytokines

Abnormal cytokine profile in PMF is considered to represent an inflammatory response and to contribute to clinical phenotype, bone marrow fibrosis, angiogenesis, extramedullary hematopoiesis, and constitutional symptoms. The interest in cytokines has recently arisen, as JAK inhibitors may reduce different pattern of proinflammatory cytokines.[93–95] Among 30 cytokines tested in a cohort of 90 treatment-naive patients with PMF, high levels of interleukin (IL)-8, IL-2R, IL-12, and IL-15 correlated with inferior survival independently from conventional risk stratification.[85] Investigators found that the presence of threefold increased levels of one or both IL-8 and IL-2R may predict worse survival.

Plasma immunoglobulin free light chains

Plasma immunoglobulin free light chains (FLCs) might be considered as surrogate markers of host immune response. FLC (κ or λ) values above the upper limit of normal have been documented in 33% of 240 patients with PMF.[96] Increased FLC was significantly associated with increased creatinine, and advanced age in PMF. In multivariable analysis, increased FLC predicted shortened survival independently from age, creatinine, and other conventional risk factors. No correlations were seen with leukemia-free survival, karyotype, or *JAK2, MPL,* or *IDH* mutations. In patients with PMF who were studied by cytokine profiling, the prognostic value of an increased FLC level was independent of that from circulating IL-2R or IL-8 levels.

Dynamic Models for Survival in PMF

In a non–time-dependent analysis (models at diagnosis), patients are assigned to a risk group on the basis of the assessment of risk factors at diagnosis, and are followed in the same category irrespective of the acquisition of other risk factors during disease course. According to a dynamic model, patients contribute to the estimate of survival in a score category only as long as they do not acquire further risk factors, then they shift to a higher score category. Dynamic prognostic models are based on the knowledge that the acquisition of additional risk factors during the disease course may substantially modify patients' outcome.

The DIPSS model

The DIPSS was developed on 525 patients with PMF who were regularly followed.[56] DIPSS risk factors are age older than 65 years, presence of constitutional symptoms, hemoglobin level lower than 10 g/dL, leukocyte count greater than 25×10^9/L, and circulating blast cells 1% or greater. The scoring system of DIPSS is different from IPSS (see **Table 2**). The resulting DIPSS risk categories are low (score = 0), intermediate-1 (score 1 or 2), intermediate-2 (score 3 or 4), and high (score 5 or 6). Median survival was not reached in low-risk patients; however, was 14.2 years in intermediate-1, 4 years in intermediate-2, and 1.5 years in high risk. From a practical point of view, any time a decision has to be made on the basis of an updated prognostic status, the parameters of the DIPSS model will be checked and corresponding values will be assigned. The sum of the values will allow allocating the patient into a risk category (low, intermediate-1, intermediate-2, high) and cumulative survival can be estimated. It is obvious that the corresponding cumulative probability of survival at each time point of the follow-up should be read considering the time elapsed since diagnosis. This estimate remains applicable thereafter until the patient changes risk category. The DIPPS model was also able to predict the evolution into BP.[63]

Very recently, Scott and coworkers[97] found that DIPSS categories at the time of HSCT predict posttransplant outcome in 170 patients with PMF (related = 86; unrelated donors = 84). After a median follow-up of 5.9 years, the median survivals have not been reached for DIPSS risk groups low and intermediate-1, and were 7.0 and 2.5 years for intermediate-2 and high-risk patients, respectively.

The DIPPS-plus model

This model was designed on the basis of 793 patients with PMF, of whom 428 were referred within and 365 were referred after their first year of diagnosis.[57] This composite model included as worse prognostic factors the unfavorable cytogenetics as previously grouped (complex, sole, or 2, including +8, −7/7q−, i[17q], inv [3], −5/5q−, 12p−, 11q23 rearrangements), RBC transfusion need, platelet count lower than 100 × 10^9/L, and DIPSS categories. According to the model, 1 point each was assigned to DIPSS intermediate-1 risk, unfavorable karyotype, platelets lower than 100 × 10^9/L, and RBC transfusion need, whereas DIPSS intermediate-2 and high risk were assigned 2 and 3 points, respectively (**Table 3**). On the basis of this scoring system, 4 categories were generated: low risk (0 adverse points; median survival, 185 months), intermediate-1 risk (1 adverse point; median survival, 78 months), intermediate-2 risk (2–3 adverse points; median survival, 35 months), and high risk (4–6 adverse points; median survival, 16 months). It is interesting to note that DIPSS-plus investigators found a proportion of patients in each DIPSS risk category with RBC transfusion need, unfavorable karyotype, and thrombocytopenia of 0%, 7%, and 7% for low risk; 13%, 12%, and 18% for intermediate-1 risk; 56%, 17%, and 32% for intermediate-2 risk; and 69%, 23%, and 47% for high risk, respectively. This shed light on the possibility of better stratifying patients with intermediate-risk categories.

Table 3
Score values Dynamic International Prognostic Scoring System-plus (DIPSS-plus)

Parameter	Score Value
DIPSS intermediate-1	1
DIPSS intermediate-2	2
DIPSS high risk	3
Unfavorable cytogenetic	1
Red blood cell need	1
Platelet <100 × 10^9/L	1

DIPSS-plus: score 0 for low risk, score 1 for intermediate risk-1, score 2–3 for intermediate risk-2, score 4–6 for high risk.

SUMMARY

PV and ET are dominated by a high risk of thrombosis and a late risk of clonal evolution into secondary MF and AML. For these patients, current risk prediction of thrombosis requires only 2 parameters: age older than 60 years and prior history of thrombosis. On the basis of these 2 risk factors, patients can be stratified as low risk and high risk. Additionally, it might be important to obtain information from leukocyte count, bone marrow fibrosis, and mutational status (for ET only).

Concerning MF, the IPSS model at diagnosis and the DIPSS anytime during the course of the disease define survival. The IPSS and the DIPSS are based on age older than 65 years, presence of constitutional symptoms, hemoglobin level lower than 10 g/dL, leukocyte count greater than 25×10^9/L, and circulating blast cells 1% or greater. IPSS and DIPSS very well and easily define survival of patients with PMF. DIPSS-plus adds critical prognostic information and suggests paying attention to cytogenetic categories, platelet count, and RBC transfusion need. Any conclusion on *JAK2* mutation and allele burden in MPN prognostication seems premature, as data are in part conflicting and the method for quantification is not yet standardized.

REFERENCES

1. Tefferi A, Thiele J, Orazi A, et al. Proposals and rationale for revision of the World Health Organization diagnostic criteria for polycythemia vera, essential thrombocythemia, and primary myelofibrosis: recommendations from an ad hoc international expert panel. Blood 2007;110:1092–7.
2. Passamonti F, Rumi E, Arcaini L, et al. Prognostic factors for thrombosis, myelofibrosis, and leukemia in essential thrombocythemia: a study of 605 patients. Haematologica 2008;93:1645–51.
3. Campbell PJ, Scott LM, Buck G, et al. Definition of subtypes of essential thrombocythaemia and relation to polycythaemia vera based on JAK2 V617F mutation status: a prospective study. Lancet 2005;366:1945–53.
4. Passamonti F, Rumi E, Pungolino E, et al. Life expectancy and prognostic factors for survival in patients with polycythemia vera and essential thrombocythemia. Am J Med 2004;117:755–61.
5. Passamonti F, Rumi E, Caramella M, et al. A dynamic prognostic model to predict survival in post-polycythemia vera myelofibrosis. Blood 2008;111:3383–7.
6. Passamonti F, Rumi E, Arcaini L, et al. Leukemic transformation of polycythemia vera: a single center study of 23 patients. Cancer 2005;104:1032–6.
7. Beer PA, Delhommeau F, LeCouedic JP, et al. Two routes to leukemic transformation after a JAK2 mutation-positive myeloproliferative neoplasm. Blood 2010;115: 2891–900.
8. Passamonti F, Rumi E, Pietra D, et al. A prospective study of 338 patients with polycythemia vera: the impact of JAK2 (V617F) allele burden and leukocytosis on fibrotic or leukemic disease transformation and vascular complications. Leukemia 2010;24(9):1574–9 [Epub 2010 Jul 15].
9. Gangat N, Wolanskyj AP, McClure RF, et al. Risk stratification for survival and leukemic transformation in essential thrombocythemia: a single institutional study of 605 patients. Leukemia 2007;21:270–6.
10. Gangat N, Strand J, Li CY, et al. Leucocytosis in polycythaemia vera predicts both inferior survival and leukaemic transformation. Br J Haematol 2007;138:354–8.
11. Barbui T, Thiele J, Passamonti F, et al. Survival and disease progression in essential thrombocythemia are significantly influenced by accurate morphologic diagnosis: an international study. J Clin Oncol 2011;29:3179–84.

12. Passamonti F, Rumi E, Arcaini L, et al. Blast phase of essential thrombocythemia: A single center study. Am J Hematol 2009;84:641–4.

13. Bjorkholm M, Derolf AR, Hultcrantz M, et al. Treatment-related risk factors for transformation to acute myeloid leukemia and myelodysplastic syndromes in myeloproliferative neoplasms. J Clin Oncol 2011;29:2410–5.

14. Barbui T, Barosi G, Birgegard G, et al. Philadelphia-negative classical myeloproliferative neoplasms: critical concepts and management recommendations from European LeukemiaNet. J Clin Oncol 2011;29:761–70.

15. Cervantes F, Passamonti F, Barosi G. Life expectancy and prognostic factors in the classic BCR/ABL-negative myeloproliferative disorders. Leukemia 2008;22:905–14.

16. Bilgrami S, Greenberg BR. Polycythemia rubra vera. Semin Oncol 1995;22:307–26.

17. Beer PA, Erber WN, Campbell PJ, et al. How I treat essential thrombocythemia. Blood 2011;117:1472–82.

18. Landolfi R, Marchioli R, Kutti J, et al. Efficacy and safety of low-dose aspirin in polycythemia vera. N Engl J Med 2004;350:114–24.

19. Passamonti F. Prognostic factors and models in polycythemia vera, essential thrombocythemia, and primary myelofibrosis. Clin Lymphoma Myeloma Leuk 2011;11(Suppl 1):S25–7.

20. Ziakas PD. Effect of JAK2 V617F on thrombotic risk in patients with essential thrombocythemia: measuring the uncertain. Haematologica 2008;93:1412–4.

21. Dahabreh IJ, Zoi K, Giannouli S, et al. Is JAK2 V617F mutation more than a diagnostic index? A meta-analysis of clinical outcomes in essential thrombocythemia. Leuk Res 2009;33:67–73.

22. Vannucchi AM, Antonioli E, Guglielmelli P, et al. Clinical profile of homozygous JAK2 617V>F mutation in patients with polycythemia vera or essential thrombocythemia. Blood 2007;110:840–6.

23. Pardanani AD, Levine RL, Lasho T, et al. MPL515 mutations in myeloproliferative and other myeloid disorders: a study of 1182 patients. Blood 2006;108:3472–6.

24. Vannucchi AM, Antonioli E, Guglielmelli P, et al. Characteristics and clinical correlates of MPL 515W>L/K mutation in essential thrombocythemia. Blood 2008;112:844–7.

25. Beer PA, Campbell PJ, Scott LM, et al. MPL mutations in myeloproliferative disorders: analysis of the PT-1 cohort. Blood 2008;112:141–9.

26. Tefferi A, Pardanani A, Lim KH, et al. TET2 mutations and their clinical correlates in polycythemia vera, essential thrombocythemia and myelofibrosis. Leukemia 2009;23:905–11.

27. Gangat N, Tefferi A, Thanarajasingam G, et al. Cytogenetic abnormalities in essential thrombocythemia: prevalence and prognostic significance. Eur J Haematol 2009;83:17–21.

28. Reilly JT. Pathogenetic insight and prognostic information from standard and molecular cytogenetic studies in the BCR-ABL-negative myeloproliferative neoplasms (MPNs). Leukemia 2008;22:1818–27.

29. Carobbio A, Finazzi G, Antonioli E, et al. Thrombocytosis and leukocytosis interaction in vascular complications of essential thrombocythemia. Blood 2008;112:3135–7.

30. Carobbio A, Antonioli E, Guglielmelli P, et al. Leukocytosis and risk stratification assessment in essential thrombocythemia. J Clin Oncol 2008;26:2732–6.

31. Passamonti F, Rumi E, Pascutto C, et al. Increase in leukocyte count over time predicts thrombosis in patients with low-risk essential thrombocythemia. J Thromb Haemost 2009;7:1587–9.

32. Palandri F, Polverelli N, Catani L, et al. Impact of leukocytosis on thrombotic risk and survival in 532 patients with essential thrombocythemia: a retrospective study. Ann Hematol 2011;90:933–8.

33. Caramazza D, Caracciolo C, Barone R, et al. Correlation between leukocytosis and thrombosis in Philadelphia-negative chronic myeloproliferative neoplasms. Ann Hematol 2009;88:967–71.

34. Gangat N, Wolanskyj AP, Schwager SM, et al. Leukocytosis at diagnosis and the risk of subsequent thrombosis in patients with low-risk essential thrombocythemia and polycythemia vera. Cancer 2009;115:5740–5.

35. Berk PD, Goldberg JD, Donovan PB, et al. Therapeutic recommendations in poly-cythemia vera based on Polycythemia Vera Study Group protocols. Semin Hem-atol 1986;23:132–43.

36. Wilkins BS, Erber WN, Bareford D, et al. Bone marrow pathology in essential thrombocythemia: interobserver reliability and utility for identifying disease subtypes. Blood 2008;111:60–70.

37. Thiele J, Kvasnicka HM, Mullauer L, et al. Essential thrombocythemia versus early primary myelofibrosis: a multicenter study to validate the WHO classification. Blood 2011;117:5710–8.

38. Passamonti F, Thiele J, Girodon F, et al. A prognostic model to predict survival in 867 World Health Organization-defined essential thrombocythemia at diagnosis: a study by the International Working Group on Myelofibrosis Research and Treat-ment. Blood 2012;120(6):1197–201.

39. Kralovics R, Passamonti F, Buser AS, et al. A gain-of-function mutation of JAK2 in myeloproliferative disorders. N Engl J Med 2005;352:1779–90.

40. Scott LM, Tong W, Levine RL, et al. JAK2 exon 12 mutations in polycythemia vera and idiopathic erythrocytosis. N Engl J Med 2007;356:459–68.

41. Passamonti F, Elena C, Schnittger S, et al. Molecular and clinical features of the myeloproliferative neoplasm associated with JAK2 exon 12 mutations. Blood 2011;117:2813–6.

42. Lasho TL, Pardanani A, Tefferi A. LNK mutations in JAK2 mutation-negative eryth-rocytosis. N Engl J Med 2010;363:1189–90.

43. Suessmuth Y, Elliott J, Percy MJ, et al. A new polycythaemia vera-associated SOCS3 SH2 mutant (SOCS3F136L) cannot regulate erythropoietin responses. Br J Haematol 2009;147:450–8.

44. Ernst T, Chase AJ, Score J, et al. Inactivating mutations of the histone methyl-transferase gene EZH2 in myeloid disorders. Nat Genet 2010;42:722–6.

45. Delhommeau F, Dupont S, Della Valle V, et al. Mutation in TET2 in myeloid cancers. N Engl J Med 2009;360:2289–301.

46. Olcaydu D, Rumi E, Harutyunyan A, et al. The role of the JAK2 GGCC haplotype and the TET2 gene in familial myeloproliferative neoplasms. Haematologica 2011;96:367–74.

47. Kiladjian JJ, Chevret S, Dosquet C, et al. Treatment of polycythemia vera with hydroxyurea and pipobroman: final results of a randomized trial initiated in 1980. J Clin Oncol 2011;29:3907–13.

48. Passamonti F, Malabarba L, Orlandi E, et al. Polycythemia vera in young patients: a study on the long-term risk of thrombosis, myelofibrosis and leukemia. Haema-tologica 2003;88:13–8.

49. Passamonti F, Maffioli M, Caramazza D. New generation small-molecule inhibitors in myeloproliferative neoplasms. Curr Opin Hematol 2012;19:117–23.

50. Marchioli R, Finazzi G, Specchia G, et al. A large-scale trial testing the intensity of CYTOreductive Therapy to Prevent Cardiovascular Events in Patients with Polycy-themia Vera. Thrombosis 2011;2011:794240.

51. Landolfi R, Di Gennaro L, Barbui T, et al. Leukocytosis as a major thrombotic risk factor in patients with polycythemia vera. Blood 2007;109:2446–52.
52. Vannucchi AM, Antonioli E, Guglielmelli P, et al. Prospective identification of high-risk polycythemia vera patients based on JAK2(V617F) allele burden. Leukemia 2007;21:1952–9.
53. Hernandez-Boluda JC, Pereira A, Cervantes F, et al. A polymorphism in the XPD gene predisposes to leukemic transformation and new nonmyeloid malignancies in essential thrombocythemia and polycythemia vera. Blood 2012;119(22): 5221–8 [Epub 2012 Apr 11].
54. Barbui T, Thiele J, Passamonti F, et al. Initial bone marrow reticulin fibrosis in polycythemia vera exerts an impact on clinical outcome. Blood 2012;119(10): 2239–41 [Epub 2012 Jan 13].
55. Cervantes F, Dupriez B, Pereira A, et al. New prognostic scoring system for primary myelofibrosis based on a study of the International Working Group for Myelofibrosis Research and Treatment. Blood 2009;113:2895–901.
56. Passamonti F, Cervantes F, Vannucchi AM, et al. A dynamic prognostic model to predict survival in primary myelofibrosis: a study by the IWG-MRT (International Working Group for Myeloproliferative Neoplasms Research and Treatment). Blood 2010;115:1703–8.
57. Gangat N, Caramazza D, Vaidya R, et al. DIPSS plus: a refined Dynamic International Prognostic Scoring System for primary myelofibrosis that incorporates prognostic information from karyotype, platelet count, and transfusion status. J Clin Oncol 2011;29:392–7.
58. Tam CS, Abruzzo LV, Lin KI, et al. The role of cytogenetic abnormalities as a prognostic marker in primary myelofibrosis: applicability at the time of diagnosis and later during disease course. Blood 2009;113:4171–8.
59. Barosi G, Berzuini C, Liberato LN, et al. A prognostic classification of myelofibrosis with myeloid metaplasia. Br J Haematol 1988;70:397–401.
60. Reilly JT, Snowden JA, Spearing RL, et al. Cytogenetic abnormalities and their prognostic significance in idiopathic myelofibrosis: a study of 106 cases. Br J Haematol 1997;98:96–102.
61. Cervantes F, Pereira A, Esteve J, et al. Identification of 'short-lived' and 'long-lived' patients at presentation of idiopathic myelofibrosis. Br J Haematol 1997; 97:635–40.
62. Tefferi A, Mesa RA, Schroeder G, et al. Cytogenetic findings and their clinical relevance in myelofibrosis with myeloid metaplasia. Br J Haematol 2001;113: 763–71.
63. Passamonti F, Cervantes F, Vannucchi AM, et al. Dynamic International Prognostic Scoring System (DIPSS) predicts progression to acute myeloid leukemia in primary myelofibrosis. Blood 2010;116:2857–8.
64. Dupriez B, Morel P, Demory JL, et al. Prognostic factors in agnogenic myeloid metaplasia: a report on 195 cases with a new scoring system. Blood 1996;88: 1013–8.
65. Rupoli S, Da Lio L, Sisti S, et al. Primary myelofibrosis: a detailed statistical analysis of the clinicopathological variables influencing survival. Ann Hematol 1994; 68:205–12.
66. Tefferi A, Mesa RA, Pardanani A, et al. Red blood cell transfusion need at diagnosis adversely affects survival in primary myelofibrosis—increased serum ferritin or transfusion load does not. Am J Hematol 2009;84:265–7.
67. Tefferi A, Siragusa S, Hussein K, et al. Transfusion-dependency at presentation and its acquisition in the first year of diagnosis are both equally detrimental for

survival in primary myelofibrosis—prognostic relevance is independent of IPSS or karyotype. Am J Hematol 2010;85:14–7.

68. Elena C, Passamonti F, Rumi E, et al. Red blood cell transfusion-dependency implies a poor survival in primary myelofibrosis irrespective of IPSS and DIPSS. Haematologica 2011;96:167–70.

69. Morel P, Duhamel A, Hivert B, et al. Identification during the follow-up of time-dependent prognostic factors for the competing risks of death and blast phase in primary myelofibrosis: a study of 172 patients. Blood 2010;115:4350–5.

70. Patnaik MM, Caramazza D, Gangat N, et al. Age and platelet count are IPSS-independent prognostic factors in young patients with primary myelofibrosis and complement IPSS in predicting very long or very short survival. Eur J Haematol 2010;84:105–8.

71. Pereira A, Bruguera M, Cervantes F, et al. Liver involvement at diagnosis of primary myelofibrosis: a clinicopathological study of twenty-two cases. Eur J Haematol 1988;40:355–61.

72. Chelloul N, Briere J, Laval-Jeantet M, et al. Prognosis of myeloid metaplasia with myelofibrosis. Biomedicine 1976;24:272–80.

73. Mesa RA, Hanson CA, Rajkumar SV, et al. Evaluation and clinical correlations of bone marrow angiogenesis in myelofibrosis with myeloid metaplasia. Blood 2000;96:3374–80.

74. Barosi G, Viarengo G, Pecci A, et al. Diagnostic and clinical relevance of the number of circulating CD34(+) cells in myelofibrosis with myeloid metaplasia. Blood 2001;98:3249–55.

75. Arora B, Sirhan S, Hoyer JD, et al. Peripheral blood CD34 count in myelofibrosis with myeloid metaplasia: a prospective evaluation of prognostic value in 94 patients. Br J Haematol 2005;128:42–8.

76. Alchalby H, Lioznov M, Fritzsche-Friedland U, et al. Circulating CD34(+) cells as prognostic and follow-up marker in patients with myelofibrosis undergoing allo-SCT. Bone Marrow Transplant 2012;47(1):143–5. http://dx.doi.org/10.1038/bmt.2011.17 [Epub 2011 Feb 28].

77. Rumi E, Passamonti F, Bernasconi P, et al. Validation of cytogenetic-based risk stratification in primary myelofibrosis. Blood 2010;115:2719–20.

78. Hussein K, Pardanani AD, Van Dyke DL, et al. International prognostic scoring system—independent cytogenetic risk categorization in primary myelofibrosis. Blood 2010;115:496–9.

79. Caramazza D, Begna KH, Gangat N, et al. Refined cytogenetic-risk categorization for overall and leukemia-free survival in primary myelofibrosis: a single center study of 433 patients. Leukemia 2011;25:82–8.

80. Vaidya R, Caramazza D, Begna KH, et al. Monosomal karyotype in primary myelofibrosis is detrimental to both overall and leukemia-free survival. Blood 2011;117(21):5612–5 [Epub 2011 Mar 30].

81. Guglielmelli P, Barosi G, Specchia G, et al. Identification of patients with poorer survival in primary myelofibrosis based on the burden of JAK2V617F mutated allele. Blood 2009;114:1477–83.

82. Tefferi A, Lasho TL, Huang J, et al. Low JAK2V617F allele burden in primary myelofibrosis, compared to either a higher allele burden or unmutated status, is associated with inferior overall and leukemia-free survival. Leukemia 2008;22:756–61.

83. Barosi G, Bergamaschi G, Marchetti M, et al. JAK2 V617F mutational status predicts progression to large splenomegaly and leukemic transformation in primary myelofibrosis. Blood 2007;110:4030–6.

84. Guglielmelli P, Biamonte F, Score J, et al. EZH2 mutational status predicts poor survival in myelofibrosis. Blood 2011;118:5227–34.
85. Tefferi A, Vaidya R, Caramazza D, et al. Circulating interleukin (IL)-8, IL-2R, IL-12, and IL-15 levels are independently prognostic in primary myelofibrosis: a comprehensive cytokine profiling study. J Clin Oncol 2011;29:1356–63.
86. Campbell PJ, Griesshammer M, Dohner K, et al. V617F mutation in JAK2 is associated with poorer survival in idiopathic myelofibrosis. Blood 2006;107:2098–100.
87. Alchalby H, Badbaran A, Zabelina T, et al. Impact of JAK2V617F-mutation status, allele burden and clearance after allogeneic stem cell transplantation for myelofibrosis. Blood 2010;116(18):3572–81 [Epub 2010 May 20].
88. Tefferi A, Lasho TL, Patnaik MM, et al. JAK2 germline genetic variation affects disease susceptibility in primary myelofibrosis regardless of V617F mutational status: nullizygosity for the JAK2 46/1 haplotype is associated with inferior survival. Leukemia 2010;24:105–9.
89. Tefferi A, Meyer RG, Wyatt WA, et al. Comparison of peripheral blood interphase cytogenetics with bone marrow karyotype analysis in myelofibrosis with myeloid metaplasia. Br J Haematol 2001;115:316–9.
90. Hussein K, Huang J, Lasho T, et al. Karyotype complements the International Prognostic Scoring System for primary myelofibrosis. Eur J Haematol 2009;82: 255–9.
91. Hidaka T, Shide K, Shimoda H, et al. The impact of cytogenetic abnormalities on the prognosis of primary myelofibrosis: a prospective survey of 202 cases in Japan. Eur J Haematol 2009;83:328–33.
92. Gale RP, Barosi G, Barbui T, et al. What are RBC-transfusion-dependence and -independence? Leuk Res 2011;35:8–11.
93. Verstovsek S, Mesa RA, Gotlib J, et al. A double-blind, placebo-controlled trial of ruxolitinib for myelofibrosis. N Engl J Med 2012;366:799–807.
94. Verstovsek S, Kantarjian H, Mesa RA, et al. Safety and efficacy of INCB018424, a JAK1 and JAK2 inhibitor, in myelofibrosis. N Engl J Med 2010;363:1117–27.
95. Harrison C, Kiladjian JJ, Al-Ali HK, et al. JAK inhibition with ruxolitinib versus best available therapy for myelofibrosis. N Engl J Med 2012;366:787–98.
96. Pardanani A, Lasho TL, Finke CM, et al. Polyclonal immunoglobulin free light chain levels predict survival in myeloid neoplasms. J Clin Oncol 2012;30: 1087–94.
97. Scott BL, Gooley TA, Sorror ML, et al. The Dynamic International Prognostic Scoring System for myelofibrosis predicts outcomes after hematopoietic cell transplantation. Blood 2012;119(11):2657–64 [Epub 2012 Jan 10].

Systemic Mastocytosis
Disease Overview, Pathogenesis, and Treatment

Animesh Pardanani, MBBS, PhD

KEYWORDS

- Mast cell disease • Myeloproliferative neoplasm • KITD816V

KEY POINTS

- The clinical presentation of mastocytosis is diverse, and patients may not fit the classical description.
- Diagnosis requires a bone marrow examination, including immunohistochemical stains for mast cell tryptase or CD117.
- The treatment of adult systemic mastocytosis is highly individualized.

DISEASE OVERVIEW, CLASSIFICATION, AND DIAGNOSIS

The discovery of mast cells in 1878 is credited to Paul Ehrlich, who first described cells that stained with metachromatic dyes, such as toluidine blue, which he termed mast cells (MCs). MCs are myeloid lineage cells that arise from bone marrow (BM) precursors, more specifically from CD34+ and KIT+ hematopoietic progenitors.[1-5] Mastocytosis is a stem cell–derived clonal myeloproliferation characterized by the abnormal growth and accumulation of neoplastic MCs in one or more organs; it is 1 of 8 subcategories of myeloproliferative neoplasms (MPNs) per the 2008 World Health Organization (WHO) classification of tumors of hematopoietic and lymphoid tissues.[6] The clinical presentation of mastocytosis is diverse, and patients may not fit the classical description; namely, a variably long history of urticaria pigmentosa (UP), followed by the insidious onset of flushing, cramping abdominal pain, diarrhea, and bone pain.[7-9] Other disease manifestations include osteopenia, hepatosplenomegaly, and abnormalities of blood and BM. Unlike pediatric cases, most adults with UP-like skin lesions have systemic disease (ie, systemic mastocytosis [SM]) at presentation, a condition generally confirmed by means of a BM biopsy.[10] The 2008 WHO system[6] classifies mastocytosis into the following categories (**Box 1**): (1) cutaneous mastocytosis (limited to the skin; variants include UP, diffuse cutaneous mastocytosis, and solitary mastocytoma of the skin), (2) extracutaneous mastocytoma (unifocal

---

The author has no competing financial interests.

Division of Hematology, Department of Medicine, Mayo Clinic, 200 First Street Southwest, Rochester, MN 55905, USA

E-mail address: Pardanani.animesh@mayo.edu

Hematol Oncol Clin N Am 26 (2012) 1117–1128

http://dx.doi.org/10.1016/j.hoc.2012.08.001

hemonc.theclinics.com

Box 1
World Health Organization classification of mastocytosis

1. Cutaneous mastocytosis (CM):
   a. Urticaria pigmentosa (UP)/Maculopapular CM
   b. Diffuse CM
   c. Solitary mastocytoma of skin

2. Indolent systemic mastocytosis
   a. Smoldering SM
   b. Isolated BM mastocytosis

3. Systemic mastocytosis with an associated clonal hematological non-MC lineage disease (SM-AHNMD)

4. Aggressive systemic mastocytosis (ASM)
   a. Lymphadenopathic mastocytosis with eosinophilia

5. Mast cell leukemia (MCL)

6. Mast cell sarcoma (MCS)

7. Extracutaneous mastocytoma

From Horny HP, Metcalfe DD, Bennett JM, et al. Mastocytosis. In: Swerdlow SH, Campo E, Harris NL, et al, editors. WHO classification of tumors of hematopoietic and lymphoid tissues. 4th edition. Lyon (France): International Agency for Research and Cancer (IARC); 2008. p. 54–63; with permission.

---

nondestructive MC tumor with low-grade cellular atypia), (3) MC sarcoma (destructive unifocal MC tumor with poorly differentiated MCs, and tendency to metastasize and/or evolve into MCL), and (4) SM. The latter is subclassified into 4 subcategories: indolent SM (ISM; no evidence of extracutaneous organ dysfunction), aggressive SM (ASM; presence of extracutaneous organ dysfunction), SM associated with another clonal hematological non-MC lineage disease (SM-AHNMD), and MC leukemia (MCL).

Diagnosis requires a BM examination, including immunohistochemical stains for MC tryptase or CD117 (KIT receptor) (**Box 2, Fig. 1**). Histologic diagnostic criteria for non-BM, extracutaneous organ involvement in SM have not been established as of yet. MCs may not be readily recognized by standard dyes, such as Giemsa, particularly when MCs exhibit significant hypogranulation or abnormal nuclear morphology. In contrast, tryptase is a sensitive marker and identifies virtually all MCs regardless of maturation or activation stage, or tissue of localization; however, neither tryptase nor CD117 immunostaining are able to distinguish between normal and neoplastic MCs.[11] Neoplastic MCs generally express CD25 and/or CD2 (particularly the former), and detection of abnormal expression of at least 1 of the 2 antigens counts as a minor diagnostic criterion per the WHO system (see **Box 2**).[6] Consequently, immunostaining studies enhance the morphologic and immunophenotypic distinction between normal (round and CD25-negative) and abnormal (spindle-shaped and CD25-positive) MCs, respectively.[12,13] The pathognomonic BM histologic finding is presence of multifocal, dense MC aggregates, frequently in perivascular and/or paratrabecular locations. These aggregates may be relatively monomorphic, composed mainly of fusiform MCs, or may be polymorphic with MCs admixed with lymphocytes, eosinophils, neutrophils, histiocytes, endothelial cells, and fibroblasts.[14] Eosinophils are most commonly found distributed at the periphery of MC aggregates, but increased

---

Box 2
Criteria for the diagnosis of systemic mastocytosis

Major

a. Multifocal, dense infiltrates of MCs ($\geq$15 MCs in aggregates) detected in sections of bone marrow and/or other extracutaneous organs

Minor

a. In biopsy sections of BM or other extracutaneous organs, more than 25% of the MCs in the infiltrate are spindle shaped or have atypical morphology or, of all MCs in BM aspirate smears, more than 25% are immature or atypical

b. Detection of an activating point mutation at codon 816 of *KIT* in BM, blood, or other extracutaneous organ

c. MCs in BM, blood, or other extracutaneous organ express CD2 and/or CD25 in addition to normal MC markers

d. Serum total tryptase persistently exceeds 20 ng/mL (unless there is an associated clonal myeloid disorder, in which case this parameter is not valid)

From Horny HP, Metcalfe DD, Bennett JM, et al. Mastocytosis. In: Swerdlow SH, Campo E, Harris NL, et al, editors. WHO classification of tumors of hematopoietic and lymphoid tissues. 4th edition. Lyon (France): International Agency for Research and Cancer (IARC); 2008. p. 54–63; with permission.

---

eosinophils may also be seen in noninfiltrated areas.[15] Identification of the *KIT*D816V mutation and elevated serum tryptase level (>20 ng/mL) count as a minor diagnostic criteria per the WHO system (see **Box 2**).[6] Elevated serum tryptase levels have been documented in patients with non-SM myeloid malignancies, including acute myeloid leukemia (AML),[16,17] myelodysplastic syndrome (MDS),[18] and chronic myeloid leukemia (CML)[19]; thus, non-SM myeloid disorders need to be excluded before elevated serum tryptase levels can be considered in support of a diagnosis of SM. Furthermore, levels of total serum tryptase may also be transiently elevated during anaphylaxis or a severe allergic reaction.[20]

PATHOGENESIS

MCs retain surface KIT expression at high levels on maturation, and the interaction between the KIT and SCF has been shown to promote the proliferation, maturation, adhesion, chemotaxis, and survival of MCs.[21] Consequently, gain-of-function mutations in *KIT*, particularly the D816V mutation, have been found to occur in most adult patients with SM, irrespective of WHO SM subtype.[22] Other less common (<5%) somatic *KIT* mutations identified in adult SM include V560G,[23,24] D815K,[25] D816Y,[22,25–27] insVI815-816,[22] D816F,[25,27] D816H,[28] and D820G.[29] Recent studies have suggested that pediatric mastocytosis is also clonal in nature, and is associated with germline or acquired activating *KIT* mutations.[30–32] In one study that screened for *KIT* mutations in skin lesional DNA, 42% of cases harbored missense mutations targeting *KIT*D816; in 44% of cases, heterogeneous genetic alterations were found to mainly involve exons 8 and 9, which encode the fifth immunoglobulin (D5) domain and the extracellular region near the transmembrane domain. Similar to *KIT*D816V, every mutation in exons 8 and 9 that was functionally interrogated was found to constitutively activate KIT kinase activity. Other rare germline *KIT* mutations that target the transmembrane domain and that are associated with familial mastocytosis include F522C and A533D.[33,34]

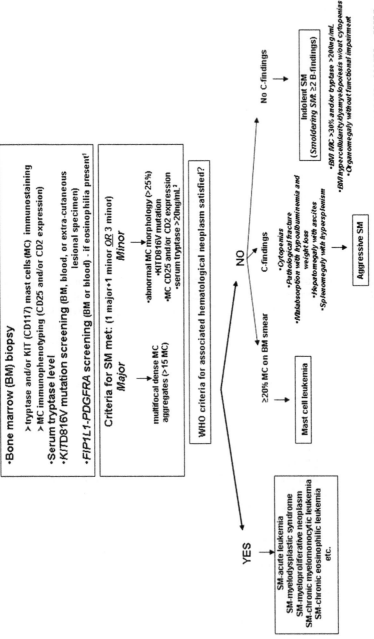

Fig. 1. Diagnostic algorithm for systemic mastocytosis.

The issue as to whether other genetic events, in addition to activating *KIT* mutations, are necessary for neoplastic transformation of MCs, and for full expression of the mastocytosis phenotype, remains to be clarified. This is illustrated by the divergent natural history of childhood-onset and adult-onset mastocytosis; although both are associated with activating *KIT* mutations, the former predominantly exhibits cutaneous-limited disease that spontaneously regresses with age In contrast, adult-onset mastocytosis is characterized by a persistent multiorgan involvement, often with a concurrent non-MC hematologic neoplasm. Experimental data from murine models have not been conclusive in this regard; in transgenic mice expressing human *KIT*D816V in mature MCs (driven by the chymase promoter), only a subset (30%) of mice developed a limited form of mastocytosis (some with cutaneous-limited disease) at an older age (12–18 months).[35] The incomplete disease penetrance in this model suggested that additional somatic mutations are necessary for full MC transformation, or that processing and intracellular trafficking of human KITD816V is abnormal in murine cells, thereby compromising signaling by the mutant receptor in this cross-species setting. In another transgenic mouse model, conditional expression of murine KITD814V was driven by the *KIT* promoter. When mutant KIT was expressed in somatic cells of adult mice, the animals developed marked mastocytosis with 100% penetrance at a young age, with infiltrates of mast cells in the skin and other organs, most frequently lymph nodes and colon.[36] This phenotype reproduced some of the features of human aggressive SM and approximately half of the mice developed a non-MC lineage hematologic neoplasm, most frequently a leukemic disease derived from an immature B-cell precursor. The severity of mast cell disease was markedly attenuated when KITD814V expression in this model was limited to more mature MCs. Although half of the mice developed MC tumors, the disease occurred significantly later and progressed much slower; there is concern, however, that the attenuated phenotype may reflect low transgene expression in this model. Cumulatively, the data suggest that the effects of constitutive KIT signaling depend on the developmental stage of the cell targeted by the gain-of-function mutation. As has been noted in patients with mastocytosis,[22] mutations targeting undifferentiated progenitors result in multilineage involvement and expression of a severe systemic disease phenotype; in contrast, mutations that target committed MC progenitors or mature MCs result in milder forms of the disease.

Recently, a high level of expression of microphthalmia-associated transcription factor (MITF), a transcription factor critical for MC development, was demonstrated in BM biopsy specimens from SM patients. Upregulation of MITF expression was found to be dependent on KIT signaling in both normal and malignant MCs. Because MITF mRNA levels did not change significantly with KIT signaling, it suggested post-transcriptional regulation of MITF expression. An array screen from MC identified miR-539 and miR-381 to be downregulated by KIT signaling; the 2 miRNAs were shown to repress MITF expression through conserved binding sites in the MITF 3′-untranslated region. These data suggest that MITF overexpression may be an important contributor to cell proliferation in mastocytosis and illustrate the role of additional genetic defects that may cooperate with *KIT* mutations in contributing to the fully transformed MC phenotype. It should be pointed out, however, that high MITF expression is not found in all cases of mastocytosis and the critical gene targets of MITF implicated in MC proliferation remain to be identified.

TET2 (TET oncogene family member 2) is a putative tumor suppressor gene located at chromosome 4q24. *TET2* mutations were first described in patients with *JAK2*V617F-positive MPN.[37] Subsequently, the same mutations were found in *JAK2*V617F-negative MPN.[38] *TET2* mutations have since been described in other myeloid malignancies, including SM, MDS, and AML.[39–41] In one study, *TET2* mutation frequency in SM was 29% and *TET2* mutations were associated with monocytosis. In this preliminary analysis, *TET2* mutations cosegregated with *KIT*D816V but did not appear to have an independent impact on survival. Overall, the pathogenetic role and/or prognostic impact of *TET2* mutations in SM currently remain unclear.

RISK-STRATIFICATION AND TREATMENT

The treatment of adult SM is highly individualized and the most practical first step in risk stratifying newly diagnosed patients is their categorization per the 2008 WHO classification system.[6] Overall, the life expectancy of adult patients with SM appears to be shorter as compared with age-matched and gender-matched controls, with the excess deaths in this group occurring within the first 3 to 5 years after diagnosis.[7,9] There is significant heterogeneity within the WHO subgroups, however; in one study, patients with ISM comprised the largest subgroup and were significantly younger at presentation (median age 49 years) and had a higher prevalence (more than two-thirds) of UP-like skin lesions, MC mediator release symptoms (MCMRS), and gastrointestinal symptoms, but had significantly less constitutional symptoms or hepatosplenomegaly (<20%), as compared with patients with ASM and SM-AHNMD.[7,42] Their median survival was 198 months, which was not significantly different from that of the age-matched and sex-matched US control population. Advanced age was the primary determinant of inferior survival; the overall risk of transformation to acute leukemia or ASM was low (<1% and 3%, respectively) but was significantly higher in smoldering SM (18%). SM-AHNMD was the second most common SM subgroup; the vast majority of these patients ($\sim$90%) had an associated myeloid neoplasm.[7,43] Overall median survival in SM-AHNMD was 24 months. Patients with SM with an associated MPN had a significantly longer median survival (31 months) as compared with those with associated chronic myelomonocytic leukemia (15 months), MDS (13 months), or acute leukemia (11 months). Leukemic transformation was observed in 13% of patients with SM-AHNMD overall, and was significantly more frequent in SM-MDS (29%). Presence of eosinophilia had no independent prognostic value. ASM was the third most common subgroup[7]; approximately half of the patients displayed constitutional symptoms and hepatosplenomegaly, a quarter displayed lymphadenopathy, severe anemia (hemoglobin <10 g/dL), or thrombocytopenia (platelets <100 $\times$ 10^9/L), and roughly 40% had leukocytosis and/or markedly elevated serum tryptase levels (>200 ng/mL). Overall median survival in ASM was 41 months and leukemic transformation occurred in 5% of patients. MCL was seen in 1% of cases; the prognosis was dismal with median survival of only 2 months.[7]

In addition to WHO SM subtype, inferior survival has shown to be associated with advanced age, history of weight loss, anemia, thrombocytopenia, hypoalbuminemia, and excess BM blasts.[7]

Overall, treatment of SM is guided only to a limited extent by specific molecular findings. In general, the promise of truly "targeted therapy" in the vast majority of patients with SM (similar to imatinib therapy in CML) has yet to be realized. For the rare patients with SM with a transmembrane KIT mutation (eg, F522C or K509I), dramatic clinical responses to imatinib therapy can be observed.[33,44] For most patients with WHO-defined SM, however, drug therapy is largely palliative; the experience with allogeneic stem cell transplantation is too limited to comment on.[45] Presence of MCMRS (eg, pruritus, urticaria, angioedema, flushing, nausea, vomiting, abdominal pain, diarrhea, episodic anaphylactoid attacks), organ dysfunction caused by direct MC infiltration (eg, hypersplenism, pathologic fracture), or symptomatic skin disease are the main indications for treatment. Management of MCMRS includes avoidance of triggering factors and use of histamine antagonists and cromolyn sodium. Phototherapy is sometimes useful for skin disease, including UP. Treatment with cytoreductive agents that are typically used in the setting of ASM and SM-AHNMD may be necessary for refractory cases of both MCRMS and skin disease.[46–49] Other supportive measures include the judicious use of red blood cell transfusions and treatment of osteoporosis.

The following cytoreductive agents are frequently used for mastocytosis therapy in clinical practice:

1. Interferon (IFN)-α: IFN-α is commonly regarded as the first-line cytoreductive therapy in symptomatic SM. It has been shown to improve skin, gastrointestinal, and systemic symptoms associated with MC degranulation. IFN-α can also have a favorable impact on skeletal disease through its ability to improve bone density.[48–60] The frequency of major response is approximately 20% to 30%, and concurrent administration of prednisone may improve the efficacy (up to 40% major response rate) and tolerability of IFN-α therapy.[49,61] Response to treatment may be delayed up to a year or longer.[49,56] IFN-α treatment is frequently (up to 50%) complicated by toxicities, including flulike symptoms, bone pain, fever, cytopenias, depression, and hypothyroidism; consequently, a significant proportion of patients discontinue treatment because of adverse events.[49,62,63] IFN-α treatment is generally continued as long as a response is observed and there are no intolerable adverse effects.

   In one study,[62] 47 patients received IFN-α with or without prednisone; the median weekly dose was 15 MU per week (range 3.5–30 MU per week) and the initial dosage of prednisone ranged from 20 to 60 mg per day with a slow tapering over weeks or months in some patients. In 40 evaluable patients, the overall response rate (ORR) was 53% (ISM and ASM 60%; SM-AHNMD 45%). Overall median duration of response was 12 months (range, 1–67 months). Responses were not significantly different when comparing patients who did or did not receive prednisone. Absence of systemic mediator-related symptoms was significantly associated with inferior response to IFN-α; 41% versus 77%, respectively. Major toxicities included fatigue, depression, and thrombocytopenia.

2. 2-chlorodeoxyadenosine (cladribine or 2-CdA): The cumulative data indicate that 2-CdA has therapeutic activity in all subtypes of SM, including in MCL.[64–69] The 2-CdA is generally reserved for treatment of patients who require rapid MC debulking, and/or who are refractory or intolerant to IFN-α.[67–69] Potential toxicities of 2-CdA therapy include significant and occasionally prolonged myelosuppression, as well as immunosuppression with increased risk of opportunistic infections.

   In one study,[62] 2-CdA was administered to 26 patients (8 as first-line); the dosage was 5 mg/m^2 per day or 0.13 to 0.17 mg/kg per day for 5 days as a 2-hour intravenous infusion, and median number of treatment cycles was 3 (range 1–9). Treatment response was evaluable in 22 patients and the ORR was 55% (ORR in ISM, ASM, and SM-AHNMD was 56%, 50%, and 55%, respectively). Median duration of response was 11 months (range, 3–74 months). Presence of circulating immature myeloid cells was significantly associated with inferior response to 2-CdA (0% vs 75%). Major toxicities were myelosuppression and infection. In the overall cohort (n = 80), treatment response was not significantly different based on *KIT*D816V or *TET2* mutational status.

3. Imatinib mesylate (IM): IM demonstrates in vitro efficacy against wild-type KIT and certain transmembrane (F522C) and juxta-membrane (V560G) KIT mutants, but not

the common kinase (D816V) domain mutants.[33,70–72] Notably, not every juxta-membrane mutation is sensitive to IM (eg, V559I).[73] Although IM has been approved by the Food and Drug Administration for SM therapy (labeled indication is treatment of adult patients with ASM without the *KIT*D816V mutation or with unknown *KIT* mutational status), it has a limited role in the treatment of unselected patients with SM, as most patients likely harbor the IM-resistant *KIT*D816V mutation. The rare SM cases that harbor an IM-sensitive *KIT* mutation, or those who are *KIT*D816-unmutated, may be appropriate candidates for IM treatment.

In one study,[62] IM was administered to 19 patients with SM (*FIP1L1-PDGFRA* patients were excluded for this analysis); the median starting dose was 400 mg per day (range 100–400 mg per day), and the maintenance dose in respond-ing patients ranged from 200 to 400 mg per day. In 22 evaluable patients, the ORR was 18% (ORR in ISM, ASM, and SM-AHNMD was 14%, 50%, and 9%, respectively), and median duration of response was 19.6 months (range, 9–69 months). Most (86%) IM-treated patients were *KIT*D816V positive; ORR in mutation-positive and mutation-negative patients was 17% and 33%, respectively. None of the 6 patients with SM associated with eosinophilia responded to IM treatment; all were *KIT*D816V-positive. Major toxicities included diarrhea and peripheral edema; 2 patients developed interstitial pneumonitis.

4. Hydroxyurea (HU): HU is most useful in treating SM-AHNMD, in which its clinical benefit stems from its myelosuppressive activity. HU does not however exhibit any selective MC inhibitory activity.

In one study,[62] HU use was largely restricted to patients with SM-AHNMD (n = 28) at a dosage ranging from 500 mg every other day to 2000 mg per day. Twenty-six patients were evaluable for response with ORR of 19%, reflected by control of thrombocytosis, leukocytosis, and/or hepatosplenomegaly. Median duration of response was 31.5 months (range, 5–50 months); the major toxicity was myelosuppression.

5. Investigational therapies: Investigational therapies include dastanib, midostaurin (PKC412), and masatinib mesylate (AB1010), which are further described in the review article by Pardanani.[74]

REFERENCES

1. Kirshenbaum AS, Goff JP, Dreskin SC, et al. IL-3-dependent growth of basophil-like cells and mastlike cells from human bone marrow. J Immunol 1989;142: 2424–9.
2. Kirshenbaum AS, Kessler SW, Goff JP, et al. Demonstration of the origin of human mast cells from CD34+ bone marrow progenitor cells. J Immunol 1991;146:1410–5.
3. Kirshenbaum AS, Goff JP, Semere T, et al. Demonstration that human mast cells arise from a progenitor cell population that is CD34(+), c-kit(+), and expresses aminopeptidase N (CD13). Blood 1999;94:2333–42.
4. Agis H, Willheim M, Sperr WR, et al. Monocytes do not make mast cells when cultured in the presence of SCF. Characterization of the circulating mast cell progenitor as a c-kit+, CD34+, Ly-, CD14-, CD17-, colony-forming cell. J Immunol 1993;151:4221–7.
5. Rottem M, Kirshenbaum AS, Metcalfe DD. Early development of mast cells. Int Arch Allergy Appl Immunol 1991;94:104–9.
6. Horny HP, Metcalfe DD, Bennett JM, et al. Mastocytosis. In: Swerdlow SH, Campo E, Harris NL, editors. WHO classification of tumors of hematopoietic

and lymphoid tissues. 4th edition. Lyon (France): International Agency for Research and Cancer (IARC); 2008. p. 54–63.

7. Lim KH, Tefferi A, Lasho TL, et al. Systemic mastocytosis in 342 consecutive adults: survival studies and prognostic factors. Blood 2009;113:5727–36.

8. Patnaik MM, Rindos M, Kouides PA, et al. Systemic mastocytosis: a concise clinical and laboratory review. Arch Pathol Lab Med 2007;131:784–91.

9. Travis WD, Li CY, Bergstralh EJ, et al. Systemic mast cell disease. Analysis of 58 cases and literature review. Medicine (Baltimore) 1988;67:345–68.

10. Czarnetzki BM, Kolde G, Schoemann A, et al. Bone marrow findings in adult patients with urticaria pigmentosa. J Am Acad Dermatol 1988;18:45–51.

11. Jordan JH, Walchshofer S, Jurecka W, et al. Immunohistochemical properties of bone marrow mast cells in systemic mastocytosis: evidence for expression of CD2, CD117/Kit, and bcl-x(L). Hum Pathol 2001;32:545–52.

12. Horny HP, Valent P. Histopathological and immunohistochemical aspects of mastocytosis. Int Arch Allergy Immunol 2002;127:115–7.

13. Pardanani A, Kimlinger T, Reeder T, et al. Bone marrow mast cell immunophenotyping in adults with mast cell disease: a prospective study of 33 patients. Leuk Res 2004;28:777–83.

14. Brunning RD, McKenna RW, Rosai J, et al. Systemic mastocytosis. Extracutaneous manifestations. Am J Surg Pathol 1983;7:425–38.

15. Horny HP, Parwaresch MR, Lennert K. Bone marrow findings in systemic mastocytosis. Hum Pathol 1985;16:808–14.

16. Sperr WR, Jordan JH, Baghestanian M, et al. Expression of mast cell tryptase by myeloblasts in a group of patients with acute myeloid leukemia. Blood 2001;98: 2200–9.

17. Sperr WR, Hauswirth AW, Valent P. Tryptase: a novel biochemical marker of acute myeloid leukemia. Leuk Lymphoma 2002;43:2257–61.

18. Sperr WR, Stehberger B, Wimazal F, et al. Serum tryptase measurements in patients with myelodysplastic syndromes. Leuk Lymphoma 2002;43:1097–105.

19. Samorapoompichit P, Kiener HP, Schernthaner GH, et al. Detection of tryptase in cytoplasmic granules of basophils in patients with chronic myeloid leukemia and other myeloid neoplasms. Blood 2001;98:2580–3.

20. Schwartz LB, Metcalfe DD, Miller JS, et al. Tryptase levels as an indicator of mast-cell activation in systemic anaphylaxis and mastocytosis. N Engl J Med 1987;316: 1622–6.

21. Valent P, Spanblochl E, Sperr WR, et al. Induction of differentiation of human mast cells from bone marrow and peripheral blood mononuclear cells by recombinant human stem cell factor/kit-ligand in long-term culture. Blood 1992;80:2237–45.

22. Garcia-Montero AC, Jara-Acevedo M, Teodosio C, et al. KIT mutation in mast cells and other bone marrow hematopoietic cell lineages in systemic mast cell disorders: a prospective study of the Spanish Network on Mastocytosis (REMA) in a series of 113 patients. Blood 2006;108:2366–72.

23. Buttner C, Henz BM, Welker P, et al. Identification of activating c-kit mutations in adult-, but not in childhood-onset indolent mastocytosis: a possible explanation for divergent clinical behavior. J Invest Dermatol 1998;111:1227–31.

24. Furitsu T, Tsujimura T, Tono T, et al. Identification of mutations in the coding sequence of the proto-oncogene c-kit in a human mast cell leukemia cell line causing ligand-independent activation of c-kit product. J Clin Invest 1993;92:1736–44.

25. Sotlar K, Escribano L, Landt O, et al. One-step detection of c-kit point mutations using peptide nucleic acid-mediated polymerase chain reaction clamping and hybridization probes. Am J Pathol 2003;162:737–46.

26. Beghini A, Cairoli R, Morra E, et al. In vivo differentiation of mast cells from acute myeloid leukemia blasts carrying a novel activating ligand-independent C-kit mutation. Blood Cells Mol Dis 1998;24:262–70.

27. Longley BJ Jr, Metcalfe DD, Tharp M, et al. Activating and dominant inactivating c-KIT catalytic domain mutations in distinct clinical forms of human mastocytosis. Proc Natl Acad Sci U S A 1999;96:1609–14.

28. Pullarkat VA, Pullarkat ST, Calverley DC, et al. Mast cell disease associated with acute myeloid leukemia: detection of a new c-kit mutation Asp816His. Am J Hematol 2000;65:307–9.

29. Pignon JM, Giraudier S, Duquesnoy P, et al. A new c-kit mutation in a case of aggressive mast cell disease. Br J Haematol 1997;96:374–6.

30. Bodemer C, Hermine O, Palmerini F, et al. Pediatric mastocytosis is a clonal disease associated with D816V and other activating c-KIT mutations. J Invest Dermatol 2010;130:804–15.

31. Yanagihori H, Oyama N, Nakamura K, et al. c-kit Mutations in patients with childhood-onset mastocytosis and genotype-phenotype correlation. J Mol Diagn 2005;7:252–7.

32. Verzijl A, Heide R, Oranje AP, et al. C-kit Asp-816-Val mutation analysis in patients with mastocytosis. Dermatology 2007;214:15–20.

33. Akin C, Fumo G, Yavuz AS, et al. A novel form of mastocytosis associated with a transmembrane c-kit mutation and response to imatinib. Blood 2004;103:3222–5.

34. Tang X, Boxer M, Drummond A, et al. A germline mutation in KIT in familial diffuse cutaneous mastocytosis. J Med Genet 2004;41:e88.

35. Zappulla JP, Dubreuil P, Desbois S, et al. Mastocytosis in mice expressing human Kit receptor with the activating Asp816Val mutation. J Exp Med 2005;202: 1635–41.

36. Gerbaulet A, Wickenhauser C, Scholten J, et al. Mast cell hyperplasia, B cell malignancy, and intestinal inflammation in mice with conditional expression of a constitutively active kit. Blood 2011;117(6):2012–21.

37. Delhommeau F, Dupont S, Della Valle V, et al. Mutation in TET2 in myeloid cancers. N Engl J Med 2009;360:2289–301.

38. Tefferi A, Pardanani A, Lim KH, et al. TET2 mutations and their clinical correlates in polycythemia vera, essential thrombocythemia and myelofibrosis. Leukemia 2009;23:905–11.

39. Tefferi A, Levine RL, Lim KH, et al. Frequent TET2 mutations in systemic mastocytosis: clinical, KITD816V and FIP1L1-PDGFRA correlates. Leukemia 2009;23: 900–4.

40. Tefferi A, Lim KH, Abdel-Wahab O, et al. Detection of mutant TET2 in myeloid malignancies other than myeloproliferative neoplasms: CMML, MDS, MDS/MPN and AML. Leukemia 2009;23:1343–5.

41. Langemeijer SM, Kuiper RP, Berends M, et al. Acquired mutations in TET2 are common in myelodysplastic syndromes. Nat Genet 2009;41:838–42.

42. Pardanani A, Lim KH, Lasho TL, et al. WHO subvariants of indolent mastocytosis: clinical details and prognostic evaluation in 159 consecutive adults. Blood 2010; 115:150–1.

43. Pardanani A, Lim KH, Lasho TL, et al. Prognostically relevant breakdown of 123 patients with systemic mastocytosis associated with other myeloid malignancies. Blood 2009;114:3769–72.

44. Zhang LY, Smith ML, Schultheis B, et al. A novel K509I mutation of KIT identified in familial mastocytosis—in vitro and in vivo responsiveness to imatinib therapy. Leuk Res 2006;30:373–8.

45. Nakamura R, Chakrabarti S, Akin C, et al. A pilot study of nonmyeloablative allogeneic hematopoietic stem cell transplant for advanced systemic mastocytosis. Bone Marrow Transplant 2006;37:353–8.

46. Casassus P, Caillat-Vigneron N, Martin A, et al. Treatment of adult systemic mastocytosis with interferon-alpha: results of a multicentre phase II trial on 20 patients. Br J Haematol 2002;119:1090–7.

47. Kluin-Nelemans HC, Jansen JH, Breukelman H, et al. Response to interferon alfa-2b in a patient with systemic mastocytosis. N Engl J Med 1992;326:619–23.

48. Butterfield JH. Response of severe systemic mastocytosis to interferon alpha. Br J Dermatol 1998;138:489–95.

49. Hauswirth AW, Simonitsch-Klupp I, Uffmann M, et al. Response to therapy with interferon alpha-2b and prednisolone in aggressive systemic mastocytosis: report of five cases and review of the literature. Leuk Res 2004;28:249–57.

50. Butterfield JH, Tefferi A, Kozuh GF. Successful treatment of systemic mastocytosis with high-dose interferon-alfa: long-term follow-up of a case. Leuk Res 2005; 29:131–4.

51. Kolde G, Sunderkotter C, Luger TA. Treatment of urticaria pigmentosa using interferon alpha. Br J Dermatol 1995;133:91–4.

52. Lehmann T, Beyeler C, Lammle B, et al. Severe osteoporosis due to systemic mast cell disease: successful treatment with interferon alpha-2B. Br J Rheumatol 1996;35:898–900.

53. Lehmann T, Lammle B. IFNalpha treatment in systemic mastocytosis. Ann Hematol 1999;78:483–4.

54. Takasaki Y, Tsukasaki K, Jubashi T, et al. Systemic mastocytosis with extensive polypoid lesions in the intestines; successful treatment with interferon-alpha. Intern Med 1998;37:484–8.

55. Weide R, Ehlenz K, Lorenz W, et al. Successful treatment of osteoporosis in systemic mastocytosis with interferon alpha-2b. Ann Hematol 1996;72:41–3.

56. Lippert U, Henz BM. Long-term effect of interferon alpha treatment in mastocytosis [comment]. Br J Dermatol 1996;134:1164–5.

57. Petit A, Pulik M, Gaulier A, et al. Systemic mastocytosis associated with chronic myelomonocytic leukemia: clinical features and response to interferon alfa therapy. J Am Acad Dermatol 1995;32:850–3.

58. Worobec AS, Kirshenbaum AS, Schwartz LB, et al. Treatment of three patients with systemic mastocytosis with interferon alpha-2b. Leuk Lymphoma 1996;22: 501–8.

59. Brunel V, Tadrist Z, Cailleres S, et al. Interferon alpha and pamidronate: a useful combination in the treatment of osteoporosis and systemic mastocytosis. Presse Med 1998;27:64 [in French].

60. Czarnetzki BM, Algermissen B, Jeep S, et al. Interferon treatment of patients with chronic urticaria and mastocytosis. J Am Acad Dermatol 1994;30:500–1.

61. Delaporte E, Pierard E, Wolthers BG, et al. Interferon-alpha in combination with corticosteroids improves systemic mast cell disease. Br J Dermatol 1995;132: 479–82.

62. Lim KH, Pardanani A, Butterfield JH, et al. Cytoreductive therapy in 108 adults with systemic mastocytosis: outcome analysis and response prediction during treatment with interferon-alpha, hydroxyurea, imatinib mesylate or 2-chlorodeoxyadenosine. Am J Hematol 2009;84:790–4.

63. Simon J, Lortholary O, Caillat-Vigneron N, et al. Interest of interferon alpha in systemic mastocytosis. The French experience and review of the literature. Pathol Biol (Paris) 2004;52:294–9.

64. Bohm A, Sonneck K, Gleixner KV, et al. In vitro and in vivo growth-inhibitory effects of cladribine on neoplastic mast cells exhibiting the imatinib-resistant KIT mutation D816V. Exp Hematol 2010;38:744–55.

65. Gleixner KV, Mayerhofer M, Aichberger KJ, et al. PKC412 inhibits in vitro growth of neoplastic human mast cells expressing the D816V-mutated variant of KIT: comparison with AMN107, imatinib, and cladribine (2CdA) and evaluation of cooperative drug effects. Blood 2006;107:752–9.

66. Penack O, Sotlar K, Noack F, et al. Cladribine therapy in a patient with an aleukemic subvariant of mast cell leukemia. Ann Hematol 2005;84:692–3.

67. Tefferi A, Li CY, Butterfield JH, et al. Treatment of systemic mast-cell disease with cladribine. N Engl J Med 2001;344:307–9.

68. Kluin-Nelemans HC, Oldhoff JM, Van Doormaal JJ, et al. Cladribine therapy for systemic mastocytosis. Blood 2003;102:4270–6.

69. Pardanani A, Hoffbrand AV, Butterfield JH, et al. Treatment of systemic mast cell disease with 2-chlorodeoxyadenosine. Leuk Res 2004;28:127–31.

70. Zermati Y, De Sepulveda P, Feger F, et al. Effect of tyrosine kinase inhibitor STI571 on the kinase activity of wild-type and various mutated c-kit receptors found in mast cell neoplasms. Oncogene 2003;22:660–4.

71. Akin C, Brockow K, D'Ambrosio C, et al. Effects of tyrosine kinase inhibitor STI571 on human mast cells bearing wild-type or mutated c-kit. Exp Hematol 2003;31: 686–92.

72. Ma Y, Zeng S, Metcalfe DD, et al. The c-KIT mutation causing human mastocytosis is resistant to STI571 and other KIT kinase inhibitors; kinases with enzymatic site mutations show different inhibitor sensitivity profiles than wild-type kinases and those with regulatory-type mutations. Blood 2002;99:1741–4.

73. Nakagomi N, Hirota S. Juxtamembrane-type c-kit gene mutation found in aggressive systemic mastocytosis induces imatinib-resistant constitutive KIT activation. Lab Invest 2007;87:365–71.

74. Pardanani A. Systemic mastocytosis in adults: 2012 update on diagnosis, risk stratification, and management. Am J Hematol 2012;87:401–11.

Index

Note: Page numbers of article titles are in **boldface** type.

A

Acquired uniparental disomy. *See* Uniparental disomy.
AKT inhibitors, in therapy for myeloproliferative neoplasms, 967
Alleles, rare germline, 1043–1044
Allogeneic stem cell transplant, in therapy for myeloproliferative neoplasms, 972–973
Animal models, of myeloproliferative neoplasms, **1065–1081**
    bone marrow microenvironment in, 1075–1076
    murine, 1066–1075
      BCR-ABL, 1066–1068
      c-CBL, 1074
      JAK2V617F, 1068–1073
      LNK, 1074
      MPLW515L, 1073
      other genetic lesions, 1074
      TET2, 1073
    signaling pathways activated in vivo in mice, 1024–1025
    use of JAK2V617F models in preclinical development of therapies, 1075
ASXL1 mutations, role in pathogenesis of myeloproliferative neoplasms, **1053–1064**
    biologic role in hematopoiesis, 1057–1060
    clinical importance in patients with, 1060–1061
    discovery of, 1057
   specific to JAK2V617F-negative primary myelofibrosis and essential thrombocythemia,
    1003–1004

B

BCR-ABL mutation, murine model of myeloproliferative neoplasms, 1066–1068
Beta-catenin antagonist, in therapy for myeloproliferative neoplasms, 971–972

C

c-CBL mutations, murine model of, 1074
   specific to JAK2V617F-negative primary myelofibrosis and essential thrombocythemia,
    1004–1006
CBL mutations, associated with activated signaling in myeloproliferative neoplasms,
   1022–1023
Chromatin, noncanonical JAK2 signaling to, 1027–1028
Chromosomal aberrations, acquired, in myeloproliferative neoplasms, 1043–1044
CYT387, results of JAK2 inhibitors in myelofibrosis, 1091–1092
Cytokines, signaling induction by secreted, 1028–1029

D

Disomy, uniparental. *See* Uniparental disomy.
Disordered signaling. *See* Signaling, disordered.

Hematol Oncol Clin N Am 26 (2012) 1129–1135
http://dx.doi.org/10.1016/S0889-8588(12)00168-2
0889-8588/12/$ – see front matter © 2012 Elsevier Inc. All rights reserved.

hemonc.theclinics.com

United States Postal Service

Statement of Ownership, Management, and Circulation
(All Periodicals Publications Except Requester Publications)

1. Publication Title	2. Publication Number	3. Filing Date
Hematology/Oncology Clinics of North America	0 0 2 - 4 7 3	9/14/12

4. Issue Frequency	5. Number of Issues Published Annually	6. Annual Subscription Price
Feb, Apr, Jun, Aug, Oct, Dec	6	$353.00

7. Complete Mailing Address of Known Office of Publication (Not printer) (Street, city, county, state, and ZIP+4®)

Elsevier Inc.
360 Park Avenue South
New York, NY 10010-1710

Contact Person
Stephen R. Bushing

Telephone (Include area code)
215-239-3688

8. Complete Mailing Address of Headquarters or General Business Office of Publisher (Not printer)

Elsevier Inc., 360 Park Avenue South, New York, NY 10010-1710

9. Full Names and Complete Mailing Addresses of Publisher, Editor, and Managing Editor (Do not leave blank)

Publisher (Name and complete mailing address)

Kim Murphy, Elsevier, Inc., 1600 John F. Kennedy Blvd. Suite 1800, Philadelphia, PA 19103-2899

Editor (Name and complete mailing address)

Patrick Manley, Elsevier, Inc., 1600 John F. Kennedy Blvd. Suite 1800, Philadelphia, PA 19103-2899

Managing Editor (Name and complete mailing address)

Barbara Cohen - Kligerman, Elsevier, Inc., 1600 John F. Kennedy Blvd. Suite 1800, Philadelphia, PA 19103-2899

10. Owner (Do not leave blank. If the publication is owned by a corporation, give the name and address of the corporation immediately followed by the names and addresses of all stockholders owning or holding 1 percent or more of the total amount of stock. If not owned by a corporation, give the names and addresses of the individual owners. If owned by a partnership or other unincorporated firm, give its name and address as well as those of each individual owner. If the publication is published by a nonprofit organization, give its name and address.)

Full Name	Complete Mailing Address
Wholly owned subsidiary of	1600 John F. Kennedy Blvd., Ste. 1800
Reed/Elsevier, US holdings	Philadelphia, PA 19103-2899

11. Known Bondholders, Mortgagees, and Other Security Holders Owning or Holding 1 Percent or More of Total Amount of Bonds, Mortgages, or Other Securities. If none, check box ☐ None

Full Name	Complete Mailing Address
N/A	

12. Tax Status (For completion by nonprofit organizations authorized to mail at nonprofit rates) (Check one)
The purpose, function, and nonprofit status of this organization and the exempt status for federal income tax purposes:
☐ Has Not Changed During Preceding 12 Months
☐ Has Changed During Preceding 12 Months (Publisher must submit explanation of change with this statement)

PS Form 3526, September 2007 (Page 1 of 3 (Instructions Page 3)) PSN 7530-01-000-9931 PRIVACY NOTICE: See our Privacy policy in www.usps.com

---

13. Publication Title	14. Issue Date for Circulation Data Below
Hematology/Oncology Clinics of North America	August 2012

15. Extent and Nature of Circulation		Average No. Copies Each Issue During Preceding 12 Months	No. Copies of Single Issue Published Nearest to Filing Date
a. Total Number of Copies (Net press run)		931	750
b. Paid Circulation (By Mail and Outside the Mail)	(1) Mailed Outside-County Paid Subscriptions Stated on PS Form 3541. (Include paid distribution above nominal rate, advertiser's proof copies, and exchange copies)	365	323
	(2) Mailed In-County Paid Subscriptions Stated on PS Form 3541 (Include paid distribution above nominal rate, advertiser's proof copies, and exchange copies)		
	(3) Paid Distribution Outside the Mails Including Sales Through Dealers and Carriers, Street Vendors, Counter Sales, and Other Paid Distribution Outside USPS®	230	247
	(4) Paid Distribution by Other Classes Mailed Through the USPS (e.g. First-Class Mail®)		
c. Total Paid Distribution (Sum of 15b (1), (2), (3), and (4))		595	570
d. Free or Nominal Rate Distribution (By Mail and Outside the Mail)	(1) Free or Nominal Rate Outside-County Copies Included on PS Form 3541	113	119
	(2) Free or Nominal Rate In-County Copies Included on PS Form 3541		
	(3) Free or Nominal Rate Copies Mailed at Other Classes Through the USPS (e.g. First-Class Mail)		
	(4) Free or Nominal Rate Distribution Outside the Mail (Carriers or other means)		
e. Total Free or Nominal Rate Distribution (Sum of 15d (1), (2), (3) and (4))		113	119
f. Total Distribution (Sum of 15c and 15e)		708	689
g. Copies not Distributed (See instructions to publishers #4 (page #3))		223	61
h. Total (Sum of 15f and g)		931	750
i. Percent Paid (15c divided by 15f times 100)		84.04%	82.73%

16. Publication of Statement of Ownership

☐ If the publication is a general publication, publication of this statement is required. Will be printed in the October 2012 issue of this publication.   ☐ Publication not required.

17. Signature and Title of Editor, Publisher, Business Manager, or Owner

Stephen R. Bushing – Inventory/Distribution Coordinator

Date
September 14, 2012

I certify that all information furnished on this form is true and complete. I understand that anyone who furnishes false or misleading information on this form or who omits material or information requested on the form may be subject to criminal sanctions (including fines and imprisonment) and/or civil sanctions (including civil penalties).

PS Form 3526, September 2007 (Page 2 of 3)

Moving?

Make sure your subscription moves with you!

To notify us of your new address, find your **Clinics Account Number** (located on your mailing label above your name), and contact customer service at:

Email: journalscustomerservice-usa@elsevier.com

800-654-2452 (subscribers in the U.S. & Canada)
314-447-8871 (subscribers outside of the U.S. & Canada)

Fax number: 314-447-8029

Elsevier Health Sciences Division
Subscription Customer Service
3251 Riverport Lane
Maryland Heights, MO 63043

*To ensure uninterrupted delivery of your subscription, please notify us at least 4 weeks in advance of move.